Endocrine and Neuropsychiatric Disorders

Editor

ELIZA B. GEER

ENDOCRINOLOGY AND METABOLISM CLINICS OF NORTH AMERICA

www.endo.theclinics.com

Consulting Editor
DEREK LEROITH

September 2013 • Volume 42 • Number 3

ELSEVIER

1600 John F. Kennedy Boulevard • Suite 1800 • Philadelphia, Pennsylvania, 19103-2899

http://www.theclinics.com

ENDOCRINOLOGY AND METABOLISM CLINICS OF NORTH AMERICA Volume 42, Number 3
September 2013 ISSN 0889-8529, ISBN-13: 978-0-323-18852-4

Editor: Pamela Hetherington

Endocrinology and Metabolism Clinics of North America (ISSN 0889-8529) is published quarterly by Elsevier Inc., 360 Park Avenue South, New York, NY 10010-1710. Months of issue are March, June, September, and December. Periodicals postage paid at New York, NY and additional mailing offices. Subscription prices are USD 313.00 per year for US individuals, USD 557.00 per year for US institutions, USD 159.00 per year for US students and residents, USD 393.00 per year for Canadian individuals, USD 681.00 per year for Canadian institutions, USD 456.00 per year for international individuals, USD 681.00 per year for international institutions, and USD 234.00 per year for international and Canadian students/residents. To receive student/resident rate, orders must be accompanied by name of affiliated institution, date of term, and the signature of program/residency coordinator on institution letterhead. Orders will be billed at individual rate until proof of status is received. Foreign air speed delivery is included in all *Clinics* subscription prices. All prices are subject to change without notice. **POSTMASTER:** Send address changes to *Endocrinology and Metabolism Clinics of North America*, Elsevier Health Sciences Division, Subscription Customer Service, 3251 Riverport Lane, Maryland Heights, MO 63043. **Customer Service: Telephone: 1-800-654-2452** (U.S. and Canada); **1-314-447-8871** (outside U.S. and Canada). **Fax: 1-314-447-8029. E-mail: journalscustomerservice-usa@elsevier.com** (for print support); **journalsonlinesupport-usa@elsevier.com** (for online support).

Reprints. For copies of 100 or more, of articles in this publication, please contact the Commercial Rights Department, Elsevier Inc., 360 Park Avenue South, New York, NY 10010-1710; phone: (+1) 212-633-3874; fax: (+1) 212-633-3820; e-mail: reprints@elsevier.com.

Endocrinology and Metabolism Clinics of North America is covered in *MEDLINE/PubMed (Index Medicus), EMBASE/Excerpta Medica, Current Contents/Clinical Medicine, Current Contents/Life Sciences, Science Citation Index, ISI/BIOMED, BIOSIS,* and *Chemical Abstracts.*

Printed and bound by CPI Group (UK) Ltd, Croydon, CR0 4YY

Transferred to digital print 2012

Contributors

CONSULTING EDITOR

DEREK LEROITH, MD, PhD
Director of Research, Division of Endocrinology, Metabolism, and Bone Diseases, Department of Medicine, Mount Sinai School of Medicine, New York, New York

EDITOR

ELIZA B. GEER, MD
Assistant Professor, Division of Endocrinology, Diabetes, and Bone Disease, Departments of Medicine and Neurosurgery, Icahn School of Medicine at Mount Sinai, New York, New York

AUTHORS

ANTHONY J. BELLA, MD, FRCSC
Greta and John Hansen Chair in Men's Health Research; Assistant Professor of Urology, Department of Surgery; Associate Scientist, Neuroscience, University of Ottawa, Ottawa, Ontario, Canada

NIKOLAOS P. DASKALAKIS, MD, PhD
Postdoctoral Fellow, Traumatic Stress Studies Division; Professor, Department of Psychiatry; Postdoctoral Fellow, Laboratory of Molecular Neuropsychiatry, Department of Psychiatry, Icahn School of Medicine at Mount Sinai, New York; Postdoctoral Fellow, Mental Health Care Center, PTSD Program and Laboratory of Clinical Neuroendocrinology and Neurochemistry, James J. Peters Veterans Affairs Medical Center, Bronx, New York

CHAO DENG, PhD
Associate Professor and Head, Antipsychotic Research Laboratory, School of Health Sciences, Illawarra Health and Medical Research Institute, University of Wollongong, Wollongong, New South Wales, Australia

ANNA Z. FELDMAN, MD
Fellow, Division of Endocrinology, Department of Medicine, Beth Israel Deaconess Medical Center, Harvard Medical School, Boston, Massachusetts

ELIZA B. GEER, MD
Assistant Professor, Division of Endocrinology, Diabetes, and Bone Disease, Departments of Medicine and Neurosurgery, Icahn School of Medicine at Mount Sinai, New York, New York

BRIAN D. GREENWALD, MD
Medical Director, JFK Johnson Rehabilitation Center for Head Injuries; Clinical Associate
Professor, Department of Physical Medicine and Rehabilitation, UMDNJ-Robert Wood
Johnson Medical School, JFK Johnson Rehabilitation Institute, Edison, New Jersey

JAMES V. HENNESSEY, MD
Associate Professor of Medicine, Division of Endocrinology, Department of Medicine,
Beth Israel Deaconess Medical Center, Harvard Medical School, Boston, Massachusetts

JONATHAN JUN, MD
Assistant Professor, Division of Pulmonary and Critical Care Medicine, Johns Hopkins
University School of Medicine, Baltimore, Maryland

EFRAT KRAVITZ, PhD
The Joseph Sagol Neuroscience Center, Sheba Medical Center, Ramat Gan, Israel

AMY LEHRNER, PhD
Postdoctoral Fellow, Traumatic Stress Studies Division, Department of Psychiatry;
Laboratory of Molecular Neuropsychiatry, Department of Psychiatry, Icahn School of
Medicine at Mount Sinai, New York; Mental Health Care Center, PTSD Program and
Laboratory of Clinical Neuroendocrinology and Neurochemistry, James J. Peters
Veterans Affairs Medical Center, Bronx, New York

OMAR MESARWI, MD
Postdoctoral Fellow, Division of Pulmonary and Critical Care Medicine, Johns Hopkins
University School of Medicine, Baltimore, Maryland

HEINO F.L. MEYER-BAHLBURG, Dr rer nat
Research Scientist, New York State Psychiatric Institute; Professor of Clinical Psychology
(in Psychiatry), Columbia University, New York, New York

KAREN KLAHR MILLER, MD
Associate Professor of Medicine, Harvard Medical School and Neuroendocrine Unit,
Massachusetts General Hospital, Boston, Massachusetts

GIESJE NEFS, PhD
Department of Medical and Clinical Psychology, Center of Research on Psychology in
Somatic Diseases (CoRPS), Tilburg University, Tilburg, The Netherlands

ARIE NOUWEN, PhD
Professor, School of Health and Social Sciences, Middlesex University, London,
United Kingdom

JAN POLAK, MD, PhD
Postdoctoral Fellow, Division of Pulmonary and Critical Care Medicine, Johns Hopkins
University School of Medicine, Baltimore, Maryland

VSEVOLOD Y. POLOTSKY, MD, PhD
Associate Professor, Division of Pulmonary and Critical Care Medicine, Johns Hopkins
University School of Medicine, Baltimore, Maryland

FRANÇOIS POUWER, PhD
Professor, Department of Medical and Clinical Psychology; Program Leader, Diabetes
and Hypertension, Center of Research on Psychology in Somatic Diseases (CoRPS),
Tilburg University, Tilburg, The Netherlands

NADIA RACHDAOUI, PhD
Assistant Research Professor, Rutgers Endocrine Research Program, Department of Animal Sciences, Rutgers University, New Brunswick, New Jersey

DIPAK K. SARKAR, PhD, DPhil
Distinguished Professor, Rutgers Endocrine Research Program, Department of Animal Sciences, Rutgers University, New Brunswick, New Jersey

JAMES SCHMEIDLER, PhD
Department of Psychiatry, Mount Sinai School of Medicine, New York, New York

MICHAL SCHNAIDER BEERI, PhD
The Joseph Sagol Neuroscience Center, Sheba Medical Center, Israel; Department of Psychiatry, Mount Sinai School of Medicine, New York, New York

RANY SHAMLOUL, MD, PhD
Department of Andrology, Cairo University, Cairo, Egypt; Department of Surgery, Division of Urology, University of Ottawa; Ottawa Hospital Research Institute, Ottawa, Ontario, Canada

RUPENDRA T. SHRESTHA, MD
Hospitalist, Division of Hospital Medicine, Department of Medicine, Beth Israel Deaconess Medical Center-Milton, Milton, Massachusetts

MONICA N. STARKMAN, MD, MS
Associate Professor Emerita, Department of Psychiatry, University of Michigan Medical Center, Ann Arbor, Michigan

NINA K. SUNDARAM, MD
Clinical Fellow, Division of Endocrinology, Diabetes, and Bone Disease, Mount Sinai Medical Center, New York, New York

RACHEL YEHUDA, PhD
Director and Professor, Traumatic Stress Studies Division, Department of Psychiatry; Laboratory of Molecular Neuropsychiatry, Department of Psychiatry; Professor, Department of Neuroscience, Icahn School of Medicine at Mount Sinai, New York; Mental Health Care Center, PTSD Program and Laboratory of Clinical Neuroendocrinology and Neurochemistry, James J. Peters Veterans Affairs Medical Center, Bronx, New York

ADHAM ZAAZAA, MD, PhD, FECSM
Department of Andrology, Cairo University, Cairo, Egypt

HANY SHAMLOUL, MD, PhD

Department of Medicine, Division of Endocrinology and Metabolism, Rabin Medical Center, Milton, Milton, Massachusetts

Contents

administration may elicit a hypomanic syndrome with mood, sleep and cognitive disruptions. Treatment options are discussed. Brain imaging and neuropsychological studies indicate elevated cortisol and other glucocorticoids are especially deleterious to hippocampus and frontal lobe. The research findings also shed light on neuropsychiatric abnormalities in conditions that have substantial subgroups exhibiting elevated and dysregulated cortisol: aging, major depressive disorder and Alzheimer disease.

Type 2 diabetes, like dementia, disproportionately affects the elderly. Diabetes has consistently been associated with risk of dementia, mild cognitive impairment, and cognitive decline suggesting that cognitive compromise is a deleterious manifestation of diabetes. This review summarizes observational studies and clinical trials of diabetes medications and their respective associations and effects on cognitive outcomes. Despite biological plausibility, results from most human clinical trials have failed to show any efficacy in treating Alzheimer disease symptomatology and pathology. Clinical trials targeting vascular-related outcomes, diabetic patients, or cognitively normal elderly at risk for dementia, may provide greater cognitive benefits.

Regulation of Psychiatric on Endocrine Systems

Post-traumatic stress disorder (PTSD) is a serious, multisystem disorder with multiple medical comorbidities. This article reviews the current literature on the endocrine aspects of PTSD, specifically hypothalamic-pituitary-adrenal axis alterations indicative of low cortisol and increased glucocorticoid sensitivity, and the proposed mechanisms whereby these alterations increase risk or reflect pathophysiology. Discussion includes novel treatment innovations and directions for future research.

A key feature of anorexia nervosa, a disease primarily psychiatric in origin, is chronic starvation, which results in profound neuroendocrine dysregulation, including hypogonadism, relative growth hormone resistance, and hypercortisolemia. A recent area of investigation is appetite hormone dysregulation. Whether such dysregulation is compensatory or plays a role in the pathophysiology of anorexia nervosa is incompletely understood. The primary therapy for anorexia remains psychiatric, and endocrine abnormalities tend to improve with weight restoration, although residual endocrine dysfunction can occur. In addition, therapies directed at specific complications have been a particular focus of research.

Effect of External Influences (Drugs, Trauma, Sleep) on Endocrine Function

ENDOCRINOLOGY AND METABOLISM CLINICS OF NORTH AMERICA

Foreword

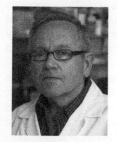

Derek LeRoith, MD, PhD
Consulting Editor

An area that is often overlooked by endocrinologists, the bidirectional impact of endocrine disorders and the brain, is discussed in this issue compiled by Dr Geer.

The first four articles discuss the regulation of endocrine systems on psychiatric disorders. One of the most challenging aspects of endocrinology is patients with somatic disorders of sex development and gender dysphoria. As described by Dr Meyer-Bahlburg, the approach to these patients must be interdisciplinary, since both psychiatric and hormonal considerations are paramount. Individuals requesting help with gender assignments or alterations often require surgical procedures in addition to hormonal therapies. The hormonal therapies in many cases require suppression of normal endocrine functions and then treatment with hormonal therapy to enhance the desired gender phenotype.

Drs Feldman, Shrestha, and Hennessey discuss the common neuropsychiatric symptoms seen in patients with hypothyroidism and hyperthyroidism. Experimental research has clearly demonstrated effects of thyroid hormones on brain development and nervous system function and, not surprisingly, thyroid dysfunction leads to nervous system symptoms. While many of the systems are reversible upon appropriate therapy of thyroid dysfunction, some may persist. Importantly, the authors stress that using thyroid hormone for neuropsychiatric disorders in the absence of laboratory evidence of dysfunction lacks evidence and should be avoided.

Dr Starkman describes the neuropsychiatric manifestations of Cushing disease and syndrome. Common symptoms include depression, anxiety, sleep disturbances, and cognitive disorders to mention just a few. It seems most likely that many of these changes are related to the increased cortisol levels in Cushing and, after appropriate treatment, there is often improvement but not always total disappearance of these disorders. Interestingly, imaging has demonstrated hippocampal abnormalities that may be secondary to hypercorticolism and it will be important to determine whether these changes can ever recover after successful therapy.

Diabetes is clearly related to an increase in dementia. As Drs Kravitz, Schmeidler, and Schnaider Beeri describe, this association includes Alzheimer, vascular dementia, and mild cognitive decline. There is evidence that insulin resistance maybe an etiologic factor in the effects of diabetes on cognitive decline and Alzheimer. Interestingly some

Endocrinol Metab Clin N Am 42 (2013) xiii–xv
http://dx.doi.org/10.1016/j.ecl.2013.06.007
0889-8529/13/$ – see front matter © 2013 Published by Elsevier Inc.

recent clinical trials have tested the administration of insulin intranasally and demonstrated some improvement in cognition. Whether this is an effect of insulin on b-amyloid protein requires further investigation. There are other studies on PPARγ agonists that have been successful in animals but not in humans and there are suggestions that the GLP-1 agonists and metformin may be of value. However, at present the possibility is that treating patients at risk may be more effective than those with established disorders.

The next three articles focus on the role of psychiatric disorders on the endocrine system. In their article on posttraumatic stress disorder (PTSD), Daskalakis, Lehrner, and Yehuda describe the derangements of the hypothalamic-adrenal axis (HPA) and how these may impact the pathophysiology and potential therapeutics of PTSD. While catecholamines were elevated as expected, surprisingly, cortisol levels and glucocorticoid (GC) signaling were reduced, also reflected by the increased levels of corticotropin-releasing hormone and pro-inflammatory cytokines. The hypothesis is that at the time of stress this reduced GC response may influence the degree of PTSD. While acute or chronic administration of GCs may affect PTSD, the authors conclude that more studies are required on the HPA axis and the enzymatic regulation of GCs and will require newer technologies for the detection of biomarkers that would help in therapeutic approaches.

Anorexia nervosa is a psychiatric disorder that affects the endocrine system. The marked reduction in caloric intake has profound effects on many tissues. Neuroendocrine dysregulation leads to GH resistance, hypercorticolism, and hypothalamic amenorrhea, effects that can cause delayed puberty in adolescent girls and inability to reach peak bone mass. As Dr Miller describes, it is mostly seen in women. Studies have suggested that reduced levels of leptin and kisspeptin may be involved in the development of amenorrhea, though administration of these proteins may not be feasible. Other hormones such as PYY and ghrelin, both appetite-regulating hormones from the gut, are elevated in patients with anorexia nervosa. While these and other studies are of interest in helping to understand the pathophysiology, they maybe secondary effects. Importantly, while the therapy needs to be undertaken by psychiatrist, consultation with the endocrinologist is obviously extremely important.

While it is clear that diabetes is associated with depression, the reverse is not always appreciated by the clinician. Drs Pouwer, Nefs, and Nouwen discuss how depression may affect the diabetic patient, having an impact on self-care by the patient and how in longitudinal studies this has been shown to affect long-term outcomes with an increase in diabetic complications. Once again, the endocrinologist needs to be cognisant of the issue and consider therapeutic options, to allow for maximal diabetes management.

In the final five articles, the role of external factors, including drugs and trauma, on the endocrine system, are reviewed. In an article regarding weight gain, insulin resistance, and even the development of type 2 diabetes secondary to antipsychotic medications, Dr Deng discusses both the clinical relevance and the potential mechanisms. While it is clear that many antipsychotic drugs increase appetite and/or reduce satiety to varying degrees, presumably via effects on the hypothalamus, there is also growing evidence that the peripheral effects on insulin resistance and induction of diabetes may be independent, to some degree, on the weight gain. The antipsychotic agents' effects on central serotonin 5-HT$_{2C}$, histamine H1, dopamine D2, and muscarinic receptors have all been invoked as important players for various aspects of the side effects, elegantly described in this article.

As discussed in the article by Drs Sundaram, Geer, and Greenwald, the pituitary is an extremely vulnerable anatomical structure and prone to involvement following both mild and severe traumatic brain injury, which may occur in one in four cases. In particular, the gonadotrophs and somatotrophs are often the first cells to be affected, perhaps due to their location, and later the corticotrophs and thyrotrophs, given their unique blood supply. Independent of this temporal dysfunction, posterior pituitary functional loss may also be seen in an equivalent number of cases. Appropriate screening and initiation of therapy should be performed for months and even years after the trauma as pituitary endocrine deficits, which significantly impact recovery, may be seen acutely, and may even develop at much later stages.

There are many medical problems associated with drug addiction, including hormonal abnormalities, sexual dysfunction being one of them. Indeed, almost 80% of young drug abusers describe sexual dysfunction and this side effect is often the reason for them "kicking" the habit. Drs Zaazaa and Shamloul describe the pathophysiology of drug addiction in their article and then enlarge on the specific dysfunction caused by drug addiction, including alcohol, cannabis, cocaine, amphetamines, and psychotropics. Clearly the therapeutic regimen is to cease using the drugs, but endocrinologists will often be referred patients with sexual dysfunction and diagnosing drug abuse should be at the top of the differential diagnosis.

The article by Drs Rachdaoui and Sarkar includes more discussion regarding the effects of alcohol on the endocrine system. They describe the interplay between the nervous system, the immune system, and the endocrine system and how alcohol disturbs this normal homeostasis. There are acute and chronic effects on the hypothalamic-pituitary axis that may be mediated by vasopressin and the endogenous opioid system. Similarly, alcohol affects the male and female hypothalamic-pituitary-gonadal axis, the pituitary-thyroid axis, the GH-IGF axis, as well as pancreatic function. These multiple potential endocrine effects need careful evaluation in patients displaying chronic alcoholism.

Finally, a fascinating area of discussion revolves around the role of altered sleep and sleep apnea on body weight and type 2 diabetes. While it is clear that overweight and obese individuals may suffer from sleep apnea for reasons related to physical obstruction of airways as well as possible effects on the hypothalamus, the question is whether the reverse is true. Drs Mesarwi, Polak, Jun, and Polotsky discuss the reduction in the number of hours we sleep that has been documented over the past few decades. Since sleep is a critical time for whole metabolic restoration, they posit that the lack of sleep may have effects both centrally and peripherally that could lead to obesity, insulin resistance, and diabetes. While the mechanisms need to be determined, the effects seem to be more frequently occurring and becoming clinically extremely relevant to the practicing endocrinologist.

I believe that the articles included in this issue written by leaders in the field have practical implications for the readers and the practicing endocrinologists. Dr Geer and the authors should be applauded for an excellent job and we thank them.

Derek LeRoith, MD, PhD
Division of Endocrinology, Metabolism, and Bone Diseases
Department of Medicine
Mount Sinai School of Medicine
One Gustave L. Levy Place
Box 1055, Altran 4-36
New York, NY 10029, USA

E-mail address:
derek.leroith@mssm.edu

Preface

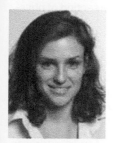

Eliza B. Geer, MD
Editor

The endocrine and neuropsychiatric systems are closely intertwined. The master regulator of the endocrine systems, the hypothalamic-pituitary unit, which includes neural and endocrine structures, serves to integrate external environmental, nutritional, and circadian cues with internal metabolic and emotional signals. Thus it is the prototypical example of the sameness of the mind and body.

The enclosed issue of *Endocrinology and Metabolism Clinics of North America* illustrates critical relationships between endocrine and neuropsychiatric disorders. The first four articles highlight the regulation of the endocrine on the neuropsychiatric systems: the formative role of sex steroids in development of gender identity and transgenderism; the regulation of thyroid hormones on neuropsychiatric function; the effects of endogenous and exogenous glucocorticoid exposure on cognitive and psychiatric states; and finally, the effect of diabetes on cognitive function. The subsequent three articles investigate the opposite direction: the regulation of psychiatric disorders on endocrine systems. These articles include reviews of the effect of posttraumatic stress disorder on the function of the hypothalamic-pituitary-adrenal axis; endocrine consequences of anorexia nervosa; and the role of depression on glycemic control and outcomes in patients with diabetes. The final five articles depict effects of external influences (medications, drugs, sleep disorders, and trauma) on endocrine function. These articles include reviews of the effects of antipsychotic medications on weight and insulin sensitivity; the impact of traumatic brain injury on pituitary endocrine function; effects of alcohol and other drugs in the endocrine systems and sexual function; and finally, the role of sleep and sleep deprivation on insulin sensitivity and risk for obesity.

The enclosed comprehensive and interdisciplinary articles beautifully illustrate the complex interplay between cognitive, emotional, and metabolic signals. These topics depict the need for careful orchestration of the endocrine and neuropsychiatric systems for the homeostasis and ultimate survival of any organism. Finally, the contributing authors reveal the profound effect neuropsychiatric states can exert on a body's

Endocrinol Metab Clin N Am 42 (2013) xvii–xviii
http://dx.doi.org/10.1016/j.ecl.2013.06.008
0889-8529/13/$ – see front matter © 2013 Published by Elsevier Inc.

metabolic regulation, and the diseases that result from damage or dysregulation between these systems. I hope that the enclosed reviews contribute to the development of future collaborative and interdisciplinary research on the critical intersection of physiology, psychology, and behavior.

Eliza B. Geer, MD
Division of Endocrinology, Diabetes, and Bone Diseases
Departments of Medicine and Neurosurgery
Icahn School of Medicine at Mount Sinai
One Gustave L. Levy Place, Box 1055
New York, NY 10029, USA

E-mail address:
eliza.geer@mssm.edu

Sex Steroids and Variants of Gender Identity

Heino F.L. Meyer-Bahlburg, Dr rer nat

KEYWORDS

- Disorders of sex development • Gender assignment • Gender dysphoria
- Gender identity • Sex steroids • Transgenderism

KEY POINTS

- In somatic disorders of sex development (DSD), gender dysphoria (GD) and patient-initiated gender change vary with syndrome, syndrome severity, and initial assignment of gender.
- Data on long-term gender and sexuality outcome of DSD have recently led to considerable changes in policies of gender assignment and gender-confirming surgery.
- The prenatal androgen milieu appears to be more closely associated with later gendered behavior than with gender identity.
- GD without DSD may be associated with atypical brain anatomy or function, but abnormalities of systemic hormone levels or receptor functions have not been established.
- More research is needed on the short-term and long-term effects of treatment with puberty-suppressing medications and cross-sex hormones on brain and behavior.

INTRODUCTION

For most individuals, their gender identity as "boy" or "girl," "man" or "woman," develops in line with the gender they were assigned at birth, which, in turn, is usually based on the appearance of their genital sex as "male" or "female." Individuals may have some notion as to what extent they fit or do not fit their society's ideal of a masculine man or feminine woman, but they do not doubt that they are one or the other gender. Only a small minority of people with normally formed male or female genitalia experience their gender development as being at variance with their assigned gender. People with a severe gender-identity variant may come to clinicians' attention and receive diagnoses such as "Transsexual" in International Classification of Diseases

Funding Sources: NIMH; previously NCRR, NICHD.
Conflict of Interest: Nil.
New York State Psychiatric Institute, Columbia University, 1051 Riverside Drive, Unit 15, New York, NY 10032, USA
E-mail address: meyerb@nyspi.columbia.edu

Endocrinol Metab Clin N Am 42 (2013) 435–452
http://dx.doi.org/10.1016/j.ecl.2013.05.011
0889-8529/13/$ – see front matter © 2013 Elsevier Inc. All rights reserved.

endo.theclinics.com

(ICD)-10,[1] "Gender Identity Disorder" in *Diagnostic and Statistical Manual of Mental Disorders* (4th edition, text revision) (DSM-IV-TR),[2] or "Gender Dysphoria" (GD) in DSM-5 (see **Box 1** for gender terms).[3] Recent years have seen a marked increase of referrals of gender-dysphoric individuals to specialty clinics in Europe and North America.[4] At the same time, the general transgender spectrum has widened considerably and now includes many more or less fluid identity categories between male and female, such as "genderqueer." Many of these less strongly gender-atypical individuals do not see any need for psychiatric or other medical assistance.[5]

In individuals born with a reproductive system that is not clearly male or female and, therefore, labeled as "ambiguous genitalia" or "intersex" (now subsumed under the broader category of "Disorders of Sex Development"),[6] the assignment of gender is typically based on a more complex process involving various diagnostic tests and prognostic interpretations of the research available on long-term gender outcomes. The empirical evidence, on which such assignment decisions are based, is still somewhat limited. Given the additional fact that many patients with DSD are aware of their genital ambiguity, it is not surprising that later GD and patient-initiated

---

Box 1
Gender terms

1. Gender behaviors

   a. Also known as gender-role behaviors, gender-related behaviors, sex-dimorphic behaviors, gendered behaviors

   b. Defined as behaviors, traits, interests, and attitudes whereby the genders differ in a given place, culture, and historical era

2. Gender identity

   a. Also known as core gender identity (and, sometimes and unfortunately, "sexual identity," which more commonly is used as a short form for "sexual orientation identity," that is, identity as "gay," "lesbian," "straight," or "bisexual")

   b. Defined as the basic sense of being a girl or boy, woman or man, or, rarely, of being some other category, eg, "neither-nor," "third gender," or "intersex"

3. Gender dysphoria

   a. Also known as "Gender Identity Disorder" (DSM-IV-TR)

   b. Defined as cognitive/affective discontent with the assigned gender

   c. Definition of Gender Dysphoria as diagnostic category in DSM-5: "A marked incongruence between one's experienced/expressed gender and assigned gender, of at least 6 months duration" [as manifested by at least 6 of 8 indicators in children and 2 of 6 indicators in adults] and "associated with clinically significant distress or impairment in social, school/occupational, or other important areas of functioning"

4. Transsexual

   a. Defined as an individual who, in the binary gender system of male and female, identifies with the "other" gender than the one she or he was assigned to

5. Transgender

   a. Widely used as an umbrella term to cover all gender-atypical identities

6. Genderqueer

   a. Defined as an identity that is not constrained by the common binary systems of gender (male and female) and sexual orientation (heterosexual and homosexual)

gender change occur more frequently in such individuals than in the general population.[7]

In several countries, the legal systems have recently begun to recognize that not all individuals fall neatly into one or the other of the two traditional categories of sex or gender. For instance, in 2005 India permitted emasculinated male-to-female (MtF) transgender individuals, called *hijras*, to list their gender on passports as "E" (for Eunuch).[8] As of 2010, the Australian Recognized Details Certificate permits the entry "Sex Not Specified," initially for a 47,XXY individual who underwent sex reassignment surgery including castration, did not take hormone replacement therapy, and had a gender-neutral identity.[9] In January of 2013, the German parliament passed a law requiring that the sex category on birth certificates be left open in cases of DSD, for whom the sex could not be determined.[10]

GD and patient-initiated gender change in general as well as the question of initial gender assignment in cases of intersex newborns confront clinicians with a complex challenge involving genetic, endocrine, surgical, psychiatric, cultural, legal, and ethical questions and are, therefore, preferably managed by multidisciplinary teams.[6] The participating endocrinologist contributes expertise in the assessment of both function and dysfunction of the endocrine system, and the effects of endocrine treatment. This article is designed to update the reader on the current status of knowledge regarding the contribution of the sex steroids to long-term gender-identity outcome.

DISORDERS OF SEX DEVELOPMENT
Policies of Gender Assignment

From the essentialist perspective prevalent before the 1950s, sex was understood as a basically binary system, even in societies that allowed social niches of a small minority of people who did not fit in somatically or behaviorally, and there was no systematic distinction between sex and gender. In cases of genital ambiguity, a "true-sex policy"[11] applied; that is, one had to identify the key biological criterion of sex and determine its prevailing gender as the basis for the assignment of gender to the newborn: in antiquity the external genitalia; in the late nineteenth century the gonadal histology; and in the mid-twentieth century the karyotype. The detailed documentation of people whose gender identity was well formed but at odds with the assumed key biological criteria led the psychologist, John Money, and his team at Johns Hopkins Hospital, in collaboration with the pediatric endocrinologist Lawson Wilkins, to introduce a policy[12,13] that took into consideration the (assumed) effects of social-rearing factors and the sexual function expected with the best surgical and hormonal treatment available at the time ("optimal-gender policy"[11]).

This work took place a few years before systematic research on nonhuman mammals began elucidating the role of sex hormones in the sexual differentiation of brain and behavior during a hormone-sensitive phase of early (fetal and/or neonatal) development, which gave rise to the organization-activation theory of sexual differentiation (Phoenix and colleagues,[14] 1959; see later discussion). When Money's team (and, subsequently, others) was able to show similar effects also in humans, some animal researchers proposed a "true-brain-sex policy,"[11] whereby the assignment of sex was to be based on the assumed androgenization of the brain as inferred from the degree of genital masculinization and/or endogenous peripheral androgen production.[15] In recent years, actual clinical practice has increasingly followed an eclectic policy evolving from the international Consensus Conference on Intersex in Chicago, 2005,[6] which is based on the combination of inferred brain androgenization, prognosis of the functional outcome of genital surgery and hormone treatment (including their impact on fertility), and evidence from long-term follow-up of gender outcome in relation to a specific syndrome and syndrome severity. Increasingly, human-rights issues are also being taken into consideration.[16,17]

Factors Contributing to the Development of Gendered Behavior

Over the past half century extensive research in humans and animals has led to a gradual recognition of how complex the entire process of the sexual differentiation of body, brain, behavior, and identity really is. Our understanding of this process today is still far from complete. In the now classic animal-research–based organization-activation theory of sexual differentiation, the bipotential gonadal anlagen differentiate early during pregnancy into either testes or ovaries under the influence of a cascade of genes. Shortly afterward, the newly formed testes begin the production of fetal androgen, whereas the ovaries stay dormant. The subsequent sexual differentiation of body, brain, and behavior depends on the amount of steroid sex hormones available in the fetal and/or neonatal circulation. In precocial species such as the guinea pig, much of the sexual differentiation of the brain appears to take place prenatally; in altricial species such as the rat, it takes place late prenatally and early postnatally.[18] Other species differences concern the role of estrogens and androgens. In rats, for instance, prenatal and perinatal estrogens defeminize (ie, diminish the later expression of female-typical behavior) and prenatal/perinatal androgens masculinize (ie, enhance the later expression of male-typical behavior), whereas in primates prenatal androgens both defeminize and masculinize later behavior.[18,19]

Money's team was the first to demonstrate that prenatal androgens were also associated with masculinization of postnatal gender-related behavior in humans. This association was shown first in girls with a history of prenatal exposure to exogenous (androgen-derived) 19-nor progestins that had moderately masculinized their genitalia,[20] and then in girls and women with excessive endogenous androgen production resulting from classic congenital adrenal hyperplasia (CAH).[21,22] Despite variable behavioral masculinization, most of these girls and women developed and maintained a female gender identity. In the meantime, many teams have replicated the findings on CAH in different countries and cultures, although with considerable variability dependent on sample composition in terms of CAH variants, sample size, psychological domains studied, and assessment methods used.[23] The masculinization extends to all domains of gendered behavior whereby healthy males and females typically differ: childhood play, affiliation with male versus female peers, physical-activity level, physical strength, aggression, adolescent leisure-time activities, sports participation, career preferences, voice characteristics in adulthood, habitual body positions and movement patterns, romantic/erotic attraction toward women, and maternalism.[23]

The reverse, namely reduction of masculine behavior, is seen in 46,XY individuals whose prenatal androgen synthesis is deficient, as, for instance, in 46,XY gonadal dysgenesis, or in those who have androgen insensitivity syndrome (AIS) caused by genetic defects of the androgen receptor or its cofactors. In individuals with 46,XY complete AIS, for instance, the gonads are testicular and produce normal or high-normal amounts of testosterone and antimullerian hormone, but the external genitalia appear normal-female at birth.[24] Therefore, such newborns are usually not recognized as DSD but are assigned and reared as females, although they lack a uterus and fallopian tubes, and the vagina may be reduced to a dimple. As shown in several studies, again initiated by Money and his team[25] and later replicated by others,[26,27] gendered behavior in girls and women with complete AIS does not differ from that of healthy female controls. This finding indicates that the androgen-receptor defect prevents the masculinizing effects of androgens also on brain and behavior. By contrast, 46,XY individuals with less severe hypomasculinization and genital ambiguity severe enough that they are still assigned and raised female at birth tend to show variable masculinization of behavior in comparison with non-DSD female controls.[28,29]

That androgens likely contribute causally to the atypical gender behaviors associated with such DSD syndromes is best illustrated by the findings on 46,XX CAH. Several studies have shown that patients with the more severe salt-wasting subtype, who have more severe deficiencies of 21-hydroxylase, cortisol, and aldosterone, produce more adrenal androgens, and usually show more marked genital masculinization than the simple virilizing subtype, and also show more behavioral masculinization.[23] Even the mildest subtype, Nonclassic CAH, which is not associated with genital ambiguity at birth, shows slightly but significantly increased behavioral masculinization,[30,31] and the genotype with the most extreme 21-hydroxylase deficiency, namely the null mutation, is even more masculinized somatically and behaviorally than the other salt-wasting variants.[32] Although some published data on 46,XY DSD with hypomasculinization also suggest dose-response relationships between prenatal androgens and later gendered behavior,[33] systematic analyses of such data have yet to be conducted.

The role of estrogens in the sexual differentiation of brain and behavior in humans is less well understood. During fetal life the ovaries are dormant, but in both sexes estrogens are released from the placenta into the fetoplacental unit. Their contribution to the sexual differentiation of brain and behavior in humans is unknown. Follow-up studies of gendered behavior in female offspring from pregnancies that were treated with the potent nonsteroidal estrogen diethylstilbestrol (DES) did not show masculinization of various facets of gendered behavior.[34] However, in another study from the author's team prenatally DES-exposed women experienced increased bisexuality,[35] a finding that was not replicated elsewhere.[36] As mentioned earlier, 46,XY individuals with complete AIS produce estrogens in amounts sufficient for breast development (in the absence of androgen effects), but their gendered behavior usually does not differ from that of female controls.[25–27] The few scattered reports on individual (very rare) cases of 46,XY men with normal external genitalia but deficient estrogen production resulting from aromatase deficiency[37,38] or with estrogen insensitivity owing to a genetic defect of the estrogen receptor[39] suggest that their gendered behavior falls into the normal range of men, although possibly with low libido in the case of the aromatase-deficient men.

Furthermore, fetal C-17 progesterone is unlikely to contribute to behavioral masculinization, because exogenous C-17 progestagens, which are closely related to C-17 progesterone, demasculinize.[40] By contrast, exogenous C-19 progestagens masculinize the behavior of girls,[20] as mentioned earlier.

Thus, in humans as well as other primates, androgens appear to be the primary steroid hormone driving the sexual differentiation of brain and behavior. Indeed, fetal testosterone levels as measured in amniotic fluid, for instance, are much higher in males than in females.[24] As male infants also show a neonatal testosterone surge between about 2 weeks and 5 months of age, the question arises as to whether these postnatal androgens rather than the prenatal ones cause, or at least contribute to, the sexual differentiation of brain and behavior. The early publications by Money's team[21,22] showed that marked behavioral masculinization can be seen in girls and women with either late onset of the then newly introduced glucocorticoid replacement treatment, which also suppresses androgen excess, or onset of glucocorticoid treatment at birth. This finding implies a prenatal effect of androgen, as has been shown in other mammals. In line with these findings, later studies[41] showed that masculinization of play behavior in girls with CAH was significantly associated with the diagnosis of the more severe, salt-wasting subtype of CAH, early age at CAH diagnosis, and degree of genital masculinization at birth—all indicating androgen excess during prenatal development—rather than with later bone-age advance, concurrent or cumulative high levels of 17-hydroxyprogesterone, or accelerated growth velocity in early childhood, which all would point to postnatal androgen excess attributable to insufficient hormonal control by postnatal treatment.

Unfortunately, the available human observational studies in this area are not yet able to match the rigor of recent experimental work in animals. Such animal studies led to the distinction of 3 organizational phases of hormone effects on brain development: the prenatal/perinatal phase, puberty, and, in females, pregnancy.[42] Even more detailed studies in Syrian hamsters led to the conclusion that the sensitivity of the central nervous system (CNS) to organizational effects of sex hormones gradually decreases from prenatal development to young adulthood.[43] Only the fact that gonadal hormone production is dormant between the perinatal phase and puberty underlies the appearance of distinct phases of sexual differentiation of brain and behavior (early vs late in development). To the extent this applies to humans as well (and there is no reason to assume that it does not), one would expect that exposure to postnatal androgen excess may further contribute to CNS organization, although progressively less so with advancing age.

A related question frequently arises for the urological surgeon in decisions on the timing of gonadectomy in 46,XY DSD. Does the removal of (at least partially functional) testes before the end of the neonatal testosterone surge affect the later gender outcome? Related experimental studies in rhesus monkeys (Macaca mulatta) have shown no striking effects of neonatal surgical or (transient) chemical castration on either juvenile or adult male behavior, although puberty may be somewhat delayed.[44] In the human DSD literature several cases of newborns with 46,XY cloacal exstrophy have been documented, in whom neonatal castration in the context of female gender assignment did not prevent later patient-initiated gender change to male.[45] Such data underline the assumed importance of prenatal hormones for human psychosexual differentiation, although firm conclusions will require more systematic and definitive data.

Studies on 46,XX CAH show increased variability of gendered behavior with increasing syndrome severity in terms of endocrine criteria or molecular genotype.[30] The likely explanation of this decreasing correlation of genotype with behavioral phenotype as a function of increased prenatal androgen levels rests with the role of other genes in the sexual differentiation of the brain. Whereas about 2 dozen genes are known or suspected to be involved in the differentiation of the gonads,[46] the sexual differentiation of the brain involves several hundred steroid-responsive genes in the mouse,[47] and probably even more in the human, given the higher degree of complexity of the human brain. In addition, some genes affect brain differentiation independently of steroid hormones.[48] Thus, the organization-activation hypothesis had to be substantially revised.[49,50] The rapid advances of genetic techniques for automated screening of large numbers of genes and gene products are likely to provide new approaches to the sexual differentiation of brain and behavior in humans for use in both research and clinical decision making.[51]

Apart from biological factors, a vast body of research in developmental psychology has identified a variety of cognitive and social factors that contribute to psychosexual differentiation (**Box 2**).[52] However, there is no proof that such psychosocial factors on their own can cause long-term gender-behavior shifts as strong as seen in individuals with severe DSD or even full change of gender.

| **Box 2** |
| **Cognitive and social factors in psychosexual differentiation** |

- Verbal gender labeling (eg, "boy," "girl")
- Nonverbal gender cueing (eg, gender-specific clothing styles, colors, and haircuts)
- Differential reinforcement (positive, negative) of gender-typical behavior
- Categorizing other people by gender: fuzzy concepts/stereotypes/gender schemas (including affective evaluation)
  - Physical
  - Behavioral
- Categorizing self by gender: self-concept, self-schema (including gender identity)
  - Physical (body image)
  - Behavioral (masculinity, femininity)
- Observational learning/imitation (gender-selective)
- Self-socialization (by gender)

Factors Contributing to the Development of Gender Identity

That the karyotype is not a firm biological determinant of gender identity has been amply demonstrated by the existence of 46,XY female-identified and 46,XX male-identified persons in individuals both with or without a peripheral DSD. Moreover, the association of prenatal sex hormones with gender outcome is not uniform. In the best studied DSD syndrome, 46,XX CAH, most individuals with the severe form, salt-wasting CAH, are living and identified as women, despite markedly masculinized behavior. The (group-level) dose-response relationship between degree of prenatal androgen excess and gendered behavior[30,31] could not be extended to a dimensional measure of gender identity.[53] In addition, a few individuals of complete androgen insensitivity with male identity have been described in recent years.[54–59]

On the other hand, gender identity as male or female does not develop randomly. A set of reviews of the world literature on gender identity in DSD patients produced in preparation for the International Consensus Conference on Intersex Management in Chicago[7,45,60–62] shows wide variations in GD and patient-initiated gender change dependent on the syndrome, syndrome severity, and gender assigned at birth (**Table 1**). Particularly high rates of GD and patient-initiated gender change were found in 46,XY patients with high levels of prenatal androgen exposure, as is characteristic of the syndromes of penile agenesis, cloacal exstrophy of the bladder, and 5α-reductase-2 deficiency.[45,60] Such findings have led to a reduction of the assignment of newborns of 46,XY DSD with plausibly high prenatal androgenization of the brain to the female gender. Nevertheless, gender assignment still appears to be the primary determinant of gender outcome in 46,XY cases with hypoandrogenization in the middle range of the respective scales.[29]

Recent psychological research on the complexities of normative development of gender identity has led to a reconceptualization of gender identity as a complex construct that includes several experiential and cognitive components (eg, Egan and Perry[63]): the individual's sense of compatibility with the assigned gender (self-perceived gender typicality and degree of contentedness with the assigned gender); the felt social pressure to conform to the assigned gender; and intergroup bias, that is, the degree to which one feels that one's own gender is superior to the other. Thus,

Table 1
Patient-initiated gender change or gender dysphoria as a function of syndrome and initial gender assignment based on reviews of the world literature

Syndrome	Gender Change or Gender Dysphoria (%)		Reference
	F to M	M to F	
46,XX CAH	5.2	12.1	61
46,XY 5α-R2-D	63–66	0	60
46,XY 17β-HSD3-D	64	0	60
46,XY CAIS	0[a]	—[b]	62
46,XY PAIS	7	14	62
46,XY micropenis	0	3	62
46,XY nonhormonal DSD[c]	35	0.3	45

Abbreviations: 5α-R2-D, 5α-reductase-2 deficiency; 17β-HSD3-D, 17β-hydroxysteroid dehydrogenase-3 deficiency; CAH, congenital adrenal hyperplasia; CAIS, complete androgen insensitivity syndrome; DSD, disorder of sex development; F, female; M, male; PAIS, partial androgen insensitivity syndrome.

[a] Two cases added now: one questionable F to M requesting reassignment to M in early adolescence, possibly under coercion by family, in India[57,58]; one F to M transitioning in his twenties, in Belgium.[59]

[b] One case added now: one M with some possible early masculinization of the external genitalia, but later completely androgen-insensitive, ending in suicide at age 26 years, in the United States.[54–56]

[c] Including penile agenesis, cloacal exstrophy of the bladder, traumatic loss of the penis in infancy (followed in some by imposed reassignment to female during infancy).

the binary concept of (core) gender identity is an oversimplification. Moreover, a recent study has shown that the "certainty of belonging to the assigned gender" of patients with DSD varies considerably with the degree of atypicality of their biological condition, even if they publicly continue to live in their assigned gender.[64] It is plausible, therefore, that psychological and social factors may variably motivate individuals with low "certainty" to seek better adjustment and a better quality of life by socially transitioning to the other gender or some nonstereotypical intermediate identity such as "intersex" or "genderqueer."

Given that men and women show marked differences in neuroanatomy and that we know from animal research that such differences are due to the action of genes and sex hormones, one hopes that, at some point in the future, brain imaging will be of help in decisions on gender assignment. Unfortunately, brain-imaging work on patients with DSD is just beginning and has as not yet produced results that can be used for such decisions.[23] In addition, the sexual differentiation of the brain advances after birth for years while the gonads are dormant.[65] Thus, it is currently unclear as to whether at some point in the future neuroanatomy norms can be established for newborns that would allow the use of brain imaging for gender-assignment decisions in newborns with DSD.

The use of the degree of genital masculinization as an estimate of the degree of brain masculinization has its own complications. Genital staging such as Prader staging for 46,XX CAH,[66] Quigley staging for 46,XY AIS,[67] or the clinical score of Ahmed and colleagues[68] is not really applicable to such conditions as 46,XX CAH after prenatal dexamethasone treatment (whereby in cases of inconsistent adherence the development of the internal reproductive tract and clitoral growth can be very discrepant), 5α-reductase-2 deficiency (whereby the deficiency of dihydrotestosterone reduces or blocks the masculinization of the external genitalia, but testosterone still has strong masculinizing effects on brain and behavior), or penile agenesis (whereby the penile anlage has been lost owing to nonhormonal factors). Moreover, the growth of the clit-orophallus does not depend exclusively on androgens. It is also unclear as to what extent the hormones involved in the differentiation of the reproductive tract (testos-terone, dihydrotestosterone, antimullerian hormone, estrogens) have comparable organizational effects on the CNS. Furthermore, the few studies reporting correlations of Prader stage at birth with later gendered behavior for 46,XX girls or women with CAH list correlation coefficients ranging from low and nonsignificant for boy/girl-typical play[69] and interest in infants[70] to $\rho = .40, .41,$ and $.50$ for masculine interest/behavior and appearance[71] to $\rho = .67$ and $.78$ for indices of boy-typical play,[41] thus leaving much variance unaccounted for. Finally, patient-initiated later gender change in 46,XX CAH raised females has been documented for a wide range of Prader stages (3–5), although most women at any point of those stages remain female identified.[61,72]

At this stage of our knowledge of the psychological development of persons with DSD, a definitive biological predetermination of gender identity seems unlikely. Not a single biological factor, but multiple factors—biological, psychological, and social—influence the development of gender identity.

Clinical Implications

From this perspective, the gender assignment of the newborn with a DSD should take into account everything we know about the likely sex-steroid effects on the brain in the syndrome at hand, the hormonal and surgical treatment possibilities, and the known long-term gender outcome, given an initial assignment as male or female, in the given cultural context, so as to minimize the risk of later GD and patient-initiated gender change.

Gender reassignment may become a question in infancy, when an initial diagnosis by a primary care provider is replaced later by a different, more definitive expert diag-nosis at a tertiary care medical facility that supports a different gender. In infancy, such gender reassignment can be imposed on the patient, provided the parents can be convinced of its appropriateness. However, after infancy, any gender reassignment, be it because of a new diagnosis, another physician's different policy, or some gender-atypical behavior expressed by the child, should be postponed until the child is mature enough for a thorough psychological assessment of gender development, which may require several years of development.[73]

TRANSGENDERISM
GD Without DSD

The ultimate challenge for the gender clinician is patients with GD but without a DSD, originally introduced to modern medicine as "transsexualism"; that is, people who felt the need to change from one gender to the other both socially and medically (by treat-ment with cross-sex hormones and genital surgery). In DSM-5,[3] GD was chosen as the new term and its core definition was changed from "a strong and persistent cross-gender identification and persistent discomfort with his or her sex or sense of inappropriateness in the gender role of that sex" to "a marked incongruence between one's experienced/expressed gender and assigned gender." (This redefinition also facilitated the inclusion of patients who developed GD in the context of a DSD as a subtype.)

Those non-DSD patients who present with marked gender-atypical behavior and cross-gender wishes from early on, appear at preschool age behaviorally quite similar to markedly gender-atypical persons with DSD. However, the follow-up studies done to date show that only a small fraction of them actually persisted and underwent a full social transition to the desired gender in later adolescence or adulthood.[74] The majority "desisted" from the cross-gender path and lived their adult lives as lesbians or gays without leaving their natal gender. Whether their long-term gender trajectories will change with the current fashion for early social transition (increasingly as early as elementary school age) remains to be seen.

Apart from the non-DSD patients with early onset of GD, there are others whose GD begins much later: in late childhood, adolescence, or even adulthood, often in the absence of any cross-gender behaviors that were noticed by others during early or middle childhood. Many of these individuals, especially natal males, will develop as a heterosexual (relative to their natal sex), may even get married, and have children before their sex change. For a large subset of these late-onset natal male patients, their cross-gender trajectory appears to have started out with fetishistic cross-dressing in adolescence and sexual arousal associated with seeing or imagining themselves dressed as a woman, termed autogynephilia.[75,76] The cross-gender desire of patients with late-onset GD may become as strong as those with early onset, and also most of the late-onset ones who transition to the desired gender will remain in it for the rest of their lives, although their (low) regret rates tend to be somewhat higher than those with early onset.[77]

Factors Contributing to the Development of Non-DSD GD

Although patients with DSD are excluded from the diagnosis of (non-DSD) GD, the search for biological explanations of the latter continues. The karyotype is typically in line with the genital sex. In natal males with non-DSD GD, no systemic sex-hormone abnormality has been found, but about one-third of natal females appear to have increased systemic androgen levels in the hirsute range, that is, far below the normal male range and far below the range of most females with classic CAH, so that a causal role of the modestly increased androgens in the development of GD seems doubtful.[78]

In recent years, several investigators have performed studies of peripheral sex-steroid–related nucleotide polymorphisms of steroid receptors or steroid-enzyme genes, but the results have been inconsistent or negative.[79–83] Thus, the evidence at this point is entirely insufficient to categorize people with non-DSD GD as a form of CNS-limited intersexuality.[84]

Tantalizing results have come from neuroanatomic and neurofunctional studies. A group of postmortem studies of the brains of persons with non-DSD GD have shown shifts in the size of the central portion of the bed nucleus of the stria terminalis[85,86] and the uncinate nucleus[87] that are in line with expectations based on sex-hormone–dependent sex differences in other mammals. Most of the transsexuals whose brains were studied had been treated with cross-sex hormones. In the context of post-mortem studies of brains from several control groups, the investigators plausibly argued that the differences found in the transsexuals could not be fully explained by variations in adult levels of sex hormones, so that early developmental factors, possibly including the prenatal hormonal milieu, may well have played a role. Some findings from live brain-imaging studies of transsexuals who had never been treated with cross-sex hormones show a similar trend. Luders and colleagues[88] found a larger volume of regional gray matter in the right (and possibly the left) putamen of MtF transsexuals than in that of control men, although otherwise regional gray matter variation of the MtF was more similar to the pattern found in men than in women. Rametti and colleagues,[89] using diffusion tensor imaging, concluded that in untreated MtF transsexuals the white-matter microstructure pattern falls halfway between that of non-GD men and non-GD women, whereas in untreated female-to-male (FtM) trans-sexuals the white-matter microstructure pattern is closer to the pattern found in non-GD men than in non-GD women.[90] However, in a more comprehensive magnetic resonance imaging (MRI) study of untreated MtF transsexuals, Savic and Arver[91] found multiple structural differences between the brains of MtF individuals and those from heterosexual men and women, but concluded that their data did not support the notion that the brains of MtF transsexuals are feminized. In addition, a first study using resting-state functional MRI (fMRI) for a cerebral connectivity analysis[92] did not find a difference between one FtM transsexual and a female control group. It is also impor-tant to bear in mind that all of the studies that find differences show considerable over-lap between transsexuals and controls in the distribution of neuroanatomic markers of brain dimorphisms. Thus, in this form, the markers do not yet seem to be very useful as diagnostic aids.

Remarkable gender atypicalities have also been found in recent functional studies of the brain. On positron emission tomography, (late-onset) MtF transsexuals shared a hy-pothalamic activation cluster with non-GD women when smelling 4,16-androstadien-3-one (a pheromone included in men's secretions), and with non-GD men when smelling estra-1,3,5(10),16-tetraen-3-ol (which is contained in the urine of pregnant women).[93] When viewing erotic films, MtF transsexuals showed cerebral activation patterns on fMRI similar to those of control women (ie, no specific activation) rather than to those of control men (enhanced activation in thalamus, amygdala, orbitofrontal, and insular cortex).[94] Another study using fMRI during the performance of a spatial cognition task showed that the classic mental-rotation network was activated in both MtF trans-sexuals and non-GD control men, but MtF transsexuals (both before and on estrogen treatment) showed greater activation of temporo-occipital regions than control men, and control men greater activation of the left parietal cortex (region BA 40) than MtF.[95]

As intriguing as these brain findings are, one has to remind oneself how many find-ings in the research on human sex differences have been unreplicable. As a rule of thumb, the author usually recommends not to accept any findings as probably true, unless they have been independently replicated by 3 laboratories of high quality, and this rule has not yet been met by any of the aforementioned brain-imaging results. It is particularly perplexing that many of these studies include patients with late-onset GD, because animal research on the sexual differentiation of brain and behavior as well as findings on human DSD point to the brain-organizational effects of sex hor-mones very early in development. If so, why would corresponding behavioral changes not already become visible in early childhood, as they do in patients with GD in asso-ciation with DSD and in non-DSD patients with early-onset GD? There is, therefore, ample room for speculation ranging from epigenetic mechanisms to psychodynamic interpretations, none of which have solid empirical evidence to back them up at this stage. That some genetic factors are likely to be involved is also supported by a few studies documenting familiality or increased concordance of monozygotic versus dizygotic twins for gender nonconformity[96,97] and gender-identity disorder.[98,99] Over-all, however, the evidence currently available is much too limited to reach a definitive conclusion regarding one or few biological factors that cause GD and gender change in people without a DSD. Variable multifactorial causation that is conceptualized from a biopsychosocial perspective seems to be more plausible.

Effects of Hormone Treatment

Also in need of urgent research are questions related to the effects of hormone treat-ment. One of these concerns the suppression of pubertal development by treatment, preferably with gonadotropin-releasing hormone (GnRH) analogue or, less expensively, with spironolactone.[100] In view of the frequent gender-atypical body appearance of individuals with late cross-sex hormone treatment, especially natal males, the transgender clinic in Amsterdam introduced the suppression of puberty for selected young adolescents with GD of early onset to reduce their suffering under the progression of unwanted secondary sex characteristics, while giving them more time to carefully consider their gender-trajectory options.[77] The Amsterdam team wants to have their patients experience the beginning of secondary sex characteristics and uses pubertal Tanner stage 2 as prerequisite for the start of puberty-suppression treatment, if the youngster shows aversive reactions to pubertal maturation. Multiyear follow-ups show the expected positive emotional effects and no negative medical side effects of early puberty suppression except for an arrest of the normal pubertal bone-mass increase followed by catch-up once cross-sex hormone treatment is begun.[101] The somatic effects of treatment with GnRH analogue are apparently fully reversible; that is, the gonads increase hormone production and the secondary sex characteristics resume maturation if the treatment is stopped. However, there is no information about the effects of early puberty suppression on brain development. Concerns regarding the latter are derived from animal research showing that the sexual differentiation of the brain continues in early puberty (see earlier discussion), and from recent research on humans demonstrating that the brain undergoes a major reorganization during the adolescent period.[102]

Later treatment with cross-sex hormones also initiates the development of some of the secondary sex characteristics desired by the patient with GD. Nevertheless, we do not know whether there are any unusual effects of treatment with cross-sex hormones on a brain that has presumably been exposed to the hormones characteristic of the natal sex of the individual during pregnancy, in early infancy, and again in puberty (if not suppressed). We do not even know whether the brains of people with GD differ from those of others in the production of neurosteroids,[103] which might make inappropriate the extrapolation of the effects of systemic hormone treatment on brain and behavior from non-GD people to people with GD.

Related concerns have been raised by the recent phenomenon of pregnant husbands: FtM transsexuals who underwent testosterone treatment and mastectomy but not genital surgery, and thus kept their ovaries.[104] Increasing numbers of these individuals have decided to temporarily interrupt their testosterone treatment to be able to bear a child, because their partners are unable or unwilling to do so, and to resume testosterone treatment once they have given birth. Anecdotal narratives provided in the media or on the Internet do not suggest that the resulting dramatic variations in the sex-hormone milieu directly affect gender identity, although only systematic investigations would permit firmer conclusions.

Clinical Implications

Although a satisfactory evidence-based etiology of non-DSD GD is still lacking, the common standard treatment approach for adult transsexuals with cross-sex hormones and, less commonly, sex-reassignment surgeries, and the increasingly common puberty-suppression approach to adolescents with GD, assigns a crucial role to the endocrinologist among the various subspecialties involved in the care of such individuals, as outlined in the recent guidelines of the Endocrine Society[100] and the World Professional Association for Transgender Health.[3] The endocrinologist's task differs from that of the common one of diagnosis and correction of deficient or excessive hormone levels relative to the patient's biological sex. Instead, blocking the normal pubertal maturation of the patient's secondary sex characteristics requires the suppression of (in most cases) a healthy endocrine system that complements the patient's congenital reproductive tract and assigned gender. For completion of the social transition to the other gender at later stages of development, the task involves the replacement of that healthy congenital reproductive system with a combination of iatrogenic hypogonadism and a regimen of exogenous hormone administration that helps conform the body to the patient's desired gender. In resource-rich countries, the endocrinologist typically bases the decision for this type of treatment on the patient's evaluation by a mental health professional with specialization in the area of gender management. Thus, an interdisciplinary team approach is recommended for both categories of GD.

REFERENCES

1. World Health Organization. Multiaxial version of ICD 10: clinical descriptions and diagnostic guidelines. Geneva (Switzerland): WHO; 1992.
2. American Psychiatric Association. Diagnostic and statistical manual of mental disorders. 4th edition, text revision. Washington, DC: APA; 2000.
3. American Psychiatric Association. Diagnostic and statistical manual of mental disorders. 5th edition. Washington, DC: APA; 2013.
4. Wood H, Sasaki S, Bradley SJ, et al. Patterns of referral to a gender identity service for children and adolescents (1976-2011): age, sex ratio, and sexual orientation. J Sex Marital Ther 2013;39(1):1–6.
5. Coleman E, Bockting W, Botzer M, et al. Standards of care for the health of transsexual, transgender, and gender-nonconforming people, Version 7. Int J Transgenderism 2012;13(4):165–232.
6. Hughes IA, Houk C, Ahmed SF, et al, LWPES Consensus Group, ESPE Consensus Group. Consensus statement on management of intersex disorders. Arch Dis Child 2006;91:554–63.
7. Meyer-Bahlburg HF. Gender dysphoria and gender change in persons with intersexuality: introduction. Arch Sex Behav 2005;34:371–3.
8. "Third sex" finds a place on Indian passport forms, The Telegraph, March 10, 2005. Cited in: Third gender. Wikipedia, the free encyclopedia. Available at: http://www.en.wikipedia.org/wiki/Third_gender. Accessed June 26, 2013.
9. Available at: http://www.thewest.com.au/20030111/news/perth/tw-news-perth-home-sto84205.html. Accessed January 28, 2003.
10. Available at: http://dipbt.bundestag.de/dip21/btp/17/17219.pdf. Accessed February 14, 2013.
11. Meyer-Bahlburg HF. Gender assignment in intersexuality. J Psychol Human Sex 1998;10:1–21.
12. Money J. Hermaphroditism, gender and precocity in hyperadrenocorticism: psychologic findings. Bull Johns Hopkins Hosp 1955;96(6):253–64.
13. Money J, Hampson JG, Hampson JL. Hermaphroditism: recommendations concerning assignment of sex, change of sex, and psychologic management. Bull Johns Hopkins Hosp 1955;97:284–300.
14. Phoenix CH, Goy RW, Gerall AA, et al. Organizing action of prenatally administered testosterone propionate on the tissues mediating mating behavior in the female guinea pig. Endocrinology 1959;65:369–82.
15. Diamond M, Sigmundson HK. Sex reassignment at birth. Long-term review and clinical implications. Arch Pediatr Adolesc Med 1997;151:298–304.
16. Gillam LH, Hewitt JK, Warne GL. Ethical principles for the management of infants with disorders of sex development. Horm Res Paediatr 2010;74:412–8.

17. Wiesemann C, Ude-Koeller S, Sinnecker GH, et al. Ethical principles and recommendations for the medical management of differences of sex development (DSD)/intersex in children and adolescents. Eur J Pediatr 2010;169:671–9.

18. Wallen K, Baum MJ. Masculinization and defeminization in altricial and precocial mammals: comparative aspects of steroid hormone action. In: Pfaff DW, Arnold AP, Etgen AM, et al, editors. Hormones, brain, and behavior, vol. 4. Oxford (United Kingdom): Elsevier; 2002. p. 385–423.

19. Wallen K, Hassett JM. Sexual differentiation of behaviour in monkeys: role of prenatal hormones. J Neuroendocrinol 2009;21(4):421–6.

20. Ehrhardt AA, Money J. Progestin-induced hermaphroditism: IQ and psychosexual identity in a study of ten girls. J Sex Res 1967;3(1):83–100.

21. Ehrhardt AA, Epstein R, Money J. Fetal androgens and female gender identity in the early-treated adrenogenital syndrome. Johns Hopkins Med J 1968;122: 165–7.

22. Ehrhardt AA, Evers K, Money J. Influence of androgen and some aspects of sexually dimorphic behavior in women with the late-treated adrenogenital syndrome. Johns Hopkins Med J 1968;123:115–22.

23. Meyer-Bahlburg HF. Psychoendocrinology of congenital adrenal hyperplasia. In: New MI, Lekarev O, Parsa A, et al, editors. Genetic steroid disorders. Amsterdam: Elsevier, in press.

24. Grumbach MM, Hughes IA, Conte FA. Disorders of sex differentiation. In: Larson PR, Kronenberg HM, Melmed S, et al, editors. Williams textbook of endocrinology. 10th edition. Philadelphia: W.B. Saunders; 2003. p. 842–1002.

25. Masica DN, Ehrhardt AA, Money J. Fetal feminization and female gender identity in the testicular feminizing syndrome of androgen insensitivity. Arch Sex Behav 1971;1:131–42.

26. Wisniewski AB, Migeon CJ, Meyer-Bahlburg HF, et al. Complete androgen insensitivity syndrome: long-term medical, surgical, and psychosexual outcome. J Clin Endocrinol Metab 2000;85:2664–9.

27. Hines M, Ahmed SF, Hughes IA. Psychological outcomes and gender-related development in complete androgen insensitivity syndrome. Arch Sex Behav 2003;32(2):93–101.

28. Money J, Ogunro C. Behavioral sexology: ten cases of genetic male intersexuality with impaired prenatal and pubertal androgenization. Arch Sex Behav 1974;3(3):181–205.

29. Migeon CJ, Wisniewski AB, Gearhart JP, et al. Ambiguous genitalia with perineoscrotal hypospadias in 46, XY individuals: long-term medical, surgical, and psychosexual outcome. Pediatrics 2002;110(3):e31. Available at: http://www.pediatrics.org/cgi/content/full/110/3/e31.

30. Meyer-Bahlburg HF, Dolezal C, Baker SW, et al. Gender development in women with congenital adrenal hyperplasia as a function of disorder severity. Arch Sex Behav 2006;35:667–84.

31. Meyer-Bahlburg HF, Dolezal C, Baker SW, et al. Sexual orientation in women with classical or non-classical congenital adrenal hyperplasia as a function of degree of prenatal androgen excess. Arch Sex Behav 2008;37:85–99.

32. Nordenskjöld A, Holmdahl G, Frisén L, et al. Type of mutation and surgical procedure affect long-term quality of life for women with congenital adrenal hyperplasia. J Clin Endocrinol Metab 2008;93:380–6.

33. Jürgensen M, Kleinemeier E, Lux A, et al. Psychosexual development in children with disorder of sex development (DSD)—results from the German clinical evaluation study. J Pediatr Endocrinol Metab 2010;23:565–78.

34. Lish JD, Meyer-Bahlburg HF, Ehrhardt AA, et al. Prenatal exposure to diethylstilbestrol (DES): childhood play behavior and adult gender-role behavior in women. Arch Sex Behav 1992;21:423–41.
35. Meyer-Bahlburg HF, Ehrhardt AA, Rosen LR, et al. Prenatal estrogens and the development of homosexual orientation. Dev Psychol 1995;31:12–21.
36. Titus-Ernstoff L, Perez K, Hatch EE, et al. Psychosexual characteristics of men and women exposed prenatally to diethylstilbestrol. Epidemiology 2003;14(2):155–60.
37. Morishima A, Grumbach MM, Simpson ER, et al. Aromatase deficiency in male and female siblings caused by a novel mutation and the physiological role of estrogens. J Clin Endocrinol Metab 1995;80(12):3689–98.
38. Carani C, Rochira V, Faustini-Fustini M, et al. Role of oestrogen in male sexual behaviour: insights from the natural model of aromatase deficiency. Clin Endocrinol 1999;51:517–24.
39. Smith EP, Boyd J, Frank GR, et al. Estrogen resistance caused by a mutation in the estrogen-receptor gene in a man. N Engl J Med 1994;331(16):1056–61.
40. Ehrhardt AA, Grisanti GC, Meyer-Bahlburg HF. Prenatal exposure to medroxyprogesterone acetate (MPA) in girls. Psychoneuroendocrinology 1977;2:391–8.
41. Berenbaum SA, Duck SC, Bryk K. Behavioral effects of prenatal versus postnatal androgen excess in children with 21-hydroxylase-deficient congenital adrenal hyperplasia. J Clin Endocrinol Metab 2000;85:727–33.
42. Kinsley CH, Lambert KG. Reproduction-induced neuroplasticity: natural behavioural and neuronal alterations associated with the production and care of offspring. J Neuroendocrinol 2008;20:515–25.
43. Schulz KM, Molenda-Figueira HA, Sisk CL. Back to the future: the organizational-activational hypothesis adapted to puberty and adolescence. Horm Behav 2009;55:597–604.
44. Wallen K. Hormonal influences on sexually differentiated behavior in nonhuman primates. Front Neuroendocrinol 2005;26:7–26.
45. Meyer-Bahlburg HF. Gender identity outcome in female-raised 46,XY persons with penile agenesis, cloacal exstrophy of the bladder, or penile ablation. Arch Sex Behav 2005;34:423–38.
46. Eggers S, Sinclair A. Mammalian sex determination—insights from humans and mice. Chromosome Res 2012;20:215–38.
47. Yang X, Schadt EE, Wang S, et al. Tissue-specific expression and regulation of sexually dimorphic genes in mice. Genome Res 2006;16:995–1004.
48. Pilgrim C, Reisert I. Differences between male and female brains—developmental mechanisms and implications. Horm Metab Res 1992;24(8):353–9.
49. McCarthy MM, Arnold AP. Reframing sexual differentiation of the brain. Nat Neurosci 2011;14(6):1–7.
50. Xu X, Coats JK, Yang CF, et al. Modular genetic control of sexually dimorphic behaviors. Cell 2012;148:596–607.
51. Holterhus PM. Molecular androgen memory in sex development. Pediatr Endocrinol Rev 2011;9(Suppl 1):515–8.
52. Blakemore JE, Berenbaum SA, Liben LS. Gender development. New York: Psychology Press; 2008.
53. Meyer-Bahlburg HF, Dolezal C, Baker SW, et al. Prenatal androgenization affects gender-related behavior but not gender identity in 5-12-year-old girls with congenital adrenal hyperplasia. Arch Sex Behav 2004;33:97–104.
54. Money J. Biographies of gender and hermaphroditism in paired comparisons. Amsterdam; New York: Elsevier Science Publishers B.V. (Biomedical Divisions); 1991.

55. Cadet P. Androgen insensitivity syndrome with male sex-of-living. Arch Sex Behav 2011;40:1101–2.
56. Meyer-Bahlburg HF. Androgen insensitivity syndrome with male sex-of living: comment on Cadet (2011). Arch Sex Behav 2011;40:1103–4.
57. Kulshreshtha B, Philibert P, Eunice M, et al. Apparent male gender identity in a patient with complete androgen insensitivity syndrome. Arch Sex Behav 2009; 38(6):873–5.
58. Meyer-Bahlburg HF. Concerns regarding gender change to male in a 46, XY child with complete androgen insensitivity: comment on Kulshreshtha et al. (2009). Arch Sex Behav 2009;38(6):876–7.
59. T'Sjoen G, De Cuypere G, Monstrey S, et al. Male gender identity in complete androgen insensitivity syndrome. Arch Sex Behav 2011;40:635–8.
60. Cohen-Kettenis PT. Gender change in 46, XY persons with 5α-reductase-2-deficiency and 17β-hydroxysteroid dehydrogenase-3 deficiency. Arch Sex Behav 2005;34(4):399–410.
61. Dessens AB, Slijper FM, Drop SL. Gender dysphoria and gender change in chromosomal females with congenital adrenal hyperplasia. Arch Sex Behav 2005;34:389–97.
62. Mazur T. Gender dysphoria and gender change in androgen insensitivity or micropenis. Arch Sex Behav 2005;34(4):411–21.
63. Egan SK, Perry DG. Gender identity: a multidimensional analysis with implications for psychosocial adjustment. Dev Psychol 2001;37:451–63.
64. Schweizer K, Brunner F, Schützmann K, et al. Gender identity and coping in female 46,XY adults with androgen biosynthesis deficiency (intersexuality/DSD). J Couns Psychol 2009;56(1):189–201.
65. Swaab DF, Gooren LJ, Hofman MA. The human hypothalamus in relation to gender and sexual orientation. Prog Brain Res 1992;93:205–19.
66. Prader A. Der Genitalbefund beim Pseudohermaphroditismus femininus des kongenitalen adrenogenitalen Syndroms. Helv Paediatr Acta 1954;9:231–48.
67. Quigley CA, De Bellis A, Marschke KB, et al. Androgen receptor defects: historical, clinical and molecular perspectives. Endocr Rev 1995;16:271–321.
68. Ahmed SF, Khwaja O, Hughes IA. The role of a clinical score in the assessment of ambiguous genitalia. BJU Int 2000;85:120–4.
69. Berenbaum SA, Hines M. Early androgens are related to childhood sex-typed toy preferences. Psychol Sci 1992;3:203–6.
70. Leveroni CL, Berenbaum SA. Early androgen effects on interest in infants: evidence from children with congenital adrenal hyperplasia. Dev Neuropsychol 1998;14(2/3):321–40.
71. Dittmann RW, Kappes MH, Kappes ME, et al. Congenital adrenal hyperplasia II: gender-related behavior and attitudes in female salt-wasting and simple-virilizing patients. Psychoneuroendocrinology 1990;15:421–34.
72. Meyer-Bahlburg HF, Gruen RS, New MI, et al. Gender change from female to male in classical CAH. Horm Behav 1996;30:319–32.
73. Meyer-Bahlburg HF. Gender monitoring and gender reassignment of children and adolescents with a somatic disorder of sex development. Child Adolesc Psychiatr Clin N Am 2011;20:639–49.
74. Wallien MS, Cohen-Kettenis PT. Psychosexual outcome of gender-dysphoric children. J Am Acad Child Adolesc Psychiatry 2008;47:1413–23.
75. Blanchard R. The concept of autogynephilia and the typology of male gender dysphoria. J Nerv Ment Dis 2008;177(10):616–23.

76. Lawrence AA. Men trapped in men's bodies: narratives of autogynephilic transsexualism (focus on sexuality research). New York: Springer; 2013.
77. Cohen-Kettenis PT, Pfäfflin F, editors. Transgenderism and intersexuality in childhood and adolescence. Making choices. Thousand Oaks (CA): SAGE Publications; 2003.
78. Meyer-Bahlburg HF. From mental disorder to iatrogenic hypogonadism—dilemmas in conceptualizing gender identity variants as psychiatric conditions. Arch Sex Behav 2010;39(2):461–76.
79. Bentz EK, Schneeberger C, Hefler LA, et al. A common polymorphism of the SRD5A2 gene and transsexualism. Reprod Sci 2007;14(7):705–9.
80. Bentz EK, Hefler LA, Kaufmann U, et al. A polymorphism of the CYP17 gene related to sex steroid metabolism is associated with female-to-male but not male-to-female transsexualism. Fertil Steril 2008;90:56–9.
81. Hare L, Bernard P, Sánchez FJ, et al. Androgen receptor repeat length polymorphism associated with male-to-female transsexualism. Biol Psychiatry 2009;65:93–6.
82. Henningsson S, Westberg L, Nilsson S, et al. Sex steroid-related genes and male-to-female transsexualism. Psychoneuroendocrinology 2005;30:657–64.
83. Ujike H, Otani K, Nakatsuka M, et al. Association study of gender identity disorder and sex hormone-related genes. Prog Neuropsychopharmacol Biol Psychiatry 2009;33(7):1241–4.
84. Meyer-Bahlburg HF. Transsexualism ("gender identity disorder")—a CNS-limited form of intersexuality? Adv Exp Med Biol 2011;707:75–9.
85. Zhou JN, Hofman MA, Gooren LJ, et al. A sex difference in the human brain and its relation to transsexuality. Nature 1995;378:68–70.
86. Kruijver FP, Zhou J, Pool C, et al. Male-to-female transsexuals have female neuron numbers in a limbic nucleus. J Clin Endocrinol Metab 2000;85:2034–41.
87. Garcia-Falgueras A, Swaab DF. A sex difference in the hypothalamic uncinate nucleus: relationship to gender identity. Brain 2008;131:3132–46.
88. Luders E, Sánchez FJ, Gaser C, et al. Regional gray matter variation in male-to-female transsexualism. Neuroimage 2009;46:904–7.
89. Rametti G, Carrillo B, Gómez-Gil E, et al. The microstructure of white matter in male to female transsexuals before cross-sex hormonal treatment. A DTI study. J Psychiatr Res 2011;45:949–54.
90. Rametti G, Carrillo B, Gómez-Gil E, et al. White matter microstructure in female to male transsexuals before cross-sex hormonal treatment. A diffusion tensor imaging study. J Psychiatr Res 2011;45:199–204.
91. Savic I, Arver S. Sex dimorphism of the brain in male-to-female transsexuals. Cereb Cortex 2011;21:2525–33.
92. Santarnecchi E, Vatti G, Déttore D, et al. Intrinsic cerebral connectivity analysis in an untreated female-to-male transsexual subject: a first attempt using resting-state fMRI. Neuroendocrinology 2012;96:188–93.
93. Berglund H, Lindström P, Dhejne-Helmy C, et al. Male-to-female transsexuals show sex-atypical hypothalamus activation when smelling odorous steroids. Cereb Cortex 2008;18:1900–8.
94. Gizewski ER, Krause E, Schlamann M, et al. Specific cerebral activation due to visual erotic stimuli in male-to-female transsexuals compared with male and female controls: an fMRI study. J Sex Med 2009;6:440–8.
95. Schöning S, Engelien A, Bauer C, et al. Neuroimaging differences in spatial cognition between men and male-to-female transsexuals before and during hormone therapy. J Sex Med 2010;7:1858–67.

96. Knafo A, Iervolino AC, Plomin R. Masculine girls and feminine boys: genetic and environmental contributions to atypical gender development in early childhood. J Pers Soc Psychol 2005;88(2):400–12.
97. van Beijsterveldt CE, Hudziak JJ, Boomsma DI. Genetic and environmental influences on cross-gender behavior and relation to behavior problems: a study of Dutch twins at ages 7 and 10 years. Arch Sex Behav 2006;35(6):647–58.
98. Gómez-Gil E, Esteva I, Almaraz MC, et al. Familiality of gender identity disorder in non-twin siblings. Arch Sex Behav 2010;39(2):546–52.
99. Heylens G, DeCuypere G, Zucker KJ, et al. Gender identity disorder in twins: a review of the case report literature. J Sex Med 2012;9(3):751–7.
100. Hembree WC, Cohen-Kettenis P, Delemarre-van de Waal HA, et al. Endocrine treatment of transsexual persons: an Endocrine Society clinical practice guideline. J Clin Endocrinol Metab 2009;94(9):3132–54.
101. Delemarrre-van de Waal HA, Cohen-Kettenis PT. Clinical management of gender identity disorder in adolescents: a protocol on psychological and paediatric endocrinology aspects. Eur J Endocrinol 2006;155:S131–7.
102. Giedd JN, Raznahan A, Mills KL, et al. Review: magnetic resonance imaging of male/female differences in human adolescent brain anatomy. Biol Sex Differ 2012;3(1):19.
103. Melcangi RC, Panzica G, Garcia-Segura LM. Neuroactive steroids: focus on human brain. Neuroscience 2011;191:1–5.
104. Male pregnancy. Wikipedia, the free encyclopedia. Available at: http:www.en.wikipedia.org/wiki/Male_pregnancy. Accessed June 26, 2012.

Neuropsychiatric Manifestations of Thyroid Disease

Anna Z. Feldman, MD[a], Rupendra T. Shrestha, MD[b],
James V. Hennessey, MD[c],*

KEYWORDS

- Neuropsychiatric symptoms • Thyrotoxicosis • Hypothyroidism • Hyperthyroidism

KEY POINTS

- The symptoms of hypothyroidism often mimic those of depression, whereas those of hyperthyroidism include anxiety, dysphoria, emotional lability, intellectual dysfunction, mania, or depression.
- Most patients with depression have normal thyroid function, but 1% to 4% of patients with affective disorders are overtly hypothyroid while 4% to 40% may have subclinical hypothyroidism.
- Up to 52% of patients with refractory depression may have evidence of subclinical hypothyroidism, compared with 8% to 17% in an unselected population of depressed patients.
- Thyrotoxicosis may commonly present with anxiety, dysphoria, emotional lability, intellectual dysfunction, and mania, so a diagnosis of thyrotoxicosis should be considered in any patient with new onset of anxiety or mania.
- The indications for treatment of subclinical hyperthyroidism are controversial, and current guidelines do not address treatment based on neuropsychiatric symptoms, but rather for other potential morbidities.
- Iatrogenic thyrotoxicosis may be symptomatic, occurring after exposure to medications or other physician-directed disruptions of normal function of the thyroid gland.

INTRODUCTION

For more than 125 years[1] it has been recognized that thyroid disease may give rise to psychiatric disorders that can be corrected by reestablishment of normal thyroid function. More than 60 years ago we learned that patients with profound hypothyroidism may present with depressive psychosis.[2] The symptoms of hypothyroidism mimic

[a] Division of Endocrinology, Department of Medicine, Beth Israel Deaconess Medical Center, Harvard Medical School, 330 Brookline Ave, Gryzmish 6, Boston, MA 02215, USA; [b] Division of Hospital Medicine, Department of Medicine, Beth Israel Deaconess Medical Center-Milton, 199 Reedsdale Road, Milton, MA 02186, USA; [c] Division of Endocrinology, Department of Medicine, Beth Israel Deaconess Medical Center, Harvard Medical School, 330 Brookline Avenue, Gryzmish 619, Boston, MA 02215, USA
* Corresponding author.
E-mail address: jhenness@bidmc.harvard.edu

Endocrinol Metab Clin N Am 42 (2013) 453–476
http://dx.doi.org/10.1016/j.ecl.2013.05.005
0889-8529/13/$ – see front matter © 2013 Elsevier Inc. All rights reserved.

those of depression, whereas those of hyperthyroidism include anxiety, dysphoria, emotional lability, and mania.

Assuming a thyroid link to depression, ingestion of thyroid hormone was projected to benefit depressed patients. But controlled studies have not documented success with this approach,[3,4] leaving the role of thyroid hormones in the treatment of euthyroid depression in question.[5] Likewise, combinations of LT_3 and antidepressants in euthyroid patients, as well as LT_3 with levothyroxine in fully replaced hypothyroid subjects, have been explored but remain a matter of much debate.[10–12]

The prevalence of hypo- and hyperthyroidism in the US population is outlined below in **Table 1**. Surks and Hollowell[13] demonstrated that up to 14.5% of disease free older individuals have a thyrotropin (TSH) level higher than 4.5 mIU/mL, therefore the prevalence of subclinical hypothyroidism (SCH) in the elderly may be overestimated.[14] TSH values in seniors with extreme longevity are higher than expected,[15] and they also have TSH values higher than appropriate controls.[16,17] So not every elevation of TSH represents thyroid disease.

1% to 4% of patients with affective disorders are overtly hypothyroid and 4% to 40% may have SCH.[16] Many patients with refractory depression may have SCH, compared with unselected depressed patients.[18]

Thyrotoxicosis commonly presents with anxiety, dysphoria, emotional lability, intellectual dysfunction, and mania.[19] After restoration of biochemical euthyroidism, many hyperthyroid patients have persistent residual neuropsychiatric symptoms.[20,21] Patients with subclinical hyperthyroidism may be nervous, irritable,[22] and anxious in comparison with controls.[23] Some have found dementia in elderly patients with subclinical hyperthyroidism,[24] while others have failed to show this association.[25] The indications for treatment of subclinical hyperthyroidism,[26] do not consider neuropsychiatric symptoms.[27] Iatrogenic thyrotoxicosis may be symptomatic, occurring after exposure to medications[28] or other disruptions of normal thyroid gland function.[29]

RELATIONSHIP OF THYROID HORMONES WITH MOOD AND COGNITION

In most depressed subjects, the basal serum TSH, thyroxine (T_4) and triiodothyronine (T_3) are within the expected range, although in one report a third of such patients were observed to have suppressed TSH levels.[30] Depressed patients admitted to a psychiatry unit, may have an increase in serum total or free T_4 levels, which generally regresses following successful treatment.[30] 25% of patients with depression have a "blunted" TSH response to thyrotropin-releasing hormone (TRH) administration (as defined by a TSH increase of <5 μU/mL). A blunted TSH response has been observed more frequently in unipolar than in bipolar depression, but differentiating these disorders with TRH stimulation has been disappointing.[31] The blunted TSH response has

Table 1
Prevalence of hypothyroidism and hyperthyroidism in the United States population

Study	Hypothyroidism			Hyperthyroidism		
	TSH Cutoff	Subclinical	Overt	TSH Cutoff	Subclinical	Overt
Colorado Thyroid Disease Prevalence Study[6]	>5.1 mIU/mL	8.5%	0.4%	<0.3 mIU/mL	0.9%	0.1%
National Health and Nutrition Examination Survey III[7]	>4.5 mIU/mL	4.3%	0.3%	<0.1 mIU/mL	0.7%	0.5%

Data from Refs.[6–9]

been considered a "state" marker that normalizes on recovery from the depression. The mechanism for the blunted TSH response in affective disorders is not known; however, glucocorticoids, known to inhibit the hypothalamic-pituitary-thyroid axis, are elevated in depression and could be responsible.[19]

An enhanced TSH response may occur in up to 15% of depressed subjects. The majority of such patients have positive antithyroid antibodies, suggesting that latent hypothyroidism caused by autoimmune thyroiditis. Indeed in one such study, individuals with positive antithyroid peroxide antibodies were found to have symptoms of anxiety and depression more frequently than in controls.[32] Not all studies, however, have found an increased prevalence of antithyroid antibodies or apparent mild hypothyroidism in depressed subjects when compared with matched control groups.[33]

In normal subjects, the TSH level begins to increase in the evening before the onset of sleep, reaching a peak between 11 PM and 4 AM.[34] In depression, the nocturnal surge of TSH is frequently absent, resulting in a reduction in thyroid hormone secretion, supporting the view that functional central hypothyroidism might occur in some depressed subjects.[35] Sleep deprivation, which has an antidepressant effect, returns TSH circadian rhythm to normal.[36] The mechanism responsible for the impaired nocturnal increase in TSH is unknown.

Deiodinases are selenocysteine enzymes that remove iodine molecules from thyroid hormones. Three types of deiodinases have been identified. Deiodinase 1 (D1) is found mainly in liver and kidney, whereas deiodinase 2 (D2) is found in adipose tissue, brain, and pituitary gland. Both D1 and D2 result in the conversion of T_4 to T_3. Deiodinase 3 (D3) inactivates T_4 by converting it into reverse T_3 and converts T_3 to diiodothyronine (T_2). Brain derives most of its T_3 from the conversion of T_4 to T_3 from D2 enzyme activity.[37,38] Single-nucleotide polymorphisms (SNPs) have been identified in the deiodinase genes. One such polymorphism identified is related to D2 coding and is cited as the Thr92Ala polymorphism. This SNP is seen commonly in various ethnic groups.[39] This polymorphism has been studied for an association of any changes in well-being and neurocognitive functioning, as well as to potentially identify a preference for combined LT_4 and LT_3 therapy for treatment of hypothyroidism, with mixed results. No differences in symptoms were noted, and there was no benefit of adding LT_3 to levothyroxine in the 2005 study by Appelhof and colleagues.[40] Panicker and colleagues,[41] however, reported that patients with the Thr92Ala polymorphism had worse baseline General Health Questionnaire scores while on LT_4 monotherapy for hypothyroidism, but showed greater improvement on LT_4/LT_3 combination therapy for hypothyroidism compared with continued LT_4 alone. Under hypothyroid conditions, it has been proposed that the D2 enzyme with this polymorphism may deiodinate less effectively and therefore lead to diminished levels of local T_3 production and, perhaps, an increased dependence on circulating T_3 to maintain optimal brain T_3 levels.[41]

Serotonin deficiency has been proposed as a central pathologic factor in depression. In one study, brain serotonin levels correlated positively with T_3 levels in rat brain.[42] A state of relative hypothyroidism in brain with coexisting systemic euthyroidism attributable to deficient D2 has therefore been proposed.[43,44] Alternatively, D2 activity may be depressed by the elevated cortisol levels seen in depression and stress, resulting in T_4 being converted to reverse T_3 by D3 activity, leading to decreased brain T_3 and increased reverse T_3 levels.[45] Selective serotonin reuptake inhibitors (SSRIs) and tricyclic antidepressants appear to promote the activity of D2, which results in an increased conversion of T_4 to T_3 within the brain tissues.[46]

Organic anion transporting polypeptides (OATPs) are proteins capable of transporting thyroid hormone into the cell.[47] Genetic coding for OATP1C1 is located on chromosome 12p12, and the protein is a thyroid hormone (T_4 and reverse T_3)

transporter expressed at the blood-brain barrier, considered to play a key role in delivering serum T_4 to the brain. One hundred forty-one patients with primary autoimmune hypothyroidism were studied to determine the presence of this polymorphism in the gene encoding for this protein. The presence of the OATP1C1 SNP was associated with an increased frequency of hypothyroid symptoms, including fatigue and depression.[47]

Altered cerebral perfusion has been demonstrated under hypothyroid conditions. Both global[48–51] and regional[51] hypoperfusion have been demonstrated. Whereas some researchers have demonstrated partial normalization following LT_4 treatment,[49,50,52] others have found no improvement in perfusion[51] following correction of the hypothyroid state.

NEUROPSYCHIATRIC MANIFESTATIONS OF OVERT HYPOTHYROIDISM

There is a considerable overlap between the clinical manifestations of mood disorders and those of hypothyroidism, as shown in **Table 2**. In fact, many of the symptoms attributed to both hypothyroidism and depression such as poorer memory, slower thinking, and being more tired are seen in almost equal frequency when comparing those with documented hypothyroidism and non-depressed euthyroid controls.[6] An evaluation of overtly hypothyroid and euthyroid controls for the presence of classic hypothyroid symptoms, including several considered neuropsychiatric in nature, revealed no significant differences in the percentage complaining of tiredness, feeling depressed, thinking slowly, having poor memory, or having difficulty in performing math operations.[53] Individuals report fatigue as a response to the question "Do you feel tired?" with nearly equal frequency if hypothyroid or euthyroid controls.[54] Moreover, the subscale on vitality of the RAND 36-item Health Survey and the Shortened

Table 2
Common clinical features in hypothyroidism and mood disorders

	Hypothyroidism	Mood Disorders
Depression	Yes	Yes
Diminished interest	Yes	Yes
Diminished pleasure	Yes	Yes
Decreased libido	Yes	Yes
Weight loss	No	Yes
Weight gain	Yes	Sometimes
Appetite loss	Yes	Yes
Increased appetite	No	Yes
Insomnia	No	Yes
Hypersomnia	Yes	Yes
Agitation/anxiety	Occasionally	Yes
Fatigue	Yes	Yes
Poor memory	Yes	Yes
Cognitive dysfunction	Yes	Yes
Impaired concentration	Yes	Yes
Constipation	Yes	Sometimes

Data from Hennessey JV, Jackson IM. The interface between thyroid hormones and psychiatry. Endocrinologist 1996;6:214–23.

Fatigue Questionnaire, which quantify the intensity of fatigue, are similar in hypothyroid patients and non-depressed euthyroid controls.[54] Thus it is evident that the symptoms of hypothyroidism are indeed somewhat nonspecific and require further classification when present. It is therefore recommended that all patients diagnosed with psychiatric disorders be tested for thyroid hormone abnormalities[19,55] because the presence of even SCH may provide an opportunity to treat apparent depression with thyroid hormones.[56]

Severe hypothyroidism may present with melancholic depression.[57,58] Frank psychosis with hallucinations and delusions has been described, but is thankfully rare.[58] Asher described psychosis in 14 hypothyroid patients and coined the term "myxedema madness."[2] There is no clear consensus regarding diagnostic criteria for establishing the diagnosis of myxedema madness, but is has been reported that 5% to 15% of all hypothyroid patients may have some form of psychosis.[59,60] The manifestations of thought disorders vary considerably and include delusions of the paranoid, schizophrenic, or affective type.[58] Capgras syndrome (believing that one's spouse or close family member has been replaced by an identical-looking imposter),[61] visual and auditory hallucinations, perseveration, loose associations, and paranoia[60] have all been reported. These psychotic symptoms are said to be preceded by physical symptoms of hypothyroidism by months to years before manifestation.[62]

EFFECTS OF LT$_4$ TREATMENT OF HYPOTHYROIDISM

Treatment with levothyroxine improves the neuropsychiatric symptoms, although the pattern is inconsistent and complete resolution of all symptoms is variable.[63,64] Usually, normalization of TSH and circulating levels of T$_3$ can be achieved by the oral administration of LT$_4$.[65] Achievement of a TSH level in the expected range ooms to be adequate to assure restoration of physical and neuropsychiatric function, as attempts to demonstrate any further superiority of maintaining the TSH in a low normal versus a higher normal range have failed to document any advantage of a certain narrower range.[66,67] Despite achieving euthyroidism as indicated by the serum TSH, some patients may continue to complain of various hypothyroid symptoms, including a picture consistent with that of depression.[68] This particular study's finding of excessive symptoms, however, has been difficult to interpret because at baseline, those treated with T$_4$ were more likely to have additional chronic medical conditions and to be receiving more chronic medications than the comparison group.[68] The results may further be unique to this study because a portion of the TSH levels achieved with treatment would be considered to be in the mildly hypothyroid range as defined in many studies of SCH, so it is unclear whether all subjects were actually euthyroid. For this reason, a clinician following patients with TSH values in the upper end of the range that was considered euthyroid by Saravanan and colleagues[68] would likely increase the replacement dose in a patient with such complaints to return the TSH to the expected range. In addition, Saravanan's findings have been criticized because of issues of potential ascertainment bias, which might provide an alternative explanation for the results.[69] Further studies have also claimed that euthyroid patients on T$_4$ may have worse cognitive function test results compared with a reference population,[70] and others have noted higher anxiety and depression symptoms on the Hospital Anxiety and Depression Scale.[10] As it is not possible to differentiate euthyroid from hypothyroid subjects based on neuropsychiatric symptoms,[6,53,54] it is extremely problematic to then expect that all hypothyroid individuals will experience complete resolution of all subjective symptoms once rendered euthyroid. Despite this obvious caveat, the persistence of these findings has been cited to justify further research on combination of LT_3 with LT_4 to improve symptomatology.

EFFECTS OF COMBINATION T_4/T_3 THERAPY ON THE NEUROPSYCHIATRIC MANIFESTATIONS OF TREATED HYPOTHYROIDISM

Murray introduced thyroid hormone therapy to the clinical world in 1891. This therapy was from its beginning a treatment based on a combination of LT_4 and LT_3 derived from animal thyroid extracts.[71] Variability of the LT_4 and LT_3 content and ratios of animal extracts from batch to batch and brand to brand[72] led to the replacement of this "natural" combination therapy of extracts with pharmaceutically more precise synthetic T_4 and T_3.[72–74] Eventually the simplicity of T_4 monotherapy was adopted as usual therapy, and seems to provide satisfactory replacement.[75] T_4, like thyroid hormone extract dosage, was initially titrated based on clinical symptoms during the era before serum TSH assays became available. During the 1980s more sensitive TSH assays allowed titration of thyroid hormone therapy to "normal," which resulted in significant dose reductions of LT_4 dosage to as little as 100 µg per day,[76] likely indicating the excessive amounts of both LT_4 and thyroid extracts previously used. When actually euthyroid according to current biochemical parameters, some patients still complained of symptoms consistent with components of the nonspecific symptoms associated with hypothyroidism.[68,77] As patients were no longer routinely overdosed with their thyroid hormone therapy, it was proposed that the difference in outcomes (compared with historical experience with thyroid hormone extracts) might be due to the absence of significant amounts of LT_3 in the LT_4 preparations. Subsequently, multiple reports have appeared evaluating the effectiveness of combining LT_3 with T_4 to improve neuropsychological outcomes. The report of Bunevicius and colleagues,[78] for example, seemed to indicate that substituting 12.5 µg of T_3 for 50 µg of the individual's usual T_4 dose resulted in improvement in mood and neuropsychological function. These results, however, may not be widely applicable, as was evident in an analysis of the subset of this population who were being treated with T_4 for primary hypothyroidism[79] and who demonstrated no significant improvement in clinical outcome with the combination.[79] Several double-blind, randomized controlled trials designed to correct flaws observed in the initial trials have subsequently failed to reproduce the positive effects reported by Bunevicius, and do not demonstrate objective improvement in self-rated mood, well-being, or depression scales with the addition of LT_3 to LT_4 therapy.[5] Furthermore, most of these studies fail to demonstrate differences in cognitive function, quality of life, or subjective satisfaction with treatment, but some do report that anxiety scores were significantly worse in those treated with the LT_4/LT_3 combination.[80] However, more recent investigations have proposed that there may be a subset of T_4-treated patients who may benefit from LT_3 supplementation in those who experience higher depression and anxiety scores than euthyroid counterparts.[10] Preliminary evidence suggests that those patients with the D2 gene polymorphism (Thr92Ala) may have a positive response to T_3 potentiation,[41] but other research has not confirmed this observation,[40] and prospective trials in this situation have not yet been conducted.

On the other hand, there is also evidence that a further subset of patients may be predicted to not respond to LT_3 potentiation. Polymorphism in the coding for the organic anion-transporting polypeptide (OATP1C1) appears to be linked to increased depressive symptoms among those with hypothyroidism. When compared with controls, these patients do not appear to have any decrease in depressive scores when LT_3 supplementation is added to LT_4.[47] The clinical significance of this finding is yet to be determined, but may have a meaningful impact on the future of depression treatment.

At present, meta-analysis has concluded that it would not seem justified to use combined T_4 and LT_3 treatment as a general rule in hypothyroid patients who complain of depressive symptoms after biochemical euthyroidism is restored.[81] In patients with ongoing symptoms despite being euthyroid, a thorough history and physical examination along with a laboratory evaluation including a complete blood count, comprehensive metabolic panel, celiac disease testing, and obstructive sleep apnea screening, along with an endocrine workup including vitamin D levels, thyroid peroxidase antibodies, cortisol levels and, if indicated, cosyntropin stimulation testing, is recommended to rule out other causes.[82] Given the conflicting data in regard of D2 gene polymorphisms, when lifestyle changes (dietary changes, exercise, sleep hygiene) and optimal medical treatment with LT_4 including changes in brand of T_4 have failed, some investigators have recommended that a trial of combination therapy be considered,[82] but others await further evidence of predictable efficacy before making this recommendation.

NEUROPSYCHIATRIC MANIFESTATION OF SUBCLINICAL HYPOTHYROIDISM

SCH is diagnostically defined as the finding of an elevated serum TSH concentration and normal circulating free T_4 and T_3 concentrations. SCH, by definition, cannot be diagnosed by clinical findings. It has been conceptualized as a stage in the continuum of normal thyroid function to overt clinical hypothyroidism.[83] The prevalence of SCH varies with the population studied and the upper limit set for TSH measurement.[26] Various studies investigating this question have determined the presence of hypothyroidism by using a TSH upper normal cutoff ranging between 3 and 4.5 mIU/mL.[55] These differences are the result of assessing populations differing in iodine intake and the use of assays with different performance characteristics. As a result of these issues, there is considerable debate about the upper limit of TSH.[55] Elegant studies have confirmed that TSH levels increase with advancing age among those free of thyroid disease and that, therefore, the use of age-specific TSH levels would predictably reduce the apparent prevalence of SCH in the elderly population.[13] In fact, a study assessing longitudinal change in thyroid function in very elderly subjects free of thyroid disease demonstrated a 12% increase in TSH along with a 1.7% increase in free T_4 and a 13% decline in serum T_3 over a 13-year follow-up period.[14] The upper limit of the expected TSH range was observed to increase from 6.2 mIU/mL in those 80 to 84 years old to 7.96 mIU/mL in those older than 90 years, clearly demonstrating a need for age-adjusted expectations in interpreting TSH.[14]

Experts typically further classify SCH into those with a mildly elevated TSH (4.5–10 mIU/mL) and others with markedly elevated TSH (>10 mIU/mL).[27] The natural history of SCH depends on the underlying cause and the population studied.[26] The estimated annual rate of conversion from SCH to overt disease in the Whickham survey was 2.6% if thyroid autoantibodies were negative and 4.3% if antibodies to thyroid peroxidase were present.[84] In the study reported by Parle and colleagues,[85] 5.5% of the 73 patients older than 60 years presenting with an elevated TSH and normal free T_4 were found to have a normal TSH after 1 year of follow-up while 17.8% progressed to overt hypothyroidism. Somwaru and colleagues[86] showed that nearly half of patients with SCH spontaneously reverted to normal during follow-up in a 4-year study of people older than 65 years at entry. This trend was especially observed in those in whom the initial TSH elevation was minimal and titers of thyroid peroxidase (TPO) antibody were negative.[86] The risk of conversion to overt hypothyroidism during follow-up increases with the degree of TSH elevation and the positivity of thyroid autoantibodies to thyroid peroxidase, indicating low thyroid reserve.[87]

While it is well accepted that depressive symptoms and anxiety states are common in overt hypothyroidism,[19,88] studies of symptoms in SCH have found mixed results. Higher scores (indicating worse performance) on scales measuring memory, anxiety, somatic complaints, and depression have been reported in many,[64,77,89-92] but not all[93-95] studies. In a recent observational study, 63.5% of patients with SCH had depressive symptoms.[96] Larger cross-sectional studies have mostly failed to show a clear link between SCH and impaired cognition and depression.[93-95,97-99] The symptoms of depression are more frequent and severe in young or middle-aged adults with SCH.[90,100,101] In the elderly, depressive symptoms are less likely to be linked to the presence of SCH, perhaps because of the frequency of depressive symptoms in this population.[97,98]

Mild cognitive impairment with difficulties in new learning and selective attention associated with SCH has been observed in younger individuals.[99] In an elderly subgroup, cognitive impairment has been described in one small study, but these results did not reach statistical significance.[102] Larger population studies using limited neuropsychological assessment have not shown significant cognitive impairment in SCH subjects.[103]

EFFECTS OF TREATMENT OF SUBCLINICAL HYPOTHYROIDISM WITH LT$_4$

Results of studies evaluating the effects of treatment with levothyroxine on neuropsychiatric manifestation have also been mixed. Some reports suggest that normalization of thyroid function as determined by the serum TSH with L-thyroxine therapy may completely reverse these neuropsychiatric features.[52,64,104-107] On the other hand, most larger randomized trials have not shown significant improvement in psychiatric symptoms. In the report by Jorde and colleagues,[94] the elegantly controlled design was curiously burdened by screening subclinically hypothyroid individuals with symptoms consistent with the presence of hypothyroidism out of the group that was eventually treated with L-thyroxine. Neurocognitive assessment of the selected, asymptomatic, subclinically hypothyroid subjects, when compared with controls who had not been screened for symptoms consistent with hypothyroidism, was found to be no different. After randomization, the normally functioning, asymptomatic patients with SCH did not become less symptomatic nor function better than controls after achieving a euthyroid state.[94] Another recent and fairly large, well-conducted study by Parle and colleagues[95] also concluded that there was no significant improvement in the well-being of the subclinically hypothyroid treatment group. However, in this trial the initial neuropsychological test scores in both placebo and LT$_4$ groups were within the expected range before the therapeutic intervention, again leaving little opportunity to observe improvement after L-thyroxine.[95] Because of these issues, conclusive evidence supporting the appropriate course to be taken with symptomatic subjects with SCH remains elusive.

EFFECTS OF LT$_4$ TREATMENT ON PATIENTS WITH EUTHYROID DEPRESSION

Asher's report on myxedema madness[2] demonstrated that thyroid hormone deficiency resulted in depression that was reversed with administration of thyroid hormone. This finding led to his suggestion of pursuing further studies on the role of thyroid hormone therapy alone in the treatment of depression and other psychiatric diseases.[2] Initially, open studies of high-dose T$_4$ for refractory bipolar and unipolar depression were conducted in patients with psychiatric problems that were difficult to treat.[108] In the study of Bauer and colleagues,[109] supratherapeutic doses of LT_4 were used (mean 378 μg/d) for an average of 51 months in 21 patients with refractory bipolar disorder, major depressive disorder, and schizoaffective disorder. Overall, more than 80% improved clinically and with regard to recurrences, as measured by the number of episodes of hospitalization, and a score on a psychiatric morbidity index that significantly declined. Of great interest in these studies is the apparent toleration of such high doses of thyroid hormone by those with these severe psychiatric issues in comparison with normal controls, 38% or more of whom will discontinue such treatment within 8 weeks of being exposed to excessive amounts of LT_4.[108] Euthyroid individuals with typical hypothyroid symptoms considered depressed on psychological testing do not improve when treated with T_4. In fact, patients presenting with symptoms of hypothyroidism with normal thyroid function tests respond more positively to placebo.[4] Limited data on cognitive function in otherwise healthy, young, euthyroid individuals indicates no significant differences in cognitive performance after about 45 days of supraphysiologic doses of LT_4 of up to 500 μg/d with subsequent suppression of TSH.[110]

COMBINED THYROID HORMONE AND ANTIDEPRESSANT THERAPY FOR DEPRESSION

Given the fact that 30% to 45% of the patients on antidepressants do not respond to antidepressant monotherapy,[111,112] the effect of adding thyroid hormones to antidepressant regimens has been studied. Adjuvant therapy has been said to be logical when depression fails to resolve after 6 weeks of adequate antidepressant medication.[113] The role of adjuvant thyroid hormone with tricyclic antidepressants (TCAs) has been investigated for more than 35 years in euthyroid patients with depression. Further studies of open LT_4 treatment in antidepressant-resistant patients have appeared, but the lack of controlled comparisons makes outcome interpretation difficult.[114,115] One of these studies indicated that responders to the levothyroxine and antidepressant combination had significantly lower pretreatment serum T_4 and reverse T_3 levels, leading the investigators to speculate that the responders might have been subclinically hypothyroid.[116] Another open-label trial seemed to indicate that effective augmentation of an antidepressant effect could be achieved with 50 μg of L-thyroxine daily.[117] In a third open-label trial of LT_4, 100 μg LT_4/d was given to euthyroid female patients (n = 17) with treatment-resistant depression, in addition to their antidepressants. More than half (64.7%) of these patients reportedly achieved remission.[118]

Most studies using thyroid hormone as adjuvant therapy have used LT_3 rather than LT_4, and in those reports where the advantages of one over the other were assessed, LT_3 was considered superior.[119] In a randomized trial combining LT_4 or LT_3 with antidepressants, only 4 of 21 patients (19%) treated with 150 μg/d of LT_4 for 3 weeks responded, whereas 9 of 17 (53%) responded with 37.5 μg/d of LT_3.[119] Combination therapy of antidepressants with LT_4 rather than LT_3 may be indicated when SCH or rapidly cycling bipolar disease is present. Because T_4 equilibrates in tissues more slowly than T_3, treatment with LT_4 for at least 6 to 8 weeks, and preferably longer, would be necessary to determine its efficacy in this situation.[19]

LT_3 doses of 25 to 50 μg daily increase serum T_3 levels and cause suppression of serum TSH and T_4 values. Two separate therapeutic effects of LT_3 therapy have been studied: first, its ability to accelerate the onset of the antidepressant response; second, its ability to augment antidepressant responses among those considered pharmacologically resistant.[19,120]

Given that the antidepressant effect of TCAs is known to be delayed, the role of LT_3 in accelerating the therapeutic onset of these drugs has been investigated. Several reports detailing the clinical outcomes of starting LT_3 (5–40 μg daily) along with varying doses of TCAs as well as SSRIs at the outset of therapy have appeared in the literature.[121,122] The study populations were inhomogeneous, consisting of patients with various types of depression. Furthermore, there were important methodologic limitations, including small sample sizes, inadequate medication doses, lack of monitoring of serum medication levels, and variable outcomes measures.[19] As 2 relatively large, prospective, randomized, placebo-controlled studies have come to opposite conclusions, it still has not been clearly established that LT_3 accelerates the antidepressant effect of SSRIs.[123,124] A recent meta-analysis of double-blind clinical trials comparing SSRI-LT_3 treatment with SSRI alone showed no significant difference in rates of remission.[12] However, a smaller pilot study to evaluate the effectiveness of LT_3 in accelerating and potentiating the antidepressant response, using various antidepressants according to the clinician's choice, showed that LT_3 may help accelerate the antidepressant response and possibly improve overall outcomes for depressed patients.[125] Clearly the debate will continue.

An additional hypothesis is that adding small doses of LT_3 to the antidepressant therapy for patients who have little or no initial response will enhance the clinical effectiveness of the antidepressant.[19] Resistance to antidepressants is defined as inadequate remission after 2 successive trials of monotherapy with different antidepressants in adequate doses, each for 4 to 6 weeks, before changing to alternative therapies.[126] However, 8 to 12 weeks of ineffective antidepressant therapy is commonly deemed unacceptable, and strategies designed to augment the response are being sought.[127] Early studies assessing LT_3 effectiveness in augmenting the antidepressant response were neither placebo-controlled nor focused on patient populations that could be directly compared.[128–131] The first placebo-controlled, double-blind, randomized study reported results in 16 unipolar depressed outpatients who had experienced no improvement in their clinical outcomes with TCAs alone.[132] The intervention consisted of adding 25 μg of LT_3 or placebo daily for 2 weeks before the patients were crossed over to the opposite treatment for an additional 2 weeks. No beneficial effect of LT_3 was apparent.[132] The only other placebo-controlled, randomized, double-blind trial investigating this question involved 33 patients with unipolar depression treated with either desipramine or imipramine for 5 weeks before random assignment to placebo or 37.5 μg of LT_3 daily.[133] After 2 weeks of observation on LT_3, during which TCA levels were monitored, significantly more patients treated with LT_3 (10 of 17; 59%) had a positive response in comparison with placebo-treated patients (3 of 16; 19%).[133] A subsequent open clinical trial of imipramine-resistant depression, using a prolonged period of TCA treatment preceding the addition of LT_3, showed no demonstrable effect of LT_3.[134]

The SSRI group of substances (including fluoxetine, paroxetine, and sertraline) is the preferred antidepressant medication in the United States today. A large, double-blind, placebo-controlled study to determine the role of LT_3 as augmentation therapy did not demonstrate an effect of LT_3 in augmenting the response of paroxetine therapy in patients with major depressive disorder,[123] but a similar study using sertraline and LT_3 seemed to demonstrate a positive response.[124] Responders in the report by Cooper-Karaz and colleagues[124] seemed to have had lower circulating thyroid hormone levels before treatment and to have experienced a greater decrease in TSH levels as a result of the intervention. This finding may indicate that those benefiting from the addition of LT_3 may have been subtly hypothyroid and that the addition of LT_3 compensated for this deficiency.[124] A recent meta-analysis of the available data suggests that coadministration of LT_3 and SSRIs has no significant clinical effect in depressed patients when compared with SSRI alone.[12] Another recent, fairly large double-blind, placebo-controlled study to determine the role of LT_3 as augmentation therapy also did not demonstrate an effect of LT_3 in augmenting the response of paroxetine therapy in patients with major depressive disorder.[135] Controlled data assessing the clinical effects of LT_3 with selective serotonin norepinephrine reuptake inhibitors (SSNRIs) is sparse to nonexistent. Of interest, LT_3 has been reported to augment the antidepressant effect of electroconvulsive therapy.[136] However, there is little to no evidence to guide the duration of treatment with supplemental LT_3, and few studies regarding side effects of long-term LT_3 administration have been published.[137]

As personalized medicine evolves, therapies will inevitably become more directed. New research directed at D1, which is important for peripheral conversion of T_4 to T_3, suggests that certain polymorphisms of D1 may be associated with a positive response to LT_3 potentiation of SSRIs. These patients with certain alleles have inherently lower D1 activity, and therefore have naturally lower serum T_3 levels. When compared with placebo, these patients have decreased depression scores at 8 weeks with LT_3 supplementation in combination with sertraline.[138] More research is necessary to determine whether those patients with a functional D1 gene polymorphism may be more responsive to LT_3 cotreatment.

Further randomized trials and long-term follow-up are required to validate these findings and determine safety.

THYROTOXICOSIS
Neuropsychiatric Manifestations of Overt Endogenous Thyrotoxicosis and Response to Treatment

Thyrotoxicosis is usually diagnosed when a patient has a low TSH value (<0.1 mIU/L) and an increased serum T_4 concentration, or an increased T_3 concentration, along with some clinical clues for excessive thyroid hormone action.[28]

Thyrotoxicosis presents with a wide array of neuropsychiatric symptoms that range from anxiety to depression.[46] Depressive disorders occur in 31% to 69% of hyperthyroid patients while anxiety disorders occur in about 60%, and these 2 states can often occur concurrently.[139,140] Mania may also be observed in hyperthyroidism, but is less common than depression and anxiety.[139,141,142] As outlined in **Table 3**, the classic neuropsychiatric symptoms of hyperthyroidism include anxiety, dysphoria, emotional lability, intellectual dysfunction, and mania.[19] A subset of hyperthyroid patients, usually the elderly population, may present with depression, lethargy, pseudodementia, and apathy, with what is termed apathetic thyrotoxicosis, and generally is reversible with treatment.[143] Psychotic symptoms including unusual presentations such as delusional parasitosis[144] are rare in hyperthyroid patients,[141,142] but case reports and case series have been conducted.[145,146] Severe hyperthyroidism can result in thyroid storm, a condition that ranges in neuropsychiatric presentation from hyperirritability, anxiety, and confusion to apathy and coma.[147]

Neuropsychiatric complaints are commonly the presenting symptoms of hyperthyroidism, and are often mistaken for primary psychiatric illness. As a result, patients frequently wait months before seeking medical help, and once they do they are often misdiagnosed.[20] In a study of hyperthyroid patients with Graves disease, which is the most common cause of hyperthyroidism,[28] Stern and colleagues[20] found that almost half of the patients waited longer than 1 month to receive an accurate diagnosis after first seeking help. One example of misdiagnosis documented in the literature is a case report by Taylor[143] of a hyperthyroid patient who presented with agitated depression, became worse when apparently appropriate psychotropic medications were administered, but improved when antithyroid drugs were prescribed. Of interest, prior

Table 3
Clinical features common to hyperthyroidism and mood disorders

	Mood Disorders	Hyperthyroidism
Depression	Yes	Yes
Diminished interest	Yes	Yes
Diminished pleasure	Yes	No
Decreased libido	Yes	Sometimes
Weight loss	Yes	Yes
Weight gain	Sometimes	Occasionally
Appetite loss	Yes	Sometimes
Increased appetite	Yes	Yes
Insomnia	Yes	Yes
Hypersomnia	Yes	No
Agitation/anxiety	Yes	Yes
Fatigue	Yes	Yes
Poor memory	Yes	Occasionally
Cognitive dysfunction	Yes	Yes
Impaired concentration	Yes	Yes
Constipation	Sometimes	No

Data from Hennessey JV, Jackson IM. The interface between thyroid hormones and psychiatry. Endocrinologist 1996;6:214–23.

personal history of psychiatric disease and family history of psychiatric disorders have not been found to predict anxiety or depression in patients with hyperthyroidism.[139] Conversely, others have found that patients with anxiety disorders have an unusually high rate of reporting a history of hyperthyroidism.[148]

Although Trzepacz and colleagues[140] did not find any correlation between thyroid function indices and depression or anxiety in hyperthyroid patients, Suwalska and colleagues[149] found that plasma levels of free T_4 correlated with the level of anxiety in the hyperthyroid patients reported. Similarly, Kathol and Delahunt[139] found that the level of T_4 excess was correlated with the number of symptoms of anxiety, but not symptoms of depression, that hyperthyroid patients experienced, and that severe anxiety symptoms tended to occur in the younger age group of patients.

The neuropsychiatric symptoms associated with hyperthyroidism do not always resolve after treatment and restoration of euthyroid state. Bunevicius and colleagues[150] found that both euthyroid and hyperthyroid women with a history of treated hyperthyroidism and ophthalmopathy caused by Graves disease had significantly more anxiety disorders, including panic disorder, social anxiety, and generalized anxiety, than a control group with no history of thyroid disease. The average time from diagnosis of Graves disease for these women was 2.9 years, with a range from 3 months to 20 years. Similarly, Bommer and colleagues[21] found that patients with remitted hyperthyroidism had significantly more depression, anxiety, hostility, mania, and sleep disturbances compared with controls. Lu and colleagues[151] found that only 50% of hyperthyroid patients with psychiatric illness recovered completely, whereas the other half of the patients showed a chronic or unremitting psychiatric condition after normalization of thyroid function tests, with 35% recovering partially, and 15% showing no change in mental status after treatment. Stern and colleagues[20] found that subjects treated for hyperthyroidism reported residual cognitive deficits of memory, attention, planning, and productivity even after they became euthyroid. Thus, somatic complaints and psychiatric symptoms can often persist after treatment of hyperthyroidism.[20,21,152] In addition, the less time patients have been euthyroid, the more likely they are to report residual psychopathological symptoms from their hyperthyroidism.[21,152]

Neuropsychiatric Manifestations of Subclinical Endogenous Hyperthyroidism and Response to Treatment

Subclinical hyperthyroidism is diagnosed when a patient has a low serum TSH concentration (<0.1 mIU/L) without increased serum levels of T_4 or T_3.[28] Its prevalence has been found to be between 2% and 16%[153] in several community or large clinic surveys mostly involving older persons.

Subclinical hyperthyroidism may be associated with nervousness and irritability[22]; even mild thyroid dysfunction has been associated with changes in mood.[154] In their study of patients with subclinical hyperthyroidism, Sait Gonen and colleagues[23] found that patients with subclinical hyperthyroidism had significantly more anxiety compared with euthyroid controls. Biondi and colleagues[155] found that compared with controls, young and middle-aged patients with subclinical hyperthyroidism have a significantly higher prevalence of symptoms of thyroid hormone excess, including nervousness, and impaired quality of life. Bommer and colleagues[21] found that patients with a history of treated overt hyperthyroidism who remained subclinically hyperthyroid had significantly more depression, mania, hostility, anxiety, and disturbed sleep compared with controls. In addition, these symptoms were more pronounced in the subclinical group than in patients who had a history of hyperthyroidism and were now euthyroid. However, a large study by Roberts and colleagues[97] did not find an increased rate of anxiety, depression, or problems with cognition in patients older than 65 years with subclinical hyperthyroidism. As a result, it is still unclear whether subclinical hyperthyroidism is generally expected to be associated with neuropsychiatric symptoms, and it is recommended that significant mood disorders or cognitive deficits in patients with subclinical hyperthyroidism be evaluated and treated as separate disorders.[156]

Whether to treat patients with subclinical hyperthyroidism in general is uncertain,[28] and is especially controversial in younger and middle-aged patients.[157] In older patients, subclinical hyperthyroidism often prompts consideration of treatment because of the increased risk of atrial fibrillation and decreased bone density,[28] as well as, possibly, an increased risk of dementia.[24] There have been no large, long-term controlled studies showing a benefit in treating subclinical hyperthyroidism,[26] but some small studies have shown a benefit of treatment on decreasing cardiac abnormalities and improving bone density.[158,159] At present, guidelines recommend treating subclinical hyperthyroidism in the elderly, patients with osteoporosis, heart disease, or cardiac risks, or those with a persistently undetectable TSH,[27] but there are no clear recommendations for treatment based on reversing neuropsychiatric symptoms that may be associated with subclinical hyperthyroidism.

It has not been shown that clinical or subclinical hyperthyroidism is more common in older persons with psychiatric disease than in others.[28] However, Kalmijn and colleagues[24] found that patients older than 55 years with subclinical hyperthyroidism have more than a 3-fold increased risk of dementia and Alzheimer disease. The risk of dementia was especially increased in subjects with low TSH who had positive TPO antibodies. On the other hand, van der Cammen and colleagues[25] did not find an increased risk of Alzheimer disease in geriatric patients with subclinical hyperthyroidism. As a result, it is still unclear whether older patients with subclinical hyperthyroidism have an increased risk of dementia, and there is no evidence that treating subclinical hyperthyroidism has any impact on this outcome.

Approximately 20% of patients admitted to hospital with acute psychiatric presentations, including schizophrenia and major affective disorders, but rarely dementia or alcoholism, may demonstrate mild elevations in their serum T_4 levels, and less often their T_3 levels.[160] The basal TSH is usually normal but may demonstrate blunted TRH responsiveness in up to 90% of such patients. These findings do not appear to represent thyrotoxicosis, as the abnormalities spontaneously resolve within 2 weeks without specific therapy. Such phenomena may be due to central activation of the hypothalamic-pituitary-thyroid axis, resulting in enhanced TSH secretion with consequent elevation in circulating T_4 levels.[33]

Neuropsychiatric Manifestations of Iatrogenic Thyrotoxicosis and Response to Treatment

There are several medications that can cause iatrogenic hyperthyroidism, including amiodarone, iodine (any form), lithium, and levothyroxine, as well as thyroid hormone extract.[28] Amphetamines induce hyperthyroxinemia through enhanced secretion of TSH, an effect that appears to be centrally mediated.[19]

With levothyroxine excess, which can occur with hypothyroid patients taking too much medication, or intentionally in the course of treatment for thyroid cancer, symptoms of overtreatment are similar to those of endogenous hyperthyroidism. However, they may be harder to recognize because of their milder degree, and the patient's adjustment owing to their longer time interval. In addition, older patients taking β-blockers, which can decrease the amount of anxiety and tremulousness they experience, may not exhibit classic neuropsychological symptoms of iatrogenic thyrotoxicosis.[161]

Several studies have evaluated the quality of life of patients with thyroid cancer who are on suppressive levothyroxine treatment. These patients have intentional chronic iatrogenic mild or subclinical thyrotoxicosis. At least one small study found that these patients had an impaired quality of life in comparison with healthy age-matched controls.[162] Specifically, the patients scored lower on emotional, sleep, energy, and social scales, and were found to have poorer mental health compared with controls. However, another randomized controlled study found that quality of life in patients with thyroid cancer and long-term subclinical hyperthyroidism is preserved, and did not improve with restoration of euthyroidism.[163] A recent systematic review of the data concluded that suppressive levothyroxine treatment results in similar or slightly impaired quality of life in comparison with the general population.[164]

Iodine-induced hyperthyroidism can develop after a patient receives iodine-rich medications such as amiodarone, topical iodine-containing antiseptics, or an iodine load from intravenous contrast,[165] which has been noted to result in the precipitation of thyroid storm with its dramatic neuropsychiatric presentation.[166] Arlt and colleagues[167] reported the case of a patient with bipolar disorder on lithium therapy who experienced thyrotoxicosis with rapid mood swings between mania and psychotic depression after receiving iodine contrast. Iatrogenic thyrotoxicosis may also be caused by the release of preformed thyroid hormones into the circulation; medications such as amiodarone or interferon-α[168,169]; and radiation, trauma, cellular injury, or lymphocytic infiltration of the thyroid gland.[29]

Ectopic thyrotoxicosis can occur in the setting of struma ovarii, large metastatic deposits of functioning differentiated thyroid cancer, or factitious ingestion of thyroid hormone.[170] TSH-mediated hyperthyroidism is triggered by a TSH-producing pituitary adenoma or pituitary resistance to thyroid hormone, and is rare.[170]

SUMMARY

The interface between the action of thyroid hormone and neuropsychiatric function is intricate, and several mechanisms of thyroid hormone uptake into brain tissues, hormone activation, and influences on neurotransmitter generation have been identified. Clinical symptoms attributed to thyroid dysfunction have been described. Symptoms of hypothyroidism are nonspecific, and those attributed to thyrotoxicosis may be more characteristic. Neuropsychiatric manifestations triggered by thyroid dysfunction likely respond well to reestablishment of the euthyroid state, although some patients appear to have persistent complaints. Strategies to address residual symptoms in those with hypothyroidism have included restoration of a truly euthyroid state, but further adjustment to "low normal TSH" has not been demonstrated to improve the response. The addition of LT_3 to ongoing LT_4 replacement, which has resulted in adequate TSH control, has yet to be definitively shown to be advantageous. Likewise, treatment of euthyroid depression with LT_3 in addition to contemporary antidepressant therapy lacks convincing evidence of superior outcomes to justify general application. Finally, the identification of SNPs in genes coding for types 1 and 2 deiodinase as well as the organic anion-transporting polypeptide may be useful in predicting the degree of symptoms associated with thyroid dysfunction, and may be useful in predicting the response to various medications and combinations when appropriately controlled, prospective studies are completed in the future.

REFERENCES

1. Report on myxoedema. Vol Suppl 1 Transactions of the Clinical Society of London. 1888.
2. Asher R. Myxoedematous madness. Br Med J 1949;22:555–62.
3. Whybrow PC. The therapeutic use of triiodothyronine and high dose thyroxine in psychiatric disorders. Acta Med Austriaca 1994;21:47–52.
4. Pollock MA, Sturrock A, Marshall K, et al. Thyroxine treatment in patients with symptoms of hypothyroidism but thyroid function tests within the reference range: randomized double blind placebo controlled crossover trial. BMJ 2001;323(7318):891–5.
5. Sawka AM, Gerstein HC, Marriott MJ, et al. Does a combination regimen of thyroxine (T4) and 3,5,3′-triiodothyronine improve depressive symptoms better T4 alone in patients with hypothyroidism? Results of a double-blind, randomized, controlled trial. J Clin Endocrinol Metab 2003;88(10):4551–5.
6. Canaris GJ, Manowitz NR, Mayor GH, et al. The Colorado Thyroid Disease Prevalence Study. Arch Intern Med 2000;160(4):526–34.
7. Hollowell JG, Staehling NW, Flanders WD, et al. Serum TSH, T4, and thyroid antibodies in the United States population (1988 to 1994): National Health and Nutrition Survey (NHANES III). J Clin Endocrinol Metab 2002;87:489–99.
8. Boucai L, Surks MI. Reference limits of serum TSH and free T4 are significantly influenced by race and age in an urban outpatient medical practice. Clin Endocrinol (Oxf) 2009;70(5):788–93.
9. Boucai L, Hollowell JG, Surks MI. An approach for development of age-, gender-, and ethnicity-specific thyrotropin reference limits. Thyroid 2011;21(1):5–11.
10. Panicker V, Evans J, Bjoro T, et al. A paradoxical difference in relationship between anxiety, depression and thyroid function in subjects on and not on T4: findings from the HUNT study. Clin Endocrinol (Oxf) 2009;71(4):574–80.
11. Burger AG. Is there a place for a combined treatment of athyreotic patients with thyroxine and triiodothyronine? Clin Thyroidal 2012;24(2):2–4.

12. Papakostas GI, Cooper-Kazaz R, Appelhof BC, et al. Simultaneous initiation (coinitiation) of pharmacotherapy with triiodothyronine and a selective serotonin reuptake inhibitor for major depressive disorder: a quantitative synthesis of double-blind studies. Int Clin Psychopharmacol 2009;24(1):19–25.

13. Surks MI, Hollowell JG. Age-specific distribution of serum thyrotropin and anti-thyroid antibodies in the US population: implications for the prevalence of sub-clinical hypothyroidism. J Clin Endocrinol Metab 2007;92(12):4575–82.

14. Waring AC, Arnold AM, Newman AB, et al. Longitudinal changes in thyroid function in the oldest old and survival: the cardiovascular health study all-stars study. J Clin Endocrinol Metab 2012;97(11):3944–50.

15. Atzmon G, Barzilai N, Hollowell JG, et al. Extreme longevity is associated with increased serum thyrotropin. J Clin Endocrinol Metab 2009;94(4):1251–4.

16. Bauer M, Szuba MP, Whybrow PC. Assessment of thyroid function. In: Wolkowitz OM, Rothschild AJ, editors. Psychoneuroendocrinology: the scientific basis of clinical practice, vol. 1, 1st edition. Washington, DC: American Psychiatric Publishing Inc; 2003. p. 366–99.

17. Atzmon G, Barzilai N, Surks MI, et al. Genetic predisposition to elevated serum thyrotropin is associated with exceptional longevity. J Clin Endocrinol Metab 2009;94(12):4768–75.

18. Howland RH. Thyroid dysfunction in refractory depression: implications for pathophysiology and treatment. J Clin Psychiatry 1993;54(2):47–54.

19. Hennessey JV, Jackson IM. The interface between thyroid hormones and psychiatry. Endocrinologist 1996;6:214–23.

20. Stern RA, Robinson B, Thorner AR, et al. A survey study of neuropsychiatric complaints in patients with Graves' disease. J Neuropsychiatry Clin Neurosci 1996;8(2):181–5.

21. Bommer M, Eversmann T, Pickardt R, et al. Psychopathological and neuropsychological symptoms in patients with subclinical and remitted hyperthyroidism. Klin Wochenschr 1990;68(11):552–8.

22. Stoudemire A. Psychological factors affecting medical conditions. In: Sadock BJ, Sadock V, editors. Kaplan and Sadock's comprehensive textbook of psychiatry; No. II. Philadelphia: Lippincott Williams and Wilkins; 2000.

23. Sait Gonen M, Kisakol G, Savas Cilli A, et al. Assessment of anxiety in subclinical thyroid disorders. Endocr J 2004;51(3):311–5.

24. Kalmijn S, Mehta KM, Pols HA, et al. Subclinical hyperthyroidism and the risk of dementia. The Rotterdam study. Clin Endocrinol (Oxf) 2000;53(6):733–7.

25. van der Cammen TJ, Mattace-Raso F, van Harskamp F, et al. Lack of association between thyroid disorders and Alzheimer's disease in older persons: a cross-sectional observational study in a geriatric outpatient population. J Am Geriatr Soc 2003;51(6):884.

26. Franklyn JA. The thyroid—too much and too little across the ages. The consequences of subclinical thyroid dysfunction. Clin Endocrinol (Oxf) 2013;78(1):1–8.

27. Surks MI, Ortiz E, Daniels GH, et al. Subclinical thyroid disease: scientific review and guidelines for diagnosis and management. JAMA 2004;291(2):228–38.

28. Sawin CT. Thyroid disease in older persons. In: Braverman L, editor. Diseases of the thyroid. 2nd edition. Totowa (NJ): Humana Press; 2010. p. 95.

29. Meurisse M, Preudhomme L, Lamberty G, et al. Iatrogenic thyrotoxicosis. Causal circumstances, pathophysiology and principles of treatment. Review of the literature. Acta Chir Belg 2001;101(6):257–66.

30. Chopra IJ, Solomon DH, Huang TS. Serum thyrotropin in hospitalized psychiatric patients: evidence for hyperthyrotropinemia as measured by an ultrasensitive thyrotropin assay. Metabolism 1990;39(5):538–43.
31. Hein MD, Jackson IM. Thyroid function in psychiatric illness. Gen Hosp Psychiatry 1990;12:232–44.
32. Carta MG, Loviselli A, Hardoy MC, et al. The link between thyroid autoimmunity (antithyroid peroxidase autoantibodies) with anxiety and mood disorders in the community: a field of interest for public health in the future. BMC Psychiatry 2004;4:25.
33. Fava M, Labbate LA, Abraham ME, et al. Hypothyroidism and hyperthyroidism in major depression revisited. J Clin Psychiatry 1995;56(5):186–92.
34. Salvador J, Dieguez C, Scanlon MF. The circadian rhythms of thyrotropin and prolactin secretion. Chronobiol Int 1988;5:85–93.
35. Souetre E, Salvati E, Wehr TA, et al. Twenty-four hour profiles of body temperature and plasma TSH in bipolar patients during depression and during remission and normal control subjects. Am J Psychiatry 1988;145:1133–7.
36. Kasper S, Sack DA, Wehr TA, et al. Nocturnal TSH and prolactin secretion during sleep deprivation and prediction of antidepressant response in patients with major depression. Biol Psychiatry 1988;24:631–41.
37. Bianco AC, Salvatore D, Gereben B, et al. Biochemistry, cellular and molecular biology, and physiological roles of the iodothyronine selenodeiodinases. Endocr Rev 2002;23(1):38–89.
38. Gereben B, Zavacki AM, Ribich S, et al. Cellular and molecular basis of deiodinase-regulated thyroid hormone signaling. Endocr Rev 2008;29(7):898–938.
39. Mentuccia D, Proietti-Pannunzi L, Tanner K, et al. Association between a novel variant of the human type 2 deiodinase gene Thr92Ala and insulin resistance: evidence of interaction with the Trp64Arg variant of the beta-3-adrenergic receptor. Diabetes 2002;51(3):880–3.
40. Appelhof BC, Peeters RP, Wiersinga WM, et al. Polymorphisms in type 2 deiodinase are not associated with well-being, neurocognitive functioning, and preference for combined thyroxine/3,5,3'-triiodothyronine therapy. J Clin Endocrinol Metab 2005;90(11):6296–9.
41. Panicker V, Saravanan P, Vaidya B, et al. Common variation in the DIO2 gene predicts baseline psychological well-being and response to combination thyroxine plus triiodothyronine therapy in hypothyroid patients. J Clin Endocrinol Metab 2009;94(5):1623–9.
42. Cleare AJ, McGregor A, O'Keane V. Neuroendocrine evidence for an association between hypothyroidism, reduced central 5-HT activity and depression. Clin Endocrinol (Oxf) 1995;43(6):713–9.
43. Bauer M, Whybrow PC. Thyroid hormones and the central nervous system in affective illness: interactions that may have clinical significance. Integr Psychiatry 1988;6:75–100.
44. Joffe RT. A perspective on the thyroid and depression. Can J Psychiatry 1990;35(9):754–8.
45. Jackson IM. The thyroid axis and depression. Thyroid 1998;8(10):951–6.
46. Hage MP, Azar ST. The link between thyroid function and depression. J Thyroid Res 2012;2012:590648.
47. van der Deure WM, Appelhof BC, Peeters RP, et al. Polymorphisms in the brain-specific thyroid hormone transporter OATP1C1 are associated with fatigue and depression in hypothyroid patients. Clin Endocrinol (Oxf) 2008;69(5):804–11.

48. Constant EL, de Volder AG, Ivanoiu A, et al. Cerebral blood flow and glucose metabolism in hypothyroidism: a positron emission tomography study. J Clin Endocrinol Metab 2001;86(8):3864–70.
49. Kinuya S, Michigishi T, Tonami N, et al. Reversible cerebral hypoperfusion observed with Tc-99m HMPAO SPECT in reversible dementia caused by hypothyroidism. Clin Nucl Med 1999;24(9):666–8.
50. Forchetti CM, Katsamakis G, Garron DC. Autoimmune thyroiditis and a rapidly progressive dementia: global hypoperfusion on SPECT scanning suggests a possible mechanism. Neurology 1997;49(2):623–6.
51. Krausz Y, Freedman N, Lester H, et al. Regional cerebral blood flow in patients with mild hypothyroidism. J Nucl Med 2004;45(10):1712–5.
52. Bauer M, Silverman DH, Schlagenhauf F, et al. Brain glucose metabolism in hypothyroidism: a positron emission tomography study before and after thyroid hormone replacement therapy. J Clin Endocrinol Metab 2009;94(8):2922–9.
53. Canaris GJ, Steiner JF, Ridgway EC. Do traditional symptoms of hypothyroidism correlate with biochemical disease? J Gen Intern Med 1997;12(9):544–50.
54. van de Ven AC, Netea-Maier RT, de Vegt F, et al. Is there a relationship between fatigue perception and the serum levels of thyrotropin and free thyroxine in euthyroid subjects? Thyroid 2012;22(12):1236–43.
55. Garber JR, Cobin RH, Gharib H, et al. Clinical practice guidelines for hypothyroidism in adults: cosponsored by the American Association of Clinical Endocrinologists and the American Thyroid Association. Thyroid 2012;22(12):1200–35.
56. Gharib H, Tuttle RM, Baskin HJ, et al. Consensus statement: subclinical thyroid dysfunction: a joint statement on management from the American Association of Clinical Endcrinologists, the American Thyroid Association, and The Endocrine Society. J Clin Endocrinol Metab 2005;90(1):581–5.
57. Jain VK. A psychiatric study of hypothyroidism. Psychiatr Clin (Basel) 1972;5(2):121–30.
58. Schuff K, Samuels MH, Whybrow P, et al. Psychiatric and cognitive effects of hypothyroidism. In: Braverman LE, Cooper DS, editors. The thyroid a fundamental and clinical text, vol. 1, 10th edition. Philadelphia: Lippincott Williams and Wilkins; 2013. p. 596–9.
59. Hall RC. Psychiatric effects of thyroid hormone disturbance. Psychosomatics 1983;24(1):7–11, 15–8.
60. Heinrich TW, Grahm G. Hypothyroidism presenting as psychosis: myxedema madness revisited. Prim Care Companion J Clin Psychiatry 2003;5(6):260–6.
61. Madakasira S, Hall TB 3rd. Capgras syndrome in a patient with myxedema. Am J Psychiatry 1981;138(11):1506–8.
62. Azzopardi L, Murfin C, Sharda A, et al. Myxoedema madness. BMJ Case Rep 2010;2010. pii:bcr0320102841.
63. Davis JD, Tremont G. Neuropsychiatric aspects of hypothyroidism and treatment reversibility. Minerva Endocrinol 2007;32(1):49–65.
64. Gulseren S, Gulseren L, Hekimsoy Z, et al. Depression, anxiety, health-related quality of life, and disability in patients with overt and subclinical thyroid dysfunction. Arch Med Res 2006;37(1):133–9.
65. Jonklaas J, Davidson B, Bhagat S, et al. Triiodothyronine levels in athyreotic individuals during levothyroxine therapy. JAMA 2008;299(7):769–77.
66. Boeving A, Paz-Filho G, Radominski RB, et al. Low-normal or high-normal thyrotropin target levels during treatment of hypothyroidism: a prospective, comparative study. Thyroid 2011;21(4):355–60.

67. Walsh JP, Ward LC, Burke V, et al. Small changes in thyroxine dosage do not produce measurable changes in hypothyroid symptoms, well-being, or quality of life: results of a double-blind, randomized clinical trial. J Clin Endocrinol Metab 2006;91(7):2624–30.
68. Saravanan P, Chau WF, Roberts N, et al. Psychological well-being in patients on "adequate" doses of L-thyroxine: Results of a large, controlled community-based questionnaire study. Clin Endocrinol 2002;57:577–85.
69. Edwards CM, Cox JP, Robinson S. Psychological well-being of patients on L-thyroxine. Clin Endocrinol (Oxf) 2003;59(2):264–5.
70. Wekking EM, Appelhof BC, Fliers E, et al. Cognitive functioning and well-being in euthyroid patients on thyroxine replacement therapy for primary hypothyroidism. Eur J Endocrinol 2005;153(6):747–53.
71. Murray GR. Note on the treatment of myxoedema by hypodermic injections of an extract of the thyroid gland of a sheep. Br Med J 1891;2(1606):796–7.
72. Selenkow HA, Wool MS. A new synthetic thyroid hormone combination for clinical therapy. Ann Intern Med 1967;67(1):90–9.
73. Sachs BA, Wolfman L, Murthy G. Lipid and clinical response to a new thyroid hormone combination. Am J Med Sci 1968;256(4):232–8.
74. Taylor S, Kapur M, Adie R. Combined thyroxine and triiodothyronine for thyroid replacement therapy. Br Med J 1970;2(5704):270–1.
75. Brent GA, Larsen PR. Treatment of hypothyroidism. In: Braverman LE, Utiger RD, editors. Werner and Ingbar's the thyroid: a fundamental and clinical text. 8th edition. Philadelphia: Lippincott Williams and Wilkins; 2000. p. 853–60.
76. Hennessey JV, Evaul JE, Tseng YC, et al. L-thyroxine dosage: a reevaluation of therapy with contemporary preparations. Ann Intern Med 1986;105:11–5.
77. Samuels MH, Schuff KG, Carlson NE, et al. Health status, mood, and cognition in experimentally induced subclinical hypothyroidism. J Clin Endocrinol Metab 2007;92(7):2545–51.
78. Bunevicius R, Kazanavicius G, Zalinkevicius R, et al. Effects of thyroxine as compared with thyroxine plus triiodothyronine in patients with hypothyroidism. N Engl J Med 1999;340:424–9.
79. Bunevicius R, Prange AJ. Mental improvement after replacement therapy with thyroxine plus triiodothyronine: relationship to cause of hypothyroidism. Int J Neuropsychopharmacol 2000;3(2):167–74.
80. Walsh JP, Shiels L, Lim EM, et al. Combined thyroxine/liothyronine treatment does not improve well-being, quality of life, or cognitive function compared to thyroxine alone: a randomized controlled trial in patients with primary hypothyroidism. J Clin Endocrinol Metab 2003;88(10):4543–50.
81. Grozinsky-Glasberg S, Fraser A, Nahshoni E, et al. Thyroxine-triiodothyronine combination therapy versus thyroxine monotherapy for clinical hypothyroidism: meta-analysis of randomized controlled trials. J Clin Endocrinol Metab 2006; 91(7):2592–9.
82. McDermott MT. Does combination T4 and T3 therapy make sense? Endocr Pract 2012;18(5):750–7.
83. Gharib H, Tuttle RM, Baskin HJ, et al. Subclinical thyroid dysfunction: a joint statement on management from the American Association of Clinical Endocrinologists, the American Thyroid Association, and the Endocrine Society. Endocr Pract 2004;10(6):497–501.
84. Vanderpump M. Cardiovascular and cancer mortality after radioiodine treatment of hyperthyroidism. J Clin Endocrinol Metab 2007;92(6):2033–5.

85. Parle JV, Franklyn JA, Cross KW, et al. Prevalence and follow-up of abnormal thyrotrophin (TSH) concentrations in the elderly in the United Kingdom. Clin Endocrinol (Oxf) 1991;34(1):77–83.

86. Somwaru LL, Rariy CM, Arnold AM, et al. The natural history of subclinical hypothyroidism in the elderly: the cardiovascular health study. J Clin Endocrinol Metab 2012;97(6):1962–9.

87. Huber G, Staub JJ, Meier C, et al. Prospective study of the spontaneous course of subclinical hypothyroidism: prognostic value of thyrotropin, thyroid reserve, and thyroid antibodies. J Clin Endocrinol Metab 2002;87(7):3221–6.

88. Stern RA, Prange AJ. Neuropsychiatric aspects of endocrine disorders. In: Kaplan HI, Sadock BJ, editors. Comprehensive textbook of psychiatry, vol. 6. Baltimore (MD): Williams and Wilkins; 1995. p. 241–51.

89. Cooper DS, Halpern R, Wood LC, et al. L-thyroxine therapy in subclinical hypothyroidism: a double-blind, placebo-controlled trial. Ann Intern Med 1984; 101(1):18–24.

90. Monzani F, DelGerra P, Caraccion N, et al. Subclinical hypothyroidism: neurobehavioral features and beneficial effect of L-thyroxine treatment. Clin Investig 1993;71:367–71.

91. Razvi S, Ingoe L, Keeka G, et al. The beneficial effect of L-thyroxine on cardiovascular risk factors, endothelial function, and quality of life in subclinical hypothyroidism: randomized, crossover trial. J Clin Endocrinol Metab 2007;92(5):1715–23.

92. Vigario P, Teixeira P, Reuters V, et al. Perceived health status of women with overt and subclinical hypothyroidism. Med Princ Pract 2009;18(4):317–22.

93. Bell RJ, Rivera-Woll L, Davison SL, et al. Well-being, health-related quality of life and cardiovascular disease risk profile in women with subclinical thyroid disease—a community-based study. Clin Endocrinol 2007;66(4):548–56.

94. Jorde R, Waterloo K, Storhaug H, et al. Neuropsychological function and symptoms in subjects with subclinical hypothyroidism and the effect of thyroxine treatment. J Clin Endocrinol Metab 2006;91(1):145–53.

95. Parle J, Roberts L, Wilson S, et al. A randomized controlled trial of the effect of thyroxine replacement on cognitive function in community-living elderly subjects with subclinical hypothyroidism: the Birmingham Elderly Thyroid study. J Clin Endocrinol Metab 2010;95(8):3623–32.

96. Demartini B, Masu A, Scarone S, et al. Prevalence of depression in patients affected by subclinical hypothyroidism. Panminerva Med 2010;52(4):277–82.

97. Roberts LM, Pattison H, Roalfe A, et al. Is subclinical thyroid dysfunction in the elderly associated with depression or cognitive dysfunction? Ann Intern Med 2006;145(8):573–81.

98. Almeida OP, Alfonso H, Flicker L, et al. Thyroid hormones and depression: the Health in Men study. Am J Geriatr Psychiatry 2011;19(9):763–70.

99. Joffe RT, Pearce EN, Hennessey JV, et al. Subclinical hypothyroidism, mood, and cognition in older adults: a review. Int J Geriatr Psychiatry 2013;28(2):111–8.

100. Tappy L, Randin JP, Schwed P, et al. Prevalence of thyroid disorders in psychogeriatric inpatients. A possible relationship of hypothyroidism with neurotic depression but not with dementia. J Am Geriatr Soc 1987;35(6):526–31.

101. Joffe RT, Levitt AJ. Major depression and subclinical (grade 2) hypothyroidism. Psychoneuroendocrinology 1992;17(2–3):215–21.

102. Osterweil D, Syndulko K, Cohen SN, et al. Cognitive function in non-demented older adults with hypothyroidism. J Am Geriatr Soc 1992;40(4):325–35.

103. Sanavi S, Afshar R. Subacute thyroiditis following ginger (Zingiber officinale) consumption. Int J Ayurveda Res 2010;1(1):47–8.

104. Correia N, Mullally S, Cooke G, et al. Evidence for a specific defect in hippocampal memory in overt and subclinical hypothyroidism. J Clin Endocrinol Metab 2009;94(10):3789–97.

105. Zhu DF, Wang ZX, Zhang DR, et al. fMRI revealed neural substrate for reversible working memory dysfunction in subclinical hypothyroidism. Brain 2006; 129(Pt 11):2923–30.

106. Aghili R, Khamseh ME, Malek M, et al. Changes of subtests of Wechsler Memory Scale and cognitive function in subjects with subclinical hypothyroidism following treatment with levothyroxine. Arch Med Sci 2012;8(6):1096–101.

107. Yin JJ, Liao LM, Luo DX, et al. Spatial working memory impairment in subclinical hypothyroidism: an fMRI study. Neuroendocrinology 2013;97(3):260–70.

108. Bauer M, Baur H, Berghofer A, et al. Effects of supraphysiological thyroxine administration in healthy controls and patients with depressive disorders. J Affect Disord 2002;68(2–3):285–94.

109. Bauer M, Berghofer A, Bschor T, et al. Supraphysiological doses of L-thyroxine in the maintenance treatment of prophylaxis-resistant affective disorders. Neuropsychopharmacology 2002;27(4):620–8.

110. Baethge C, Reischies FM, Berghofer A, et al. Effects of supraphysiological doses of L-thyroxine on cognitive function in healthy individuals. Psychiatry Res 2002;110(2):117–23.

111. Fava M. Augmentation and combination strategies in treatment-resistant depression. J Clin Psychiatry 2001;62(Suppl 18):4–11.

112. Cowen PJ. New drugs, old problems: revisiting. pharmacological management of treatment-resistant depression. Adv Psychiatr Treat 2005;11:19–27.

113. Nemeroff CB. Augmentation regimens for depression. J Clin Psychiatry 1991; 52(Suppl):21–7.

114. Shelton RC, Winn S, Ekhatore N, et al. The effects of antidepressants on the thyroid axis in depression. Biol Psychiatry 1993;33(2):120–6.

115. Stern RA, Nevels CT, Shelhorse ME, et al. Antidepressant and memory effects of combined thyroid hormone treatment and electroconvulsive therapy: preliminary findings. Biol Psychiatry 1991;30(6):623–7.

116. Nakamura T, Nomura J. Comparison of thyroid function between responders and nonresponders to thyroid hormone supplementation in depression. Jpn J Psychiatry Neurol 1992;46(4):905–9.

117. Barak Y, Stein D, Levine J, et al. Thyroxine augmentation of fluoxetine treatment for resistant depression in the elderly: an open trial. Hum Psychopharmacol 1996;11:463–7.

118. Lojko D, Rybakowski JK. L-thyroxine augmentation of serotonergic antidepressants in female patients with refractory depression. J Affect Disord 2007; 103(1–3):253–6.

119. Joffe RT, Singer W. A comparison of triiodothyronine and thyroxine in the potentiation of tricyclic antidepressants. Psychiatry Res 1990;32(3):241–51.

120. Joffe RT. Is the thyroid still important in major depression? J Psychiatry Neurosci 2006;31(6):367–8.

121. Prange AJ, Wilson IC, Rabon AM, et al. Enhancement of imipramine antidepressant activity by thyroid hormone. Am J Psychiatry 1969;126:39–51.

122. Joffe RT, Sokolov ST, Singer W. Thyroid hormone treatment of depression. Thyroid 1995;5:235–9.

123. Applehof BC, Brouwer JP, Van Dyck R, et al. Triiodothyronine addition to paroxetine in the treatment of major depressive disorder. J Clin Endocrinol Metab 2004;89(12):6271–6.

124. Cooper-Kazaz R, Apter JT, Cohen R, et al. Combined treatment with sertraline and liothyronine in major depression: a randomized, double-blind, placebo-controlled trial. Arch Gen Psychiatry 2007;64(6):679–88.

125. Posterank M, Novak S, Stern RA, et al. A pilot effectiveness study: placebo-controlled trial of adjunctive L-triiodothyronine (T3) used to accelerate and potentiate the antidepressant response. Int J Neuropsychopharmacol 2008; 11(1):15–25.

126. Bech P. Acute therapy of depression. J Clin Psychiatry 1993;54(Suppl):18–27 [discussion: 28].

127. Nelson JC. Augmentation strategies in depression 2000. J Clin Psychiatry 2000; 61(Suppl 1):13–9.

128. Ogura C, Okuma T, Uchida Y, et al. Combined thyroid (triiodothyronine)-tricyclic antidepressant treatment in depressive states. Folia Psychiatr Neurol Jpn 1974; 28(3):179–86.

129. Banki CM. Cerebrospinal fluid amine metabolites after combined amitriptyline-triiodothyronine treatment of depressed women. Eur J Clin Pharmacol 1977; 11(4):311–5.

130. Goodwin FK, Prange AJ Jr, Post RM, et al. Potentiation of antidepressant effects by L-triiodothyronine in tricyclic nonresponders. Am J Psychiatry 1982;139(1):34–8.

131. Schwarcz G, Halaris A, Baxter L, et al. Normal thyroid function in desipramine nonresponders converted to responders by the addition of L-triiodothyronine. Am J Psychiatry 1984;141(12):1614–6.

132. Gitlin MJ, Weiner H, Fairbanks L, et al. Failure of T3 to potentiate tricyclic antidepressant response. J Affect Disord 1987;13:267–72.

133. Joffe RT, Singer W, Levitt AJ, et al. A placebo-controlled comparison of lithium and triiodothyronine augmentation of tricyclic antidepressants in unipolar refractory depression. Arch Gen Psychiatry 1993;50:387–93.

134. Thase ME, Kupfer DJ, Jarrett DB. Treatment of imipramine-resistant recurrent depression: I. An open clinical trial of adjunctive L-triiodothyronine. J Clin Psychiatry 1989;50(10):385–8.

135. Fliers E, Applehof BC, Brouwer JP, et al. Efficacy of triiodothyronine (T3) addition to paroxetine in major depressive disorder: a randomized clinical trial. Annual Meeting of the Endocrine Society. Philadelphia: The Endocrine Society; 2003. S19–2, p. 25.

136. Tremont G, Stern RA. Use of thyroid hormone to diminish the cognitive side effects of psychiatric treatment. Psychopharmacol Bull 1997;33(2):273–80.

137. Cooper-Kazaz R, Lerer B. Efficacy and safety of triiodothyronine supplementation in patients with major depressive disorder treated with specific serotonin reuptake inhibitors. Int J Neuropsychopharmacol 2008;11(5):685–99.

138. Cooper-Kazaz R, van der Deure WM, Medici M, et al. Preliminary evidence that a functional polymorphism in type 1 deiodinase is associated with enhanced potentiation of the antidepressant effect of sertraline by triiodothyronine. J Affect Disord 2009;116(1–2):113–6.

139. Kathol RG, Delahunt JW. The relationship of anxiety and depression to symptoms of hyperthyroidism using operational criteria. Gen Hosp Psychiatry 1986; 8(1):23–8.

140. Trzepacz PT, McCue M, Klein I, et al. A psychiatric and neuropsychological study of patients with untreated Graves' disease. Gen Hosp Psychiatry 1988; 10(1):49–55.

141. Rockey PH, Griep RJ. Behavioral dysfunction in hyperthyroidism. Improvement with treatment. Arch Intern Med 1980;140(9):1194–7.

142. Burch EA Jr, Messervy TW. Psychiatric symptoms in medical illness: hyperthyroidism revisited. Psychosomatics 1978;19(2):71–5.

143. Taylor JW. Depression in thyrotoxicosis. Am J Psychiatry 1975;132(5):552–3.

144. Ozten E, Tufan AE, Cerit C, et al. Delusional parasitosis with hyperthyroidism in an elderly woman: a case report. J Med Case Rep 2013;7(1):17.

145. Lazarus A, Jaffe R. Resolution of thyroid-induced schizophreniform disorder following subtotal thyroidectomy: case report. Gen Hosp Psychiatry 1986;8(1): 29–31.

146. Brownlie BE, Rae AM, Walshe JW, et al. Psychoses associated with thyrotoxicosis - 'thyrotoxic psychosis.' A report of 18 cases, with statistical analysis of incidence. Eur J Endocrinol 2000;142(5):438–44.

147. Wartofsky L. Thyrotoxic storm. In: Braverman LE, Cooper DS, editors. Werner and Ingbar's the thyroid: a fundamental and clinical text, vol. 1, 10th edition. Philadelphia: Lippincott Williams and Wilkins; 2013. p. 481–6.

148. Orenstein H, Peskind A, Raskind MA. Thyroid disorders in female psychiatric patients with panic disorder or agoraphobia. Am J Psychiatry 1988;145(11):1428–30.

149. Suwalska A, Lacka K, Lojko D, et al. Quality of life, depressive symptoms and anxiety in hyperthyroid patients. Rocz Akad Med Bialymst 2005;50(Suppl 1): 61–3.

150. Bunevicius R, Velickiene D, Prange AJ Jr. Mood and anxiety disorders in women with treated hyperthyroidism and ophthalmopathy caused by Graves' disease. Gen Hosp Psychiatry 2005;27(2):133–9.

151. Lu CL, Lee YC, Tsai SJ, et al. Psychiatric disturbances associated with hyperthyroidism: an analysis report of 30 cases. Zhonghua Yi Xue Za Zhi (Taipei) 1995; 56(6):393–8.

152. Fahrenfort JJ, Wilterdink AM, van der Veen EA. Long-term residual complaints and psychosocial sequelae after remission of hyperthyroidism. Psychoneuroendocrinology 2000;25(2):201–11.

153. Marqusee E, Haden ST, Utiger RD. Subclinical thyrotoxicosis. Endocrinol Metab Clin North Am 1998;27(1):37–49.

154. Hendrick V, Altshuler L, Whybrow P. Psychoneuroendocrinology of mood disorders. The hypothalamic-pituitary-thyroid axis. Psychiatr Clin North Am 1998; 21(2):277–92.

155. Biondi B, Palmieri EA, Fazio S, et al. Endogenous subclinical hyperthyroidism affects quality of life and cardiac morphology and function in young and middle-aged patients. J Clin Endocrinol Metab 2000;85(12):4701–5.

156. Bauer M, Samuels MH, Whybrow P. Behavioral and psychiatric aspects of thyrotoxicosis. In: Braverman LE, Cooper DS, editors. Werner and Ingbar's the thyroid: a fundamental and clinical text, vol. 1, 10th edition. Philadelphia: Lippincott, Williams and Wilkins; 2013. p. 75–480.

157. Cooper DS. Subclinical thyroid disease: a clinician's perspective. Ann Intern Med 1998;129(2):135–8.

158. Sgarbi JA, Villaca FG, Garbeline B, et al. The effects of early antithyroid therapy for endogenous subclinical hyperthyroidism in clinical and heart abnormalities. J Clin Endocrinol Metab 2003;88(4):1672–7.

159. Faber J, Jensen IW, Petersen L, et al. Normalization of serum thyrotrophin by means of radioiodine treatment in subclinical hyperthyroidism: effect on bone loss in postmenopausal women. Clin Endocrinol (Oxf) 1998;48(3):285–90.

160. Sarne D, DeGroot LJ. Effects of the environment, chemicals and drugs on thyroid function. Endocrine Education, Inc; 2002. Available at: www.thyroidmanager.org. Accessed July 9, 2013.

161. Ladenson PW. Problems in management of hypothyroidism. In: Braverman LE, editor. Diseases of the thyroid. 2nd edition. Totowa (NJ): Humana Press; 2010. p. 161–76.

162. Botella-Carretero JI, Galan JM, Caballero C, et al. Quality of life and psychometric functionality in patients with differentiated thyroid carcinoma. Endocr Relat Cancer 2003;10(4):601–10.

163. Eustatia-Rutten CF, Corssmit EP, Pereira AM, et al. Quality of life in longterm exogenous subclinical hyperthyroidism and the effects of restoration of euthyroidism, a randomized controlled trial. Clin Endocrinol (Oxf) 2006;64(3): 284–91.

164. Husson O, Haak HR, Oranje WA, et al. Health-related quality of life among thyroid cancer survivors: a systematic review. Clin Endocrinol (Oxf) 2011;75(4): 544–54.

165. Rhee CM, Bhan I, Alexander EK, et al. Association between iodinated contrast media exposure and incident hyperthyroidism and hypothyroidism. Arch Intern Med 2012;172(2):153–9.

166. Martin FI, Tress BW, Colman PG, et al. Iodine-induced hyperthyroidism due to nonionic contrast radiography in the elderly. Am J Med 1993;95(1):78–82.

167. Arlt S, Burkhardt D, Wiedemann K. Thyrotoxicosis after iodine contrast medium administration: rapid mood swing to mania and subsequent psychotic depression in a patient with bipolar disorder during lithium therapy. Pharmacopsychiatry 2008;41(4):163–5.

168. Bogazzi F, Tomisti L, Bartalena L, et al. Amiodarone and the thyroid: a 2012 update. J Endocrinol Invest 2012;35(3):340–8.

169. Hamnvik OP, Larsen PR, Marqusee E. Thyroid dysfunction from antineoplastic agents. J Natl Cancer Inst 2011;103(21):1572–87.

170. Ross DS. Management of the various causes of thyrotoxicosis. In: Braverman LE, editor. Diseases of the thyroid. 2nd edition. Totowa (NJ): Humana Press; 2010. p. 177–98.

Neuropsychiatric Findings in Cushing Syndrome and Exogenous Glucocorticoid Administration

Monica N. Starkman, MD, MS

KEYWORDS

- Elevated cortisol • Cushing disease and Cushing syndrome
- Exogenous glucocorticoid administration • Depressive disorder • Hypomania
- Cognition • Brain imaging • Management

KEY POINTS

- Individuals with active Cushing disease and syndrome develop a depressive syndrome characterized by irritable and depressed mood, decreased libido, disrupted sleep and cognitive decrements.
- Exogenous glucocorticoids most often elicit a hypomanic syndrome and subtle-to-severe cognitive decrements.
- Brain imaging studies and neuropsychologic studies indicate that hypercortisolism or supraphysiologic exogenous glucocorticoids are especially deleterious to the hippocampus and frontal lobes.
- Antidepressants have little beneficial effect in Cushing disease and Cushing syndrome until the elevated cortisol concentration is reduced by surgical/medical treatment.
- Neuropsychiatric side effects of glucocorticoid therapy are best treated by reducing the dose if possible and/or administration of atypical neuroleptic medication.

Cushing disease (CD), the major type of spontaneous Cushing syndrome (SCS), is the classic endocrine disease characterized by hypersecretion of cortisol and diminished suppression of cortisol by dexamethasone. Harvey Cushing reported the presence of "emotional disturbances" as a feature of the disease.[1] This association was later confirmed by others with case reports and by using retrospective chart reviews.[2,3]

In the 1960s, investigators discovered that a subgroup of patients with primary major depression had elevated concentrations of cortisol, disrupted circadian rhythm with inappropriate secretion at night, and early escape from suppression by dexamethasone.[4] This finding led to interest in cortisol dysregulation as a biomarker suggesting an abnormal limbic system drive on the hypothalamic-pituitary-adrenal axis in

Department of Psychiatry, University of Michigan Medical Center, 1500 East Medical Center Drive, Ann Arbor, MI 48109, USA
E-mail address: Starkman@umich.edu

Endocrinol Metab Clin N Am 42 (2013) 477–488
http://dx.doi.org/10.1016/j.ecl.2013.05.010
0889-8529/13/$ – see front matter © 2013 Elsevier Inc. All rights reserved.

endo.theclinics.com

primary depression. The potential effects of cortisol hypersecretion on the brain itself were not examined.

In the 1980s, investigators began exploring the relationship from the other direction: namely, the effects of endogenous hypercortisolism on neuropsychiatric dysfunction. Cohen[5] reported that interviews and chart reviews of SCS patients showed that depression was the predominant presentation. Starkman and colleagues[6] published the first prospective study of patients with suspected SCS who were examined before the definitive diagnosis was made or ruled out. In this study, the specific new-onset neuropsychiatric symptoms and signs of hypercortisolism and the time sequence of their appearance were defined.

The study initiated a series of longitudinal and other investigations in SCS by this group over time to test their hypothesis that dysregulation of cortisol, however elicited, plays a role in the pathogenesis and/or maintenance of the depressive syndrome in primary depression and other conditions.[7–23] SCS is powerfully informative because exposure to supra-physiologic stress-level concentrations of the natural steroid cortisol is sustained for months to years before the elusive diagnosis is made. Longitudinal studies during hypercortisolism and after treatment provide the opportunity to examine the amelioration/reversibility of symptoms as well as underlying mechanisms such as alterations in brain structure and function.

In the decades that followed, investigations into the neuropsychiatric effects of endogenous and exogenous glucocorticoids accelerated. Additional human conditions showing elevations in cortisol or disruptions in its rhythm were discovered, such as subgroups of normal elderly and patients with Alzheimer disease. This review highlights clinical presentations of hypercortisolism secondary to SCS and exogenous glucocorticoid (EGC) administration, the cognitive testing and brain imaging profiles in these conditions, and the biological processes underlying them. Problems of differential diagnosis and treatment are also discussed.

ETIOLOGY OF CUSHING DISEASE

The etiology of CD, the most common form of SCS, is both well known and still under investigation. In the majority of patients the disease results from a benign monoclonal corticotropin (ACTH)-secreting microadenoma while the rest of the gland remains normal. In approximately 10% of patients with CD there is instead generalized pituitary hyperplasia. In these cases, the primary disorder has been suggested to be in the central nervous system, with an overproduction of hypothalamic corticotropin-releasing hormone (CRH).[24] Studies analyzing episodic cortisol secretion have suggested the existence of two forms of CD, one involving CRH hypersecretion and one not.[25]

SPONTANEOUS CUSHING SYNDROME
Neuropsychiatric Findings Prior to Treatment

The description and prevalence of each symptom, as determined in the first prospective study, are given here.[6]

Mood and affect
Irritability (86%) was the most frequent symptom and was usually the first neuropsychiatric symptom to appear, beginning close to the onset of weight gain and before the appearance of other physical manifestations.

Depressed mood (77%) manifested with a range of intensity. Most patients described short spells of sadness, whereas others experienced constant hopelessness.

A common pattern was for a depressive episode to persist for 1 day, and rarely more than 3 days at a time. Depressed mood could be present on awakening or appear as a sudden mood shift during the day, indicating mood lability. Patients were depressed approximately 3 days per week. There was no regular cyclicity. When present, guilt was not self-accusatory or excessively irrational, and was often secondary to remorse about uncontrollable angry outbursts. Some patients had more chronic and persistent depressed mood. Suicidal thoughts were reported by 17%, and 5% had made a suicide attempt.

Increased crying (63%) occurred spontaneously or as a result of feeling hurt or angry at others. Social withdrawal (46%) was ascribed to shame about physical appearance, feelings of decreased focus, or overstimulation when in group settings. Although some had intervals when they did not experience pleasure, they did not describe the persistent inability to experience pleasure characteristic of patients with moderate to severe primary major depressive disorder.

A minority of patients experienced not just irritability but episodes of hyperactivity and elevated mood early in the course of the disease; they had increased ambition, motor activity, and restlessness. As the disease progressed and new physical signs appeared, this type of episode became rarer or disappeared entirely. One patient (subsequently found to have an ectopic ACTH-secreting tumor with very high cortisol concentrations) had a full-blown manic presentation.

A substantial percentage (66%) reported generalized anxiety. Patients without psychic anxiety frequently described episodic symptoms of autonomic activation such as shaking, palpitations, and sweating. (Another group reported that SCS patients developed not only generalized anxiety but also new-onset panic disorder.[26])

Biological drives and vegetative functions

Fatigue was a ubiquitous complaint, with decreased libido being the next most common symptom (70%). Decreased libido was also one of the earliest manifestations of SCS, beginning when the patient was experiencing the onset of weight gain. Appetite was altered in more than 50% of patients: increased in 34% and decreased in 20%.

Sleep was disturbed: 69% of patients awakened at least once during the night and 57% awakened earlier than desired in the morning. Less frequent was inability to fall asleep at bedtime (29%). One-third of patients reported alterations in the frequency of dreams (increased) or quality of dreams (more bizarre and vivid). Some reported inability to wake themselves out of a nightmare. In a separate study to explore these findings further, sleep EEGs showed that CD patients, when compared to healthy control subjects, manifested significantly less total sleep time, lower sleep efficiency, and shortened time to onset of rapid eye movement (REM) sleep, findings similar to those in patients with primary major depressive disorder.[14,15]

Cognition

The most frequent cognitive symptom reported was impaired memory (83%). Impaired concentration was a problem for 66%, with inattention, distractibility, and shortened attention span. Patients also reported problems with registration of new information, forgetfulness for appointments, and locations of objects. Difficulty with reasoning ability, comprehension, and processing of information were also described.

On bedside evaluation of mental status, difficulties with mental subtraction (serial 7 subtractions) were observed in close to 50%. Despite cognitive decrements, patients had no disorientation or overt clouding of consciousness. Two simple bedside mental status tests in SCS patients, involving 7 serial subtractions and recall of 3 cities after 5 minutes, were significantly correlated with sophisticated neuropsychological test results.[10]

The depressive syndrome in SCS

The aforementioned neuropsychiatric symptoms and signs indicated that SCS manifested abnormalities in all 3 domains of the depressive syndrome: mood, vegetative functions, and cognition. The majority of patients met the *Diagnostic and Statistical Manual of Mental Disorders*, 3rd edition (DSM-III) criteria for a Major Depressive Disorder, except for not excluding an organic disorder.[6] Had the subsequent revised criteria in the succeeding DSM-IV been used (which accepted only depressed but no longer irritable mood as satisfying the mood criterion), then 50% would have been so classified. Subsequent prospective investigations have reported similar findings. Using the Research Diagnostic Criteria, Haskett[27] determined that 80% of SCS patients met criteria for a major depressive disorder, with almost one-third experiencing episodes of hypomanic symptoms at some point during their disease. The mean prevalence of major depressive disorder in later studies of SCS was approximately 50% to 60%, and was similar for both CD only and SCS resulting from an adrenal adenoma.[28]

The characteristics of these manifestations of the depressive syndrome argue for a pathogenesis beyond a nonspecific response to severe physical illness.[6] Irritability and decreased libido occur early, often before patients are aware they have any physical problem other than a steady increase in weight. Depressed mood is experienced not simply as the demoralization common to patients with medical illness but also as episodic sadness and crying, often in the absence of depressive thoughts. Kelly and colleagues[29] found that 80% of patients with active CD had a psychiatric diagnosis, compared with 13% in the comparison group of pituitary-adenoma patients secreting growth hormone or prolactin. In a study comparing the prevalence of pretreatment depression in SCS with Graves disease, Sonino and Fava[30] reported a significantly higher prevalence in SCS.

Differential diagnosis and treatment

SCS is difficult to diagnose, and neuropsychiatric features can be helpful in raising or lowering the index of suspicion. Patients will usually not spontaneously mention neuropsychiatric symptoms, so these need to be specifically asked about. The author's group has found that at initial evaluation, those hypercortisolemic patients subsequently found to meet endocrine criteria for SCS manifested, at minimum, a triad consisting of irritability, middle insomnia, and decreased libido. These earliest-appearing neuropsychiatric symptoms persist as the disease progresses.

Though similar in many respects to primary major depressive disorder, certain features are characteristic in SCS. Irritability is particularly prominent, as are symptoms of adrenergic stimulation such as shaking and increased sweating. Affect is typically labile, and depressed mood frequently is not relentless but episodic, lasting for 1 to 3 days and recurring at irregular intervals. Patients feel better in the morning, not in the evening as is more typical of major depression. The ability to experience pleasure is usually present.

The best therapy for the neuropsychiatric dysfunction is prompt treatment of the hypercortisolism. Several groups have found that selective serotonin reuptake inhibitors can be administered safely, but not necessarily effectively. When patients do report a useful effect, it is usually only a partial one: only mood or only vegetative symptoms improve. Tricyclic antidepressants have very little useful effect.

Reassurance that the mental symptoms are a common feature of the disease, related to biochemical changes, and that most will usually improve over time following treatment is of relief to patients and families.

Neuropsychiatric Findings After Treatment

After treatment many of the neuropsychiatric manifestations improve. The degree and timing of improvement among the different neuropsychiatric symptoms varies.

In the longitudinal restudy of subjects initially evaluated before treatment by Starkman and colleagues,[6] 72% of subjects who had reported depressed mood reported improvement, in most cases without the addition of antidepressant medication. Depressive episodes became less frequent, shorter in duration, and less intense. Of those with decreased ability to concentrate, 80% reported increased ability to concentrate; of those with memory problems, 70% improved. Regarding middle insomnia, 62% improved. By contrast, only 28% reported an increase in libido.[11] Sonino and colleagues[30] found that about 70% of SCS patients fully recovered from their depression, whereas others had no substantial change. Dorn and colleagues[31] reported that overall psychopathology in their cohort decreased from 67% to 54% at 3 months, 36% at 6 months, and 24% at 12 months.

After treatment, there was a significant relationship between the degree of improvement in depressed mood and the degree of decrease in cortisol.[11] Improvement in cognition was also seen once cortisol decreased.[20]

Just as improvement in hypertension in SCS occurs promptly whereas remission of other physical signs takes place over a period of months to years, the same is true of neuropsychiatric symptoms. Irritability improves rapidly. Depressed mood is less likely than irritability and sleep to be among the first cluster of symptoms to improve,[11] a pattern similar to that seen in patients with primary major depressive disorder treated with antidepressants, in whom psychomotor activation and sleep improve first. For cognition, different cognitive tasks show different trajectories of improvement, and subjects of older age show less improvement.[21,32]

However, amelioration of neuropsychiatric findings is not the same as their elimination. Just as problems in bone mineralization and the metabolic syndrome continue, so some of the neuropsychiatric problems also do not remit promptly or completely.[32–34] In addition, quality-of-life studies show that more than half of treated patients with Cushing syndrome report adverse effects of the disease, including problems with mood and cognition, for years.[35,36]

After treatment, when cortisol concentrations have become normal, antidepressants can be effective if depressed mood lingers, is exacerbated, or appears for the first time. Because quality of life is reduced and neuropsychiatric decrements may linger and not remit completely, continued medical observation of these patients is important, and referrals for psychiatric and psychological assistance should be made as necessary.

Neuropsychological Testing and Brain Imaging Studies

Formal neuropsychological testing by several groups of investigators confirms that patients with active SCS have decrements in multiple domains of cognitive function.[8,32,37] In a study of patients limited to CD only, decrements in multiple functions were observed showing that both hippocampus and frontal lobes are affected.[19] This study also demonstrated that once material was learned, the percentage of retention of what was learned when tested one-half hour after learning was not different in comparison with control subjects. This pattern is different from that shown by Alzheimer disease. The study also showed that there were no significant associations between severity of depressed mood and cognitive performance, indicating that hypercortisolism affects mood and cognition independently of each other.[19]

After treatment, formal neuropsychiatric testing of SCS patients at intervals during the following 12 months showed that time from surgery was a significant determinant of improvement, and that the cognitive tasks had different trajectories for the timing of improvement. Age was also an important variable, with elderly subjects showing less improvement.[21] In a different study, posttreatment scores on cognitive tasks were independent of scores for mood disorder.[38] As in the pretreatment findings, this illustrates that these 2 domains are affected separately from each other.

Imaging studies in SCS began after animal studies demonstrated that anatomic changes elicited by prolonged stress and elevated glucocorticoid included remodeling and atrophy of key cells in the hippocampus. Starkman and colleagues[12] then hypothesized that magnetic resonance imaging might reveal similar toxic effects occurring in humans, and would be particularly evident in highly hypercortisolemic patients with active SCS. Their study showed that for 27% of patients with active CD the hippocampal formation volume fell outside the 95% confidence limits for normal subjects (volumes were smaller). Hippocampal volume was also negatively correlated with plasma cortisol. In addition, there were specific and significant correlations between hippocampal volume and scores for verbal learning and recall. Further showing the interrelationship of memory function and hippocampal volume, Resmini and colleagues[39] showed that hippocampal volume was decreased in those CD subjects whose memory scores were below the normative cutoff values.

Restudy of the patients in the imaging study by Starkman and colleagues[18] showed that after treatment there was a significant increase in hippocampal volume, with a trend for increased volume of the other structure examined, namely the caudate head. The increase in hippocampal volume but not caudate head volume was associated with improvement in learning. Bourdeau and colleagues[40] found that reimaging patients with Cushing syndrome several years after treatment showed that measures of brain volume did improve. The improved values, however, still were different from those of normal control subjects.

The arrival of functional magnetic resonance technology provides a new opportunity to examine the impact of hypercortisolism on the brain. Although such studies are just beginning,[23,41] they hold promise for further elucidating where and how hypercortisolism affects brain function.

EXOGENOUS GLUCOCORTICOIDS

Clinical use of glucocorticoids began in the 1940s, and soon thereafter individual case reports began to appear about neuropsychiatric side effects: fatigue, irritability, elevated mood, insomnia, and difficulty with attention/concentration. In time, prospective studies were performed. Progress in research has been hindered by variability in the underlying medical diseases for which the steroids are given, and differences in penetration of the blood-brain barrier and receptor affinities of different glucocorticoids used in different studies.

The frequently used term steroid psychosis leads to underestimation of the variety of neuropsychiatric presentations elicited by EGC administration. The symptom picture is not only heterogeneous among individuals, but can also differ within one individual when the drugs are administered at different time points. Manifestations during short-term administration differ from those seen over long-term administration. Cognitive and mood effects may be subtle or pronounced.

Short-Term, High-Dose Administration

Most patients treated with moderate doses will develop some degree of behavioral symptoms, generally mild and subjective. Such symptoms are typically brief experiences of hyperarousal, mild euphoria, or anxiety.

Two prospective studies by Naber and colleagues[42] and by Brown and colleagues[43] showed that hypomanic and manic symptoms are the most common mood response. In the Naber study, the prevalence of hypomania/mania was 26% and that of depression was 10%. Neurocognitive effects, particularly on declarative verbal-memory assessments, were also observed. Regarding timing of symptom appearance in this study, which used very high initial doses (140 mg/d prednisone equivalent), symptoms began within the first 3 days.[42] In the study by Brown and colleagues,[43] which used a mean initial prednisone dose of 42 mg/d, examination of patients a mean of 5 days after initiation of the drug showed significant increases from baseline on the mania scale. As regards recovery after EGC is discontinued, Brown and colleagues found that when patients were restudied 2 weeks or less after discontinuation, assessment measures returned to baseline values.

At times the most prominent symptoms are cognitive, and may be subtle.[44,45] In normal subjects given prednisone equivalents of 40 mg/d or greater, the decline in declarative memory was observed quickly, was dose dependent, and resolved within a week.[45,46] Illustrating the sensitivity of learning and memory to glucocorticoids, healthy elderly subjects who received just 4 days of stress-level exposure to cortisol had decreases in immediate and delayed verbal declarative memory (but not in nonverbal memory, sustained/selective attention, or executive function).[46]

The one factor most clearly associated with the development of neuropsychiatric side effects is dose. The Boston Collaborative Drug Surveillance Program found that of patients receiving more than 80 mg/d prednisone, 18% had severe psychiatric presentations that included psychosis. Of those receiving 41 to 80 mg/d, 4.6% had such symptoms, whereas only 2% receiving less than this amount had psychotic symptoms.[47] However, lower dose is not predictive of a trouble-free course. Symptoms are also known to develop quickly even with low doses of steroids.

Risk factors other than dose are less clear. Prior adverse response to EGC predicted future neuropsychiatric symptoms with re-exposure in some but not other studies. Female gender may be a risk factor. Age has not been reported to be a significant risk factor. A history of previous psychiatric illness predicted an increased susceptibility to psychiatric side effects in some, but not other studies. To add to the complexity, the same individual may show differing susceptibility to neuropsychiatric side effects at different times, likely secondary to differing physiologic milieus.[48-53]

Long-Term Administration

Sleep disturbance and an increase in appetite and food-seeking are among the most common side effects of long-term EGC administration.

When mood disorder occurs, it is most strongly associated with depressive symptoms. In a study by Bolanos and colleagues[54] using DSM-IV criteria in patients on relatively low doses, 50% were diagnosed with a depressive mood disorder while 5% had manic and 5% had panic-disorder diagnoses. In another study of patients who received prednisone for 30 to 60 days, their depression scores were significantly higher than those of a control group with similar clinical pictures but not receiving EGC.[55] In pediatric patients, particularly those younger than 10 years, the presentation is frequently irritability and a tendency toward aggressive behavior.[56]

Cognitive symptoms include difficulty with concentration and retaining information while reading, forgetting what they have already said, and difficulty with word finding. More severe longer-lasting cognitive disturbances, though infrequent, may begin during treatment, and are reported as largely reversible but may persist from months to years after steroid discontinuation.[57,58]

Prevention and Treatment

Most serious neuropsychiatric effects are unpredictable. There have been reports of successful efforts to prevent its occurrence using lithium, but the use of lithium is complex in patients with medical illnesses.[59] The most effective treatment is tapering the dose of steroids if possible. (In certain instances such as lupus cerebritis, an increase in psychiatric symptoms is more likely the effect of the cerebritis rather than the EGC, and increased doses may be required.) A major treatment option for EGC-induced side effects is atypical antipsychotics such as olanzapine, which also have mood-stabilizing effects. Olanzapine has been shown to be rapidly effective at doses from 2.5 to 20 mg/d, with a mean dose of 9.2 mg/d.[60,61] Blood tests to regulate blood concentrations are not required.

After neuropsychiatric symptoms improve, patients and families benefit from the explanation that the new-onset neuropsychiatric symptoms are related to EGC administration and should not recur unless it is given again, and even then possibly not. As with other acute organic brain syndromes secondary to drugs, this information reassures patients and families that they need not be on guard for a spontaneous reappearance of what otherwise seems to them a newly uncovered psychiatric disorder.

Neuropsychological Testing and Brain Imaging Studies

In patients receiving EGC, neuropsychiatric studies demonstrate decrements in declarative verbal learning and memory.[62,63] These and other cognitive decrements are not dissimilar from those seen in SCS. The few imaging studies performed reveal differing results, with some finding declines in hippocampal volume[63] and others no decline.

MECHANISMS OF CORTISOL/GLUCOCORTICOID ACTION

Receptors for glucocorticoids are present throughout the brain, and are more heavily represented in some key areas relevant to mood and cognition. Glucocorticoids have pleiotropic effects on the central nervous system. Because of space limitations, this active and exciting area of research is discussed only briefly here.

One group of effects occurs at the level of the genome, altering gene expression and protein synthesis. Another set of effects are nongenomic, acting at the cell membrane to alter its permeability to ions and to affect the release of neurotransmitters.

Glucocorticoids have numerous effects on the brain. For instance, they decrease glucose use and insulin signaling in the hippocampus, and increase neuronal vulnerability to excitotoxic amino acids and calcium. Moreover, they affect the production of nerve growth factors important to the formation of new neurons in brain areas where this occurs, such as the hippocampus; nerve growth factors are also involved in the sustenance of neurons, interneurons, and glia throughout the brain. Glucocorticoids have profound effects on brain structure itself, by mechanisms such as remodeling individual neurons. For example, elevated glucocorticoids reduce the number of spines, the sites for synaptic connections and communication with other neurons, on key hippocampal[64] and cortical[65] neurons.

Endogenous cortisol and EGC steroids do not, of course, act in a hormonal vacuum. In SCS, concentrations of other hormones such as dehydroepiandrosterone and estrogen are altered. In addition, the brain is able to produce steroids locally: neurosteroids such as progesterone and its metabolites. It is not unlikely that changing glucocorticoid concentrations alter the production and release of these as well.

SIMILARITIES BETWEEN NEUROPSYCHIATRIC FINDINGS IN SCS AND EGC

Patients with SCS differ from those receiving exogenous steroids, because they are exposed to sustained chronic elevations for months to years and are less subject to the rapid rate of change of glucocorticoid concentration that occurs during quickly titrated treatment with high-dose steroids. While there are corresponding differences in their neuropsychiatric presentations, at the same time there are informative similarities. In both SCS and exogenous steroid administration, depression is not one of the earliest manifestations. One could indeed consider the irritability and sudden mood shifts that appear early in the course of SCS as counterparts of the hypomanic syndrome seen during short-term administration of EGC. Later in the course of untreated SCS and chronic EGC administration, sustained depression is the predominant affect/mood presentation in both conditions. These similarities are not surprising, given that the brain has a limited number of final common pathways.

The glucocorticoid receptor is one of the most important mediators of the brain's response to the individual's environment, both internal and external. Chronic elevations of cortisol and/or disruption of its diurnal rhythm are already known to occur in a variety of conditions in addition to major depressive disease, such as subgroups of the normal elderly and patients with Alzheimer disease; more will likely be identified. As future research exploring mechanisms underlying the neuropsychiatric disruptions in SCS and EGC continues along and beyond the paths already opened, this new knowledge will also illuminate how lesser degrees of cortisol dysregulation affect healthy humans and those with psychiatric and somatic disease.

REFERENCES

1. Cushing H. The basophil adenomas of the pituitary body and their clinical manifestations (pituitary basophilism). Bull Johns Hopkins Hosp 1932;50: 137–95.
2. Trethowan WH, Cobb S. Neuropsychiatric aspects of Cushing's syndrome. AMA Arch Neurol Psychiatry 1952;67(3):283–309.
3. Gifford S, Gunderso JG. Cushing's disease as a psychosomatic disorder—a report of 10 cases. Medicine 1970;49(5):397–409.
4. Carroll BJ, Curtis GC, Mendels J. Neuroendocrine regulation in depression. 1. Limbic system-adrenocortical dysfunction. Arch Gen Psychiatry 1976;33(9): 1039–44.
5. Cohen SI. Cushing's syndrome: a psychiatric-study of 29 patients. Br J Psychiatry 1980;136:120–4.
6. Starkman MN, Schteingart DE, Schork MA. Depressed mood and other psychiatric manifestations of Cushing syndrome—relationship to hormone levels. Psychosom Med 1981;43(1):3–18.
7. Tucker RP, Weinstein HE, Schteingart DE, et al. EEG changes and serum cortisol levels in Cushing's syndrome. Clin Electroencephalogr 1978;9(1):32–7.
8. Whelan TB, Schteingart DE, Starkman MN, et al. Neuropsychological deficits in Cushing's syndrome. J Nerv Ment Dis 1980;168(12):753–7.
9. Starkman MN, Schteingart DE. Neuropsychiatric manifestations of patients with Cushing's syndrome—relationship to cortisol and adrenocorticotropic hormone levels. Arch Intern Med 1981;141(2):215–9.
10. Starkman MN, Schteingart DE, Schork MA. Correlation of bedside cognitive and neuropsychological tests in patients with Cushing's syndrome. Psychosomatics 1986;27(7):508–11.

11. Starkman MN, Schteingart DE, Schork MA. Cushing's syndrome after treatment—changes in cortisol and ACTH levels, and amelioration of the depressive syndrome. Psychiatry Res 1986;19(3):177–88.

12. Starkman MN, Gebarski SS, Berent S, et al. Hippocampal-formation volume, memory dysfunction, and cortisol-levels in patients with Cushing's syndrome. Biol Psychiatry 1992;32(9):756–65.

13. Starkman MN, Schteingart DE, Schork MA. Discordant changes in plasma ACTH and beta-lipotropin beta-endorphin levels in Cushing's disease patients with depression. Psychoneuroendocrinology 1992;17(6):619–26.

14. Shipley JE, Schteingart DE, Tandon R, et al. Sleep architecture and sleep-apnea in patients with Cushing's disease. Sleep 1992;15(6):514–8.

15. Shipley JE, Schteingart DE, Tandon R, et al. EEG sleep in Cushing's disease and Cushing's syndrome—comparison with patients with major depressive disorder. Biol Psychiatry 1992;32(2):146–55.

16. Cameron OG, Starkman MN, Schteingart DE. The effect of elevated systemic cortisol levels on plasma catecholamines in Cushing's syndrome patients with and without depressed mood. J Psychiatr Res 1995;29(5):347–60.

17. Kronfol Z, Starkman M, Schteingart DE, et al. Immune regulation in Cushing's syndrome: relationship to hypothalamic-pituitary-adrenal axis hormones. Psychoneuroendocrinology 1996;21(7):599–608.

18. Starkman MN, Giodani B, Gebarski SS, et al. Decrease in cortisol reverses human hippocampal atrophy following treatment of Cushing's disease. Biol Psychiatry 1999;46(12):1595–602.

19. Starkman MN, Giordani B, Berent S, et al. Elevated cortisol levels in Cushing's disease are associated with cognitive decrements. Psychosom Med 2001; 63(6):985–93.

20. Starkman MN, Giordani B, Gebarski SS, et al. Improvement in learning associated with increase in hippocampal formation volume. Biol Psychiatry 2003;53(3): 233–8.

21. Hook JN, Giordani B, Schteingart DE, et al. Patterns of cognitive change over time and relationship to age following successful treatment of Cushing's disease. J Int Neuropsychol Soc 2007;13(1):21–9.

22. Starkman MN, Giordani B, Gebarski SS, et al. Improvement in mood and ideation associated with increase in right caudate volume. J Affect Disord 2007; 101(1–3):139–47.

23. Langenecker SA, Weisenbach SL, Giordani B, et al. Impact of chronic hypercortisolemia on affective processing. Neuropharmacology 2012;62(1):217–25.

24. Krieger DT. Central nervous system and Cushing's syndrome. Mt Sinai J Med 1972;39(5):416–28.

25. Vancauter E, Refetoff S. Evidence for 2 subtypes of Cushing's disease based on the analysis of episodic cortisol secretion. N Engl J Med 1985;312(21): 1343–9.

26. Loosen PT, Chambliss B, Debold CR, et al. The psychiatric phenomenology of Cushing's disease. Pharmacopsychiatry 1992;25(4):192–8.

27. Haskett RF. Diagnostic categorization of psychiatric disturbance in Cushing's syndrome. Am J Psychiatry 1985;142(8):911–6.

28. Sonino N, Fava GA. Psychiatric disorders associated with Cushing's syndrome—epidemiology, pathophysiology and treatment. CNS Drugs 2001; 15(5):361–73.

29. Kelly WF, Checkley SA, Bender DA, et al. Cushing's syndrome and depression—a prospective-study of 26 patients. Br J Psychiatry 1983;142:16–9.

30. Sonino N, Fava GA, Belluardo P, et al. Course of depression in Cushing's syndrome—response to treatment and comparison with graves-disease. Horm Res 1993;39(5–6):202–6.
31. Dorn LD, Burgess ES, Friedman TC, et al. The longitudinal course of psychopathology in Cushing's syndrome after correction of hypercortisolism. J Clin Endocrinol Metab 1997;82(3):912–9.
32. Forget H, Lacroix A, Somma M, et al. Cognitive decline in patients with Cushing's syndrome. J Int Neuropsychol Soc 2000;6(1):20–9.
33. Martignoni E, Costa A, Sinforiani E, et al. The brain as a target for adrenocortical steroids—cognitive implications. Psychoneuroendocrinology 1992;17(4): 343–54.
34. Mauri M, Sinforiani E, Bono G, et al. Memory impairment in Cushing's disease. Acta Neurol Scand 1993;87(1):52–5.
35. Gotch PM. Cushing's syndrome from the patients perspective. Endocrinol Metab Clin North Am 1994;23(3):607–17.
36. Heald AH, Ghosh S, Bray S, et al. Long-term negative impact on quality of life in patients with successfully treated Cushing's disease. Clin Endocrinol 2004; 61(4):458–65.
37. Michaud K, Forget H, Cohen H. Chronic glucocorticoid hypersecretion in Cushing's syndrome exacerbates cognitive aging. Brain Cogn 2009;71(1):1–8.
38. Ragnarsson O, Berglund P, Eder DN, et al. Long-term cognitive impairments and attentional deficits in patients with Cushing's disease and cortisol-producing adrenal adenoma in remission. J Clin Endocrinol Metab 2012; 97(9):E1640–8.
39. Resmini E, Santos A, Gomez-Anson B, et al. Verbal and visual memory performance and hippocampal volumes, measured by 3-Tesla magnetic resonance imaging, in patients with Cushing's syndrome. J Clin Endocrinol Metab 2012; 97(2):663–71.
40. Bourdeau I, Bard C, Forget H, et al. Cognitive function and cerebral assessment in patients who have Cushing's syndrome. Endocrinol Metab Clin North Am 2005;34(2):357–69.
41. Maheu FS, Mazzone L, Merke DP, et al. Altered amygdala and hippocampus function in adolescents with hypercortisolemia: a functional magnetic resonance imaging study of Cushing syndrome. Dev Psychopathol 2008;20(4):1177–89.
42. Naber D, Sand P, Heigl B. Psychopathological and neuropsychological effects of 8-days' corticosteroid treatment. A prospective study. Psychoneuroendocrinology 1996;21(1):25–31.
43. Brown ES, Suppes T, Khan DA, et al. Mood changes during prednisone bursts in outpatients with asthma. J Clin Psychopharmacol 2002;22(1):55–61.
44. Hall RC, Popkin MK, Stickney SK, et al. Presentation of the steroid psychoses. J Nerv Ment Dis 1979;167(4):229–36.
45. Wolkowitz OM, Rubinow D, Doran AR, et al. Prednisone effects on neurochemistry and behavior—preliminary findings. Arch Gen Psychiatry 1990;47(10): 963–8.
46. Newcomer JW, Selke G, Melson AK, et al. Decreased memory performance in healthy humans induced by stress-level cortisol treatment. Arch Gen Psychiatry 1999;56(6):527–33.
47. Acute adverse reactions to prednisone in relation to dosage. Clin Pharmacol Ther 1972;13(5):694–8.
48. Wolkowitz OM, Reus VI, Canick J, et al. Glucocorticoid medication, memory and steroid psychosis in medical illness. In: Moore PM, Lahita RG, editors.

Neuropsychiatric manifestations of systemic lupus erythematosus, vol. 823. 1997. p. 81–96.

49. Brown ES. Effects of glucocorticoids on mood, memory, and the hippocampus treatment and preventive therapy. In: Judd LL, Sternberg EM, editors. Glucocorticoids and mood clinical manifestations, risk factors, and molecular mechanisms, vol. 1179. 2009. p. 41–55.

50. Fietta P, Delsante G. Central nervous system effects of natural and synthetic glucocorticoids. Psychiatry Clin Neurosci 2009;63(5):613–22.

51. Ross DA, Cetas JS. Steroid psychosis: a review for neurosurgeons. J Neurooncol 2012;109(3):439–47.

52. Wolkowitz OM, Burke H, Epel ES, et al. Glucocorticoids mood, memory, and mechanisms. In: Judd LL, Sternberg EM, editors. Glucocorticoids and mood clinical manifestations, risk factors, and molecular mechanisms. 2009. p. 19–40.

53. Dubovsky AN, Arvikar S, Stern TA, et al. The neuropsychiatric complications of glucocorticoid use: steroid psychosis revisited. Psychosomatics 2012;53(2): 103–15.

54. Bolanos SH, Khan DA, Hanczyc M, et al. Assessment of mood states in patients receiving long-term corticosteroid therapy and in controls with patient-rated and clinician-rated scales. Ann Allergy Asthma Immunol 2004;92(5):500–5.

55. Gift AG, Wood RM, Cahill CA. Depression, somatization and steroid use in chronic obstructive pulmonary-disease. Int J Nurs Stud 1989;26(3):281–6.

56. Mrakotsky C, Forbes PW, Bernstein JH, et al. Acute cognitive and behavioral effects of systemic corticosteroids in children treated for inflammatory bowel disease. J Int Neuropsychol Soc 2013;19(1):96–109.

57. Wolkowitz OM, Lupien SJ, Bigler ED. The "steroid dementia syndrome": a possible model of human glucocorticoid neurotoxicity. Neurocase 2007;13(3): 189–200.

58. Varney NR, Alexander B, Macindoe JH. Reversible steroid dementia in patients without steroid psychosis. Am J Psychiatry 1984;141(3):369–72.

59. Falk WE, Mahnke MW, Poskanzer DC. Lithium prophylaxis of corticotropin-induced psychosis. JAMA 1979;241(10):1011–2.

60. Goldman LS, Goveas J. Olanzapine treatment of corticosteroid-induced mood disorders. Psychosomatics 2002;43(6):495–7.

61. Brown ES, Chamberlain W, Dhanani N, et al. An open-label trial of olanzapine for corticosteroid-induced mood symptoms. J Affect Disord 2004;83(2–3):277–81.

62. Keenan PA, Jacobson MW, Soleymani RM, et al. Commonly used therapeutic doses of glucocorticoids impair explicit memory. Ann N Y Acad Sci 1995;761: 400–2.

63. Brown ES, Woolston DJ, Frol A, et al. Hippocampal volume, spectroscopy, cognition, and mood in patients receiving corticosteroid therapy. Biol Psychiatry 2004;55(5):538–45.

64. Magarinos AM, McEwen BS. Stress-induced atrophy of apical dendrites of hippocampal CA3C neurons—comparison of stressors. Neuroscience 1995;69(1): 83–8.

65. Liston C, Gan WB. Glucocorticoids are critical regulators of dendritic spine development and plasticity in vivo. Proc Natl Acad Sci U S A 2011;108(38): 16074–9.

Type 2 Diabetes and Cognitive Compromise
Potential Roles of Diabetes-Related Therapies

Efrat Kravitz, PhD[a], James Schmeidler, PhD[b],
Michal Schnaider Beeri, PhD[a,b],*

KEYWORDS

- Type 2 diabetes • Dementia • Cognitive decline • Alzheimer disease • Insulin
- Insulin resistance • Oral hypoglycemics

KEY POINTS

- T2D is associated with a wide range of cognitive impairments, starting from cognitive decline, through mild cognitive impairment, to frank clinical dementia.
- Observational studies suggest that diabetes is more closely and more consistently associated with vascular forms of cognitive impairments, rather than with Alzheimer-like forms. Clinical trials, however, have mostly targeted Alzheimer-related outcomes (eg, Aβ accumulation, memory deficits), with limited success.
- Mechanisms underlying diabetes complications are likely to underlie dementia in nondiabetics as well, but findings suggest decreased cognitive-related efficacy of antidiabetic medication in nondiabetics.
- Discrepancies between in vitro/in vivo findings and results from clinical trials may be explained by time of intervention. It is possible that antidiabetic medications are effective at preventing, rather than treating, cognitive compromise in at-risk diabetic and nondiabetics individuals.

Diabetes disproportionately affects the elderly. Among US residents aged 65 years and older, 26.9% had diabetes in 2010 and 50% had diabetes or prediabetes between 2005 and 2008.[1] According to the Alzheimer's association, one in nine people aged 65 years and older (11%) has AD and about one-third of people aged 85 years and older (32%) have AD; the prevalence of all forms of dementia is even higher.[2] This cooccurrence may simply reflect two simultaneous age-related events, possibly sharing one or more causal pathways, or may reflect a causative relationship between the conditions.

Funding: This study was supported by NIA grants R01 AG034087 (Beeri), the Ira T. Hirschl Award (Beeri), and by an award from the Helen Bader Foundation (Beeri).
[a] The Joseph Sagol Neuroscience Center, Sheba Medical Center, Tel Hashomer, Ramat Gan 52621, Israel; [b] Department of Psychiatry, Mount Sinai School of Medicine, One Gustave Levy Place, Box 1230, New York, NY 10029, USA
* Corresponding author. Department of Psychiatry, Mount Sinai School of Medicine, One Gustave Levy Place, Box 1230, New York, NY 10029.
E-mail address: michal.beeri@mssm.edu

Endocrinol Metab Clin N Am 42 (2013) 489–501
http://dx.doi.org/10.1016/j.ecl.2013.05.009
0889-8529/13/$ – see front matter © 2013 Elsevier Inc. All rights reserved.

DIABETES IS A RISK FACTOR FOR DEMENTIA AND COGNITIVE DECLINE

Diabetes has consistently been associated with risk of dementia, mild cognitive impairment (MCI), and cognitive decline. A systematic review of the effects of diabetes on cognitive dysfunction has suggested that the latter should be considered among the chronic consequences and disabling manifestations of diabetes.[3] Increased risks of dementia and AD were also associated with borderline diabetes, independent of the future development of diabetes.[4] Diabetes, or impaired fasting glucose, may be present in up to 80% of individuals with Alzheimer disease (AD),[5] and the 2010 NIH Consensus Development Conference Statement on Preventing Alzheimer's Disease and Cognitive Decline listed diabetes first as a risk factor.[6] This coexistence of diabetes (or diabetic markers) with cognitive dysfunctions have led some investigators to propose that AD constitutes a brain-specific form of diabetes, that is, type 3 diabetes.[7]

Our group has recently shown that diabetic elderly with the earliest signs of cognitive compromise have a faster rate of cognitive decline than nondiabetic elderly.[8] Similar associations between diabetes and cognitive compromise have been reported in numerous studies. Among the cognitive domains that have been associated with diabetes are attention, executive functions, perceptual/processing speed, verbal memory, and working memory, as well as global cognitive functioning (measured by the Mini-Mental State Examination [MMSE]).[9–16] Our recent study has also demonstrated that poor glycemic control is associated with cognitive decline even in nondiabetic individuals.[17] Such association, however, was not observed in elderly aged 85 years or older,[18] possibly due to a survivors effect. Moreover, within a population of patients who were already demented at the time of the study, diabetics showed slower global cognitive decline than nondiabetics,[19] although functional status, measured by Activities of Daily Living (ADL), continuously declined.[20] One explanation for this observation may be a floor effect, or that the medical attention that this population receives is helpful in preventing cognitive deterioration.

MCI is characterized by memory complaints without loss of function in daily activities.[21] Diabetes has been related to a 40% higher risk of MCI, both amnestic and non-amnestic.[22] Two other studies reported a trend towards increased risk of MCI in a diabetic elderly population,[23] and in a sample of postmenopausal women,[24] but these changes were statistically nonsignificant. A more recent study may shed some light on these inconsistencies: the frequency of diabetes was similar in elderly subjects with and without MCI, but MCI was associated with diabetes onset before the age of 65 years, diabetes duration of 10 years or longer, treatment with insulin, and the presence of diabetes complications.[25]

According to the DSM-IV (Text Revision),[26] dementia is characterized by the development of multiple cognitive deficits that must include memory impairment and other cognitive disturbances. Our previous research showed that individuals with diabetes in midlife had a 3-fold increased risk of dementia three decades later.[27] Increased risk of dementia in diabetic patients was also reported in other studies,[28–32] but not all.[24] Furthermore, diabetes seems to increase the risk of certain subtypes of dementia to different extents. The most common subtypes of dementia are AD and vascular dementia (VaD). According to the National Institute of Neurological and Communicative Disorders and Stroke–Alzheimer's Disease and Related Disorders Association (NINCDS-ADRDA), to fulfill research criteria for probable AD, a patient must present a significant episodic memory impairment and at least one supportive biomarker (such as medial temporal lobe atrophy).[33] VaD itself is not a single disease, but a group of syndromes based on varying vascular mechanisms. These include dementias related to multiple infarcts, small vessel ischemic disease, AD with cerebrovascular disease (sometimes known as mixed dementia), and others.[34] Diabetes was reported to increase the risk of AD by 45% to 90%,[9,28,29,35] but the risk for VaD was consistently and substantially higher, with increases ranging from 100% to 160%,[32,36,37] suggesting that diabetes is more closely associated with VaD than with AD.

These findings suggest an association between diabetes and cognitive decline. Some of the studies evaluated diabetes in midlife, decades before dementia ascertainment, supporting the notion that cognitive impairment is a consequence of diabetes.

THE EFFECTS OF DIABETES TREATMENTS ON MEMORY AND COGNITION

The research of different pharmacologic and non-pharmacologic treatments of diabetes, and the known biological mechanisms of those treatments, may help us in understanding this association. Insulin and oral hypoglycemics are the most common treatments for diabetes. Diabetes medications have been associated with improved cognitive functioning, and have been demonstrated to affect AD markers, such as neuritic plaques,[38] as well as vascular integrity.[39] The SALSA (Sacramento Area Latino Study on Aging) study reported that diabetic patients on antidiabetic monotherapy (insulin or oral), and more so on any combination therapy, had less cognitive decline, especially among those with a longer duration of the disease.[40] Our previous postmortem study examined the association between AD neuropathology and diabetes medications in several brain regions that support cognitive functioning: hippocampus, entorhinal cortex, amygdala, and several neocortical regions. In each region, the study demonstrated substantially lower neuritic plaque density for the diabetic group taking both insulin and other antidiabetic medication, compared with diabetic patients on monotherapy or on no therapy.[38] This article briefly reviews the association of some of the most common antidiabetic treatments with cognitive functioning.

The Association of Circulating/Cerebrospinal Fluid Insulin Levels and Insulin Administration with Cognition

Produced nearly exclusively by the pancreas, insulin is readily transported into the central nervous system (CNS) across the blood-brain barrier (BBB) using a saturable, receptor-mediated process. Insulin receptors are highly concentrated in the olfactory bulb, cerebral cortex, hippocampus, hypothalamus, and cerebellum.[41] Localization of insulin receptors in the hippocampus and medial temporal cortex is consistent with evidence that insulin influences memory.[42] Conditions such as insulin resistance, in which insulin is chronically elevated, may eliminate the salutary effects of insulin on cognition and other brain function.[43] Elevating insulin levels, through excess production (endogenously or provoked exogenously), excess administration of insulin, or reduced clearance typically results in downregulation of insulin signaling pathways.[44] One consequence of insulin resistance and chronic excess insulin (hyperinsulinemia) is reduced insulin transport into the brain, which ultimately produces brain-insulin deficiency,[45] and may attenuate the many beneficial influences of insulin. Support for this notion may be seen in recently published results from the PIVUS (Prospective Investigation of the Vasculature in Uppsala Seniors) study: in cognitively healthy elderly men and women aged 75 years, insulin resistance was negatively correlated with verbal cognitive performance, brain size, and temporal lobe gray matter volume.[46] These findings are similar to an earlier report on prediabetic and diabetic patients, in which greater insulin resistance was associated with reduced glucose metabolic rate in frontal, parietotemporal, and cingulate regions, compatible with an AD pattern.[47] Those individuals also showed more diffused and extensive activation patterns, and recalled fewer items on a delayed memory test.[47] Because patients with type 2 diabetes and approximately half of all adults more than 60 years of age, regardless of diabetic status, are insulin resistant,[43] studying the effects of insulin on cognition is of great importance.

Craft has pioneered the study of the role of insulin regulation in AD and cognitive decline. In normal physiological conditions, insulin administered at optimal (ie, low) doses facilitates memory, as was demonstrated by direct administration of insulin to the brain in rodents,[48] and intravenous insulin administration in humans.[49] The latter study also showed that higher levels of insulin were needed to achieve effective memory facilitation in patients with AD who were apolipoprotein E (ApoE) ε4-negative, supporting the notion of reduced sensitivity to insulin in this subgroup.[49] The investigators suggested that, for these patients, factors relating to insulin resistance may be important drivers of AD pathogenesis.

For memory-impaired adults, insulin was found to improve memory functions also when administered intranasally at an acute dosage[50] and chronic treatment for 3 weeks[51] or 4 months.[52] A recently published analysis of results from this trial further suggest sex and ApoE genotype differences in the response to the treatment: whereas women showed improved memory only when administered the lower dose, men showed cognitive improvement also for the higher dose, and this sex difference was most apparent for ApoE ε4-negative individuals.[53] Those sex-specific findings may be due to brain structural and/or functional differences between men and women. Also, the authors have suggested another interpretation, in which the central insulin sensitivity is fundamentally different between men and women: women more effectively regulate insulin metabolism in peripheral organs, and men are more sensitive to the cognitive consequences of peripheral insulin abnormalities. Therefore, men are more likely to benefit from the corrective actions of higher doses of intranasal insulin.[53] Importantly, sex differences were also observed in the association between cognitive functioning and circulating insulin: men with non-amnestic or amnestic MCI had higher fasting plasma insulin—probably due to reduced insulin clearance—than cognitively normal men, while women with amnestic MCI had lower fasting plasma insulin—possibly due to impaired insulin secretion—than cognitively normal women.[54] Taken together, these results suggest an inverted U-shaped relationship between levels of circulating insulin and cognitive impairment, with specific sex and diagnostic subtype interactions.

Insulin may exert its effects on cognition and AD risk through modulation of the β-amyloid peptide (Aβ). Aβ, a metabolite of the amyloid precursor protein (APP), aggregates in extracellular depositions, neuritic plaques, which constitute one of the hallmarks of AD pathology.[55] The close bidirectional relationship between insulin and Aβ is described in detail in a recently published review article.[56] Subchronic elevations of insulin concentrations in the CNS by intranasal administration have been associated with reduced circulating concentrations of Aβ.[51] Similar to the attenuation of the positive effects of insulin on memory facilitation, and the evidence of U-shaped relationship between the two, excessive insulin elevations through intravenous infusion increased levels of Aβ in cerebrospinal fluid (CSF), most notably in older subjects.[57] In the opposite direction, greater increases in CSF Aβ levels attenuated the insulin-mediated memory facilitation.[57] Also similar to the effect on cognition, the effect of insulin administration on plasma APP concentrations was modulated by the ApoE ε4 genotype, as the reduction in APP levels was enhanced in ApoE ε4-negative individuals, both in cognitively intact subjects[58] and patients with AD.[59] The effective insulin dose for reducing plasma APP was higher for patients with AD who were ApoE ε4 negative than for normal adults and ApoE-ε4 positive AD patients.[49] Finally, insulin administration was associated with inflammation, a key factor in the pathogenesis of AD.[60] Anti-inflammatory effects were observed with low doses of insulin,[61] but excessive hyperinsulinemia exacerbates inflammation.[62] Craft's research group[63] has demonstrated that intravenous infusion of insulin to levels associated with insulin resistance increased CSF inflammatory markers.

Peroxisome Proliferator-Activated Receptor-γ and AD

These observations led to the investigation of how therapeutic strategies, originally aimed at treating diabetes, may also benefit elderly with a wide range of cognitive impairments, including AD. Agonists to the peroxisome proliferator-activated receptor-γ (PPAR-γ) are known to improve insulin sensitivity, decrease circulating insulin, and increase insulin-mediated glucose uptake with minimal risk of hypoglycemia.[64] In addition, PPAR-γ agonists were found to inhibit inflammation, and specifically the Aβ-stimulated secretion of proinflammatory products and the Aβ-stimulated expression of the cytokine genes,[65] making them good candidates for therapeutic agents for treating AD. The beneficial effects of PPAR-γ agonists have been demonstrated in studies on transgenic AD mice, typically displaying widespread microglial activation, age-related amyloid deposits, and dystrophic neurites. Tg2576 mice that were treated with chronic oral administration of ibuprofen, an efficient activator of PPAR-γ,[66] have shown marked reduction in Aβ deposits.[67] Positive effects of PPAR-γ agonists on AD mice were also shown for two compounds, rosiglitazone and pioglitazone, which are commonly prescribed for diabetics. Rosiglitazone-treated Tg2576 mice showed age-dependent reversal of cognitive deficits,[68] but with no evidence of reduction in Aβ deposits.[69] In APPswe/PS1dE9 mice, the drug improved spatial memory, decreased insoluble $Aβ_{1-42}$, and decreased plaque number in the hippocampus.[70] Transgenic mice carrying the Swedish (K670N/M671L) and Indian (V717F) AD mutations of human APP showed rescue of memory impairments, removal of amyloid plaques in the hippocampus and entorhinal cortex, and decreased phosphorylated tau protein following rosiglitazone treatment.[71] Pioglitazone administered to the latter transgenic mice fully restored cerebrovascular reactivity, albeit it failed to improve spatial memory or to reduce Aβ plaque load.[72] In triple transgenic AD mice, however, long-term pioglitazone treatment improved cognition and decreased hippocampal Aβ and tau deposits.[73]

Despite the findings from animal studies in favor of PPAR-γ agonists for the treatment of AD symptomatology and pathology, results from human clinical trials have been rather disappointing. In a placebo-controlled, double-blind, parallel-group pilot study, rosiglitazone-treated amnestic-MCI and early AD patients showed preservation of some cognitive functions, whereas placebo-assigned subjects showed the expected memory decline.[74] This cognitive maintenance was not consistent throughout the trial period, and was not observed in all functions. Also important to note is that the study group did not include patients with moderate or severe AD. A larger trial did not observe overall cognitive benefit of rosiglitazone in patients with mild to moderate AD, although improvement was noted in ApoE ε4-negative subjects on a task of general cognitive function at the highest dose.[75] Subsequent phase III trials found no evidence of statistically or clinically significant efficacy of rosiglitazone in cognition or global function, regardless of genotype, when used as monotherapy[76] or as adjunctive therapy to acetylcholinesterase inhibitors.[77] Pioglitazone produced similar results. Trials of mild-AD patients with diabetes reported improved general cognition, improved verbal memory, and improved cerebral blood flow in the parietal lobe, following six months of treatment.[78,79] Nevertheless, a trial of nondiabetic patients meeting research criteria for probable AD showed no improvements on cognitive and functional measures.[80]

The lack of efficacy in these trials may be due to several reasons, including the complicated effects that inflammation exerts in AD pathogenesis, treatment at the wrong stage of the disease, or inappropriate dosing. Importantly, there is a debate on whether rosiglitazone effectively crosses the BBB in rodents: intraperitoneal administration to gerbils[81] or oral delivery to mice[82] resulted in effective and rapid penetration to the brain, whereas intravenous administration to rats resulted in low brain uptake[83]; the ability of pioglitazone to cross the BBB is less controversial.[84,85] In addition, human trials raised some safety concerns regarding the effects of rosiglitazone on cardiovascular functioning and heart failure in diabetic patients.[86] These findings suggest that there is continuous and consistent evidence of the beneficial effects of insulin and insulin-sensitizing therapies on cognition, however, the emphasis on insulin in treating AD should be shifted towards a different approach, possibly different type of medication, route of administration, or dementia-related target subgroups.

Is Glucagon-Like Peptide-1 a Promising Novel Approach in Treatment of AD?

One such pharmacologic approach to insulin resistance involves the use of insulinotropic glucagon-like peptide-1 (GLP-1), a hormone that facilitates insulin release under high blood sugar conditions, and does not affect blood sugar levels in nondiabetic individuals, enhances insulin signaling, and protects neurons from toxic effects.[87] GLP-1 agonists bind GLP-1 receptor that is coupled to a second messenger pathway via G proteins[88] and improve dyslipidemia, blood pressure, and other diabetes-associated vascular conditions.[89] GLP-1 is proposed to play a role in a regulatory mechanism involved in the actions of GLUT1 glucose transporters and glucose metabolism, by ensuring less fluctuation of brain glucose levels in response to alterations in plasma glucose.[90] The neuroprotective actions of GLP-1 have been demonstrated in *in vivo* and *in vitro* studies. GLP-1 has been documented to induce neurite outgrowth, reduce apoptosis, protect neurons from oxidative stress, protect synaptic plasticity and memory formation from the detrimental effects of Aβ, and reduce plaque formation and the inflammation response in the brains of mouse models of AD.[87] Intraperitoneal injection of GLP-1 receptor agonist to AD transgenic mice reduced the hippocampal amyloid burden and improved spatial memory.[91]

The Association Between AD and Metformin

Metformin is a biguanide[92] that lowers blood glucose levels by increasing hepatic and muscle cell insulin sensitivity, by decreasing intestinal glucose absorption,[93] and crosses the BBB readily.[94] Metformin improved insulin sensitivity and decreased insulin levels in individuals without diabetes[95] and was therefore proposed as a new target for research in the context of cognitive compromise. *In vitro*, metformin significantly decreased phosphorylated tau and ameliorated $A\beta_{1-42}$ levels in neuronal insulin resistance and AD-associated cell cultures.[96] Counterintuitively, in primary cortical culture models, metformin significantly increases the generation of both intracellular and extracellular Aβ species, but in combined use with insulin, metformin enhances insulin's effect in reducing Aβ levels.[97] Finally, in murine primary neurons from wild-type and human tau transgenic mice, metformin reduced tau phosphorylation.[98] *In vivo*, the association between metformin and AD-like neuropathology was examined in obese leptin-resistant mice. Metformin attenuated the increase of phosphorylated tau and the reduction of the synaptic protein synaptophysin, but did no better than saline in decreasing Aβ levels, and did not attenuate the impairments of spatial learning and memory.[99] Metformin successfully attenuated cognitive deficits of diabetic rats[100] and rats fed a high-fat diet.[101]

To date, the clinical data on the efficacy of metformin in preventing or treating AD and other dementia-related disorders in humans is not adequate. Nevertheless, a study of elderly diabetic individuals showed that metformin attenuated the decline in global cognitive function but not in verbal memory, an effect that was similar to that of a diet regime and inferior to that of a combined treatment with rosiglitazone.[102] In addition, the association between metformin and risk of dementia was examined in two large cohort-based studies and yielded contradictory results. A study of individuals aged 65 years or older found no evidence that the use of metformin is associated with a lower risk of developing AD.[103] Furthermore, the findings even suggested that long-term use of metformin may be associated with a slightly higher risk of developing AD, compared with nonuse of this drug, and such a finding was not seen with other antidiabetic drugs.[103] In contrast, a study of Taiwanese aged 50 years or older found that the use of metformin in the treatment of diabetes significantly decreased the risk of dementia, compared with no medication.[104] More research, particularly clinical placebo-controlled trials, is needed to clarify the potential benefits of metformin to cognitive health.

CONCLUSIONS

Based on current evidence, there is little doubt that diabetes and cognitive compromise are closely related. This relationship is manifested in a wide range of cognitive impairments, starting from cognitive decline, through MCI, to frank clinical dementia. The underlying mechanisms of these relationship are, however, still elusive. It seems that diabetes is more strongly and more consistently associated with vascular forms of cognitive impairment, rather than with AD-like neurodegenerative forms. Moreover, the different therapeutic strategies show some cognitive benefits, particularly intranasal insulin, which do not seem to be specific to AD: treatments seem less effective in attenuation of AD neuropathology in animal models and in alleviating cognitive dysfunctions in elderly individuals who already succumbed to AD. Clinical trials have primarily targeted AD-related outcomes (eg, Aβ accumulation, memory deficits, conversion rate to AD), while evidence suggests that vascular-related outcomes might be more promising. In addition, based on current basic science evidence, it is sensible to assume that some mechanisms underlying diabetes complications might underlie dementia in nondiabetics as well. Nevertheless, some of the findings presented suggest that diabetes medications may be more beneficial to diabetic patients than nondiabetics. Both AD and vascular neuropathology are believed to begin to develop and accumulate decades before manifestation of clinical symptoms. Thus, prevention clinical trials using diabetes medication against the development of cognitive compromise may be more effective for individuals at risk but initially cognitively normal, both diabetics and nondiabetics.

REFERENCES

1. Centers for Disease Control and Prevention. National diabetes fact sheet: national estimates and general information on diabetes and prediabetes in the United States, 2011. 2011. Available at: http://www.cdc.gov/diabetes/pubs/factsheet11.htm. Accessed March 21, 2013.
2. Alzheimer's Association. 2013 Alzheimer's disease facts and figures. Alzheimers Dement 2013;9(2):208–45.
3. Cukierman T, Gerstein HC, Williamson JD. Cognitive decline and dementia in diabetes–systematic overview of prospective observational studies. Diabetologia 2005;48(12):2460–9.

4. Xu W, Qiu C, Winblad B, et al. The effect of borderline diabetes on the risk of dementia and Alzheimer's disease. Diabetes 2007;56(1):211–6.
5. Janson J, Laedtke T, Parisi JE, et al. Increased risk of type 2 diabetes in Alzheimer disease. Diabetes 2004;53(2):474–81.
6. Daviglus ML, Bell CC, Berrettini W, et al. National Institutes of Health State-of-the-Science Conference statement: preventing Alzheimer disease and cognitive decline. Ann Intern Med 2010;153(3):176–81.
7. de la Monte SM, Tong M, Lester-Coll N, et al. Therapeutic rescue of neurodegeneration in experimental type 3 diabetes: relevance to Alzheimer's disease. J Alzheimers Dis 2006;10(1):89–109.
8. Ravona-Springer R, Luo X, Schmeidler J, et al. Diabetes is associated with increased rate of cognitive decline in questionably demented elderly. Dement Geriatr Cogn Disord 2010;29(1):68–74.
9. Arvanitakis Z, Wilson RS, Bienias JL, et al. Diabetes mellitus and risk of Alzheimer disease and decline in cognitive function. Arch Neurol 2004;61(5):661–6.
10. Gilmour H. Cognitive performance of Canadian seniors. Health Rep 2011;22(2): 27–31.
11. Gregg EW, Yaffe K, Cauley JA, et al. Is diabetes associated with cognitive impairment and cognitive decline among older women? Study of Osteoporotic Fractures Research Group. Arch Intern Med 2000;160(2):174–80.
12. Hassing LB, Grant MD, Hofer SM, et al. Type 2 diabetes mellitus contributes to cognitive decline in old age: a longitudinal population-based study. J Int Neuropsychol Soc 2004;10(4):599–607.
13. Hassing LB, Hofer SM, Nilsson SE, et al. Comorbid type 2 diabetes mellitus and hypertension exacerbates cognitive decline: evidence from a longitudinal study. Age Ageing 2004;33(4):355–61.
14. Knopman D, Boland LL, Mosley T, et al. Cardiovascular risk factors and cognitive decline in middle-aged adults. Neurology 2001;56(1):42–8.
15. Logroscino G, Kang JH, Grodstein F. Prospective study of type 2 diabetes and cognitive decline in women aged 70-81 years. BMJ 2004;328(7439):548.
16. Nandipati S, Luo X, Schimming C, et al. Cognition in non-demented diabetic older adults. Curr Aging Sci 2012;5(2):131–5.
17. Ravona-Springer R, Moshier E, Schmeidler J, et al. Changes in glycemic control are associated with changes in cognition in non-diabetic elderly. J Alzheimers Dis 2012;30(2):299–309.
18. van den Berg E, de Craen AJ, Biessels GJ, et al. The impact of diabetes mellitus on cognitive decline in the oldest of the old: a prospective population-based study. Diabetologia 2006;49(9):2015–23.
19. Sanz C, Andrieu S, Sinclair A, et al. Diabetes is associated with a slower rate of cognitive decline in Alzheimer disease. Neurology 2009;73(17): 1359–66.
20. Sanz CM, Hanaire H, Vellas BJ, et al. Diabetes mellitus as a modulator of functional impairment and decline in Alzheimer's disease. The Real.FR cohort. Diabet Med 2012;29(4):541–8.
21. Petersen RC, Smith GE, Waring SC, et al. Mild cognitive impairment: clinical characterization and outcome. Arch Neurol 1999;56(3):303–8.
22. Luchsinger JA, Reitz C, Patel B, et al. Relation of diabetes to mild cognitive impairment. Arch Neurol 2007;64(4):570–5.
23. Solfrizzi V, Panza F, Colacicco AM, et al. Vascular risk factors, incidence of MCI, and rates of progression to dementia. Neurology 2004;63(10):1882–91.

24. Yaffe K, Blackwell T, Kanaya AM, et al. Diabetes, impaired fasting glucose, and development of cognitive impairment in older women. Neurology 2004;63(4): 658–63.

25. Roberts RO, Geda YE, Knopman DS, et al. Association of duration and severity of diabetes mellitus with mild cognitive impairment. Arch Neurol 2008;65(8): 1066–73.

26. American Psychiatric Association. Diagnostic and statistical manual of mental disorders, fourth edition, text revision (DSM-IV-TR). Washington, DC: American Psychiatric Press; 2000.

27. Schnaider Beeri M, Goldbourt U, Silverman JM, et al. Diabetes mellitus in midlife and the risk of dementia three decades later. Neurology 2004;63(10): 1902–7.

28. Leibson CL, Rocca WA, Hanson VA, et al. The risk of dementia among persons with diabetes mellitus: a population-based cohort study. Ann N Y Acad Sci 1997; 826:422–7.

29. Ott A, Stolk RP, van Harskamp F, et al. Diabetes mellitus and the risk of dementia: The Rotterdam Study. Neurology 1999;53(9):1937–42.

30. Peila R, Rodriguez BL, Launer LJ. Type 2 diabetes, APOE gene, and the risk for dementia and related pathologies: the Honolulu-Asia Aging Study. Diabetes 2002;51(4):1256–62.

31. Whitmer RA, Sidney S, Selby J, et al. Midlife cardiovascular risk factors and risk of dementia in late life. Neurology 2005;64(2):277–81.

32. Xu WL, Qiu CX, Wahlin A, et al. Diabetes mellitus and risk of dementia in the Kungsholmen project: a 6-year follow-up study. Neurology 2004;63(7):1181–6.

33. Dubois B, Feldman HH, Jacova C, et al. Research criteria for the diagnosis of Alzheimer's disease: revising the NINCDS-ADRDA criteria. Lancet Neurol 2007;6(8):734–46.

34. O'Brien JT. Vascular cognitive impairment. Am J Geriatr Psychiatry 2006;14(9): 724–33.

35. Wang KC, Woung LC, Tsai MT, et al. Risk of Alzheimer's disease in relation to diabetes: a population-based cohort study. Neuroepidemiology 2012;38(4): 237–44.

36. Hassing LB, Johansson B, Nilsson SE, et al. Diabetes mellitus is a risk factor for vascular dementia, but not for Alzheimer's disease: a population-based study of the oldest old. Int Psychogeriatr 2002;14(3):239–48.

37. MacKnight C, Rockwood K, Awalt E, et al. Diabetes mellitus and the risk of dementia, Alzheimer's disease and vascular cognitive impairment in the Canadian Study of Health and Aging. Dement Geriatr Cogn Disord 2002;14(2):77–83.

38. Beeri MS, Schmeidler J, Silverman JM, et al. Insulin in combination with other diabetes medication is associated with less Alzheimer neuropathology. Neurology 2008;71(10):750–7.

39. Kalaria RN. Neurodegenerative disease: diabetes, microvascular pathology and Alzheimer disease. Nat Rev Neurol 2009;5(6):305–6.

40. Wu JH, Haan MN, Liang J, et al. Impact of antidiabetic medications on physical and cognitive functioning of older Mexican Americans with diabetes mellitus: a population-based cohort study. Ann Epidemiol 2003;13(5):369–76.

41. Banks WA, Owen JB, Erickson MA. Insulin in the brain: there and back again. Pharmacol Ther 2012;136(1):82–93.

42. Cholerton B, Baker LD, Craft S. Insulin resistance and pathological brain ageing. Diabet Med 2011;28(12):1463–75.

43. Craft S. Insulin resistance syndrome and Alzheimer disease: pathophysiologic mechanisms and therapeutic implications. Alzheimer Dis Assoc Disord 2006; 20(4):298–301.
44. White MF. Insulin signaling in health and disease. Science 2003;302(5651): 1710–1.
45. Baura GD, Foster DM, Kaiyala K, et al. Insulin transport from plasma into the central nervous system is inhibited by dexamethasone in dogs. Diabetes 1996;45(1):86–90.
46. Benedict C, Brooks SJ, Kullberg J, et al. Impaired insulin sensitivity as indexed by the HOMA score is associated with deficits in verbal fluency and temporal lobe gray matter volume in the elderly. Diabetes Care 2012;35(3):488–94.
47. Baker LD, Cross DJ, Minoshima S, et al. Insulin resistance and Alzheimer-like reductions in regional cerebral glucose metabolism for cognitively normal adults with prediabetes or early type 2 diabetes. Arch Neurol 2011;68(1):51–7.
48. Park CR, Seeley RJ, Craft S, et al. Intracerebroventricular insulin enhances memory in a passive-avoidance task. Physiol Behav 2000;68(4):509–14.
49. Craft S, Asthana S, Cook DG, et al. Insulin dose-response effects on memory and plasma amyloid precursor protein in Alzheimer's disease: interactions with apolipoprotein E genotype. Psychoneuroendocrinology 2003;28(6):809–22.
50. Reger MA, Watson GS, Green PS, et al. Intranasal insulin administration dose-dependently modulates verbal memory and plasma amyloid-beta in memory-impaired older adults. J Alzheimers Dis 2008;13(3):323–31.
51. Reger MA, Watson GS, Green PS, et al. Intranasal insulin improves cognition and modulates beta-amyloid in early AD. Neurology 2008;70(6):440–8.
52. Craft S, Baker LD, Montine TJ, et al. Intranasal insulin therapy for Alzheimer disease and amnestic mild cognitive impairment: a pilot clinical trial. Arch Neurol 2012;69(1):29–38.
53. Claxton A, Baker LD, Wilkinson CW, et al. Sex and ApoE genotype differences in treatment response to two doses of intranasal insulin in adults with mild cognitive impairment or Alzheimer's disease. J Alzheimers Dis 2013;35(4):789–97.
54. Cholerton B, Baker LD, Trittschuh EH, et al. Insulin and sex interactions in older adults with mild cognitive impairment. J Alzheimers Dis 2012;31(2):401–10.
55. Braak H, Braak E. Frequency of stages of Alzheimer-related lesions in different age categories. Neurobiol Aging 1997;18(4):351–7.
56. Craft S, Cholerton B, Baker LD. Insulin and Alzheimer's disease: untangling the web. J Alzheimers Dis 2013;33(Suppl 1):S263–75.
57. Watson GS, Peskind ER, Asthana S, et al. Insulin increases CSF Abeta42 levels in normal older adults. Neurology 2003;60(12):1899–903.
58. Boyt AA, Taddei TK, Hallmayer J, et al. The effect of insulin and glucose on the plasma concentration of Alzheimer's amyloid precursor protein. Neuroscience 2000;95(3):727–34.
59. Craft S, Asthana S, Schellenberg G, et al. Insulin effects on glucose metabolism, memory, and plasma amyloid precursor protein in Alzheimer's disease differ according to apolipoprotein-E genotype. Ann N Y Acad Sci 2000;903:222–8.
60. Rogers J, Shen Y. A perspective on inflammation in Alzheimer's disease. Ann N Y Acad Sci 2000;924:132–5.
61. Dandona P. Endothelium, inflammation, and diabetes. Curr Diab Rep 2002;2(4): 311–5.
62. Krogh-Madsen R, Plomgaard P, Keller P, et al. Insulin stimulates interleukin-6 and tumor necrosis factor-alpha gene expression in human subcutaneous adipose tissue. Am J Physiol Endocrinol Metab 2004;286(2):E234–8.

63. Fishel MA, Watson GS, Montine TJ, et al. Hyperinsulinemia provokes synchronous increases in central inflammation and beta-amyloid in normal adults. Arch Neurol 2005;62(10):1539–44.
64. Olefsky JM. Treatment of insulin resistance with peroxisome proliferator-activated receptor gamma agonists. J Clin Invest 2000;106(4):467–72.
65. Combs CK, Johnson DE, Karlo JC, et al. Inflammatory mechanisms in Alzheimer's disease: inhibition of beta-amyloid-stimulated proinflammatory responses and neurotoxicity by PPARgamma agonists. J Neurosci 2000;20(2):558–67.
66. Lehmann JM, Lenhard JM, Oliver BB, et al. Peroxisome proliferator-activated receptors alpha and gamma are activated by indomethacin and other non-steroidal anti-inflammatory drugs. J Biol Chem 1997;272(6):3406–10.
67. Lim GP, Yang F, Chu T, et al. Ibuprofen suppresses plaque pathology and inflammation in a mouse model for Alzheimer's disease. J Neurosci 2000; 20(15):5709–14.
68. Rodriguez-Rivera J, Denner L, Dineley KT. Rosiglitazone reversal of Tg2576 cognitive deficits is independent of peripheral gluco-regulatory status. Behav Brain Res 2011;216(1):255–61.
69. Pedersen WA, McMillan PJ, Kulstad JJ, et al. Rosiglitazone attenuates learning and memory deficits in Tg2576 Alzheimer mice. Exp Neurol 2006;199(2):265–73.
70. O'Reilly JA, Lynch M. Rosiglitazone improves spatial memory and decreases insoluble Abeta(1-42) in APP/PS1 mice. J Neuroimmune Pharmacol 2012;7(1): 140–4.
71. Escribano L, Simon AM, Gimeno E, et al. Rosiglitazone rescues memory impairment in Alzheimer's transgenic mice: mechanisms involving a reduced amyloid and tau pathology. Neuropsychopharmacology 2010;35(7):1593–604.
72. Nicolakakis N, Aboulkassim T, Ongali B, et al. Complete rescue of cerebrovascular function in aged Alzheimer's disease transgenic mice by antioxidants and pioglitazone, a peroxisome proliferator-activated receptor gamma agonist. J Neurosci 2008;28(37):9287–96.
73. Searcy JL, Phelps JT, Pancani T, et al. Long-term pioglitazone treatment improves learning and attenuates pathological markers in a mouse model of Alzheimer's disease. J Alzheimers Dis 2012;30(4):943–61.
74. Watson GS, Cholerton BA, Reger MA, et al. Preserved cognition in patients with early Alzheimer disease and amnestic mild cognitive impairment during treatment with rosiglitazone: a preliminary study. Am J Geriatr Psychiatry 2005; 13(11):950–8.
75. Risner ME, Saunders AM, Altman JF, et al. Efficacy of rosiglitazone in a genetically defined population with mild-to-moderate Alzheimer's disease. Pharmacogenomics J 2006;6(4):246–54.
76. Gold M, Alderton C, Zvartau-Hind M, et al. Rosiglitazone monotherapy in mild-to-moderate Alzheimer's disease: results from a randomized, double-blind, placebo-controlled phase III study. Dement Geriatr Cogn Disord 2010;30(2):131–46.
77. Harrington C, Sawchak S, Chiang C, et al. Rosiglitazone does not improve cognition or global function when used as adjunctive therapy to AChE inhibitors in mild-to-moderate Alzheimer's disease: two phase 3 studies. Curr Alzheimer Res 2011;8(5):592–606.
78. Hanyu H, Sato T, Kiuchi A, et al. Pioglitazone improved cognition in a pilot study on patients with Alzheimer's disease and mild cognitive impairment with diabetes mellitus. J Am Geriatr Soc 2009;57(1):177–9.
79. Sato T, Hanyu H, Hirao K, et al. Efficacy of PPAR-gamma agonist pioglitazone in mild Alzheimer disease. Neurobiol Aging 2011;32(9):1626–33.

80. Geldmacher DS, Fritsch T, McClendon MJ, et al. A randomized pilot clinical trial of the safety of pioglitazone in treatment of patients with Alzheimer disease. Arch Neurol 2011;68(1):45–50.

81. Sheu WH, Chuang HC, Cheng SM, et al. Microdialysis combined blood sampling technique for the determination of rosiglitazone and glucose in brain and blood of gerbils subjected to cerebral ischemia. J Pharm Biomed Anal 2011;54(4):759–64.

82. Strum JC, Shehee R, Virley D, et al. Rosiglitazone induces mitochondrial biogenesis in mouse brain. J Alzheimers Dis 2007;11(1):45–51.

83. Festuccia WT, Oztezcan S, Laplante M, et al. Peroxisome proliferator-activated receptor-gamma-mediated positive energy balance in the rat is associated with reduced sympathetic drive to adipose tissues and thyroid status. Endocrinology 2008;149(5):2121–30.

84. Grommes C, Karlo JC, Caprariello A, et al. The PPARgamma agonist pioglitazone crosses the blood-brain barrier and reduces tumor growth in a human xenograft model. Cancer Chemother Pharmacol 2013;71(4):929–36.

85. Maeshiba Y, Kiyota Y, Yamashita K, et al. Disposition of the new antidiabetic agent pioglitazone in rats, dogs, and monkeys. Arzneimittelforschung 1997; 47(1):29–35.

86. Mannucci E, Monami M, Di Bari M, et al. Cardiac safety profile of rosiglitazone: a comprehensive meta-analysis of randomized clinical trials. Int J Cardiol 2010; 143(2):135–40.

87. Holscher C. The role of GLP-1 in neuronal activity and neurodegeneration. Vitam Horm 2010;84:331–54.

88. Green BD, Gault VA, Flatt PR, et al. Comparative effects of GLP-1 and GIP on cAMP production, insulin secretion, and in vivo antidiabetic actions following substitution of Ala8/Ala2 with 2-aminobutyric acid. Arch Biochem Biophys 2004;428(2):136–43.

89. Sivertsen J, Rosenmeier J, Holst JJ, et al. The effect of glucagon-like peptide 1 on cardiovascular risk. Nat Rev Cardiol 2012;9(4):209–22.

90. Gejl M, Egefjord L, Lerche S, et al. Glucagon-like peptide-1 decreases intra-cerebral glucose content by activating hexokinase and changing glucose clearance during hyperglycemia. J Cereb Blood Flow Metab 2012;32(12): 2146–52.

91. Bomfim TR, Forny-Germano L, Sathler LB, et al. An anti-diabetes agent protects the mouse brain from defective insulin signaling caused by Alzheimer's disease-associated Abeta oligomers. J Clin Invest 2012;122(4):1339–53.

92. Bailey CJ, Turner RC. Metformin. N Engl J Med 1996;334(9):574–9.

93. Tian J, Shi J, Bailey K, et al. Association between apolipoprotein E e4 allele and arteriosclerosis, cerebral amyloid angiopathy, and cerebral white matter damage in Alzheimer's disease. J Neurol Neurosurg Psychiatry 2004;75(5): 696–9.

94. Labuzek K, Suchy D, Gabryel B, et al. Quantification of metformin by the HPLC method in brain regions, cerebrospinal fluid and plasma of rats treated with lipo-polysaccharide. Pharmacol Rep 2010;62(5):956–65.

95. Kitabchi AE, Temprosa M, Knowler WC, et al. Role of insulin secretion and sensi-tivity in the evolution of type 2 diabetes in the diabetes prevention program: effects of lifestyle intervention and metformin. Diabetes 2005;54(8):2404–14.

96. Gupta A, Bisht B, Dey CS. Peripheral insulin-sensitizer drug metformin amelio-rates neuronal insulin resistance and Alzheimer's-like changes. Neuropharma-cology 2011;60(6):910–20.

97. Chen Y, Zhou K, Wang R, et al. Antidiabetic drug metformin (GlucophageR) increases biogenesis of Alzheimer's amyloid peptides via up-regulating BACE1 transcription. Proc Natl Acad Sci U S A 2009;106(10):3907–12.
98. Kickstein E, Krauss S, Thornhill P, et al. Biguanide metformin acts on tau phosphorylation via mTOR/protein phosphatase 2A (PP2A) signaling. Proc Natl Acad Sci U S A 2010;107(50):21830–5.
99. Li J, Deng J, Sheng W, et al. Metformin attenuates Alzheimer's disease-like neuropathology in obese, leptin-resistant mice. Pharmacol Biochem Behav 2012;101(4):564–74.
100. Bhutada P, Mundhada Y, Bansod K, et al. Protection of cholinergic and anti-oxidant system contributes to the effect of berberine ameliorating memory dysfunction in rat model of streptozotocin-induced diabetes. Behav Brain Res 2011;220(1):30–41.
101. Pintana H, Apaijai N, Pratchayasakul W, et al. Effects of metformin on learning and memory behaviors and brain mitochondrial functions in high fat diet induced insulin resistant rats. Life Sci 2012;91(11–12):409–14.
102. Abbatecola AM, Lattanzio F, Molinari AM, et al. Rosiglitazone and cognitive stability in older individuals with type 2 diabetes and mild cognitive impairment. Diabetes Care 2010;33(8):1700–11.
103. Imfeld P, Bodmer M, Jick SS, et al. Metformin, other antidiabetic drugs, and risk of Alzheimer's disease: a population-based case-control study. J Am Geriatr Soc 2012;60(5):916–21.
104. Hsu CC, Wahlqvist ML, Lee MS, et al. Incidence of dementia is increased in type 2 diabetes and reduced by the use of sulfonylureas and metformin. J Alzheimers Dis 2011;24(3):485–93.

Endocrine Aspects of Post-traumatic Stress Disorder and Implications for Diagnosis and Treatment

Nikolaos P. Daskalakis, MD, PhD[a,b,c,*], Amy Lehrner, PhD[a,b,c], Rachel Yehuda, PhD[a,b,c,d]

KEYWORDS

- Stress • Sympathetic • Hypothalamic-pituitary-adrenal axis • Cortisol
- Post-traumatic stress disorder

KEY POINTS

- Rather than a heightened cortisol profile, individuals with post-traumatic stress disorder (PTSD) show reduced glucocorticoid (GC) signaling. This has been shown to be associated with increased GC responsiveness or sensitivity.
- GC alterations in PTSD may reflect complex influences and interactions that extend beyond the hypothalamic-pituitary-adrenal (HPA) axis.
- HPA axis dysregulation may be a result of pretraumatic factors, including early environmental traumas or stressors, and genetic or epigenetic influences.

INTRODUCTION

Post-traumatic stress disorder (PTSD) is a serious, multisystem disorder that can develop in trauma survivors.[1] The diagnosis is based on symptoms in 3 distinct clusters: re-experiencing, hyperarousal, and avoidance.[2] Intrusive symptoms include unwanted memories of the traumatic events, nightmares, flashbacks, and emotional

The authors have nothing to disclose.
[a] Traumatic Stress Studies Division, Department of Psychiatry, Icahn School of Medicine at Mount Sinai, One Gustave L. Levy Place, New York, NY 10029-6574, USA; [b] Laboratory of Molecular Neuropsychiatry, Department of Psychiatry, Icahn School of Medicine at Mount Sinai, One Gustave L. Levy Place, New York, NY 10029-6574, USA; [c] Mental Health Care Center, PTSD Program and Laboratory of Clinical Neuroendocrinology and Neurochemistry, James J. Peters Veterans Affairs Medical Center, 130 West Kingsbridge Road, 526 OOMH 116/A, Bronx, NY 10468, USA; [d] Department of Neuroscience, Icahn School of Medicine at Mount Sinai, One Gustave L. Levy Place, New York, NY 10029-6574, USA
* Corresponding author. Laboratory of Molecular Neuropsychiatry, Department of Psychiatry, Icahn School of Medicine at Mount Sinai, One Gustave L. Levy Place, Box 1668, New York, NY 10029-6574.
E-mail address: nikolaos.daskalakis@mssm.edu

Endocrinol Metab Clin N Am 42 (2013) 503–513
http://dx.doi.org/10.1016/j.ecl.2013.05.004
0889-8529/13/$ – see front matter © 2013 Elsevier Inc. All rights reserved.

or physical distress at reminders of the trauma. Avoidance symptoms reflect attempts of the survivor to stay away from reminders of the event and can generalize into feelings of interpersonal detachment and a restricted range of emotions, bearing a strong resemblance to depressive disorder. Hyperarousal symptoms such as difficulty sleeping, increased startle response, impaired concentration, and hypervigilance are expressions of the anxiety-like aspects of this condition.

Initially, PTSD was understood as the expected response to extreme trauma, which was assumed to be a rare occurrence. However, epidemiologic research showed that traumatic experiences were much more common than expected in the general population; 40% to 65% of people experience at least one traumatic event that could lead to PTSD.[3–5] These events include interpersonal violence such as rape or assault, motor vehicle or industrial accidents, natural disasters, or exposure to terrorism or military conflict. Although it is now well recognized that most individuals exposed to trauma do not develop PTSD,[5–7] given the prevalence of trauma exposure, PTSD is a relatively common disorder, with a lifetime prevalence about 7%.[3,6] The condition confers a significant burden on individuals, families, and the public.[3,6] The cost of PTSD in terms of lost productivity, absenteeism, and medical care annually is substantial.[8,9] Indeed, PTSD is associated with the greatest increase in medical costs of all depressive and anxiety disorders.[10]

Although conceptualized as a mental disorder, PTSD is a condition that is highly comorbid with medical conditions such as hypertension and cardiovascular illness, metabolic syndrome, chronic fatigue syndrome, fibromyalgia, gastrointestinal disorder, pain disorder, respiratory illness, and other diseases.[11–15] In fact, the mortality rate among people with PTSD is significantly higher than for those without PTSD.[16] For a combination of reasons, including the stigma associated with mental health treatment, limited availability and high cost of mental health treatment, and sociodemographic factors among those chronically affected by illness, most people with PTSD do not seek specialized mental health treatment but present to primary care. Patients with PTSD are among the highest utilizers of primary care services for a variety of somatic and medical complaints. Thus it is important to understand how PTSD presents behaviorally and medically. Specifically, there are unique hormonal differences in PTSD that may lead to different medical diagnoses if the circumstances of trauma exposure are not considered.

Unlike the extreme dysfunctions associated with common endocrine disorders (eg, diabetes, thyroid diseases), the hormonal changes in PTSD are subtle, but together they reflect a specific accommodation to traumatic experiences that results in an exaggerated response to subsequent environmental stressors. PTSD represents a failure of the stress response system to regain homeostasis, and it has been associated with lower levels of cortisol.[1] The condition is not associated with pituitary endocrine deficits as is observed in traumatic brain injury. The understanding of PTSD as a failure to recover from stress provided an important context for investigations into neuroendocrine alterations associated with the disorder. That is, PTSD is not reflective of an acute response to stress, or of a response associated with a chronic stressor, both characterized by high cortisol levels, but rather it reflects a persistent response to a challenge that is no longer present. It is likely that these changes are underpinned by epigenetic mechanisms or other molecular processes that reflect an enduring transformative change. Indeed, unlike acute stressors, watershed events that result in PTSD often leave the survivor feeling that he or she has been permanently changed. Whereas the goal in acute and even to some extent chronic stress is to help the person achieve homeostasis and recovery to a prestress state, in PTSD, the therapeutic goals involve acceptance of the transformative nature of life-altering events.

NEUROENDOCRINE RESPONSE TO STRESS

Stress is the straining force that a living organism experiences when faced with a physiologic or emotional challenge (stressor), and leads to a physiologic response to maintain homeostasis through adaptive changes (stress response or allostasis or allostatic response).[17] The sympathetic nervous system (SNS) and the hypothalamic-pituitary-adrenal (HPA) axis are the major constituents of the body's neuroendocrine response to physical and emotional threat and stress. SNS response is normally brief, mobilizing the acute fight-or-flight response.[18] The immediate response by the SNS is followed by an HPA axis response that reinstates homeostasis and induces long-lasting adaptive changes (ie, stress recovery and resilience).[19] This is orchestrated by glucocorticoids (GCs; ie, cortisol and corticosterone in people and corticosterone in rodents), the end product of the HPA axis. Basal levels of GCs occupy the high-affinity mineralocorticoid receptors (MRs), whereas under stress, GCs also bind to the low-affinity GC receptor (GR) in target tissue.[19] The resulting GC-signaling cascade induces rapid modulation of neural activity and more long-term transcriptional regulation.[20,21] The HPA axis stress response, through negative feedback inhibition by the GCs at the level of hypothalamus and pituitary, eventually terminates, and the basal HPA axis activity is restored. When stress is chronic or severe, the stress system activation might be prolonged or fail, and this might lead to an allostatic load, where the stress mediators are no longer protective and burden physiologic systems, ultimately leading to disease.[17] For example, dysregulated HPA axis activity associated with chronic stress has been linked with psychiatric, circulatory, metabolic, gastrointestinal, and immunologic diseases.[17,19,22]

ENDOCRINE ALTERATIONS IN PTSD

Biological research on PTSD initially focused on SNS and the HPA axis given the early conceptualization of PTSD as an exacerbated and unremitting extension of the normal physiologic response to threat. Catecholamines and GCs within those systems were of particular interest, as basic research findings demonstrated their synergistic effects on consolidation of fear.[23] As PTSD was hypothesized to reflect a sustained stress response, increased levels of catecholamines and cortisol were expected. Although catecholamines were found to be elevated, patients with PTSD unexpectedly showed low cortisol levels,[24] a finding that has been replicated many times.[25–28] In cross-sectional studies, PTSD patients, compared with trauma-exposed or trauma-naïve controls, displayed lower daily cortisol output, along with higher levels of norepinephrine, corticotropin-releasing hormone (CRH) and proinflammatory cytokines, reflecting reduced GC signaling.[29–35] These findings contradicted the initial model of PTSD as a chronic stress disorder and necessitated a reconceptualization of the neuroendocrine basis of PTSD.[36]

Furthermore, although this neuroendocrine research suggested that lower cortisol levels and related findings may reflect PTSD pathophysiology as the disease becomes chronic, emerging research findings indicated that these alterations may in fact reflect pretraumatic vulnerabilities to the later development of PTSD. Many of the identified genetic and environmental risk factors (eg, exposure to prior traumatic events, childhood adversity and abuse, prior psychiatric history)[37,38] converged into low production of GCs and insufficient GC signaling in the acute aftermath of trauma.[39] This notion was confirmed in prospective studies, where the previously mentioned measures before or in the acute aftermath of trauma predicted the subsequent development of PTSD.[39] For example, in an emergency room study of women seeking care immediately following a rape, women with a sexual assault history showed lower cortisol levels, and had a threefold increase in risk of developing PTSD at four months, than women with no history of sexual assault.[40] Similarly, McFarlane and colleagues found lower plasma cortisol levels among survivors of motor vehicle accidents who would later develop PTSD compared to those who did not.[41] This suggested that, at the time of trauma, reduced GC signaling compromises the inhibition of stress-induced biological responses and the induction of adaptive changes, facilitating the development of PTSD.[39,40]

GR RESPONSIVENESS

Low cortisol levels and low GC signaling predict a corresponding enhanced GR responsiveness in PTSD. Increased plasma cortisol suppression by dexamethasone (DEX) in the low-dose (0.5 mg) DEX suppression test (DST), reflecting enhanced GR responsiveness, has been observed in PTSD.[41,42] Combat veterans with PTSD also showed a larger number of GRs compared with veterans without PTSD,[43] and patients with PTSD have been found to have more GRs than those with major depressive disorder, mania, panic disorder, and schizophrenia.[44] In vitro assays using peripheral blood mononuclear cells confirmed a heightened GR sensitivity in PTSD.[43,45] The GR is part of a molecular complex that includes protein chaperones such as heat shock protein 90 (HSP90) and FK506 binding protein 5 (FKBP5). FKBP5 acts as a GR inhibitor by reducing ligand binding and the translocation of the bound GR to the nucleus. Reductions in the expression of the FKBP5 gene in civilian PTSD in the aftermath of World Trade Center attacks, consistent with enhanced GR sensitivity, have been reported.[45,46] Genetic/epigenetic variation of FKBP5 in interaction with childhood abuse confers risk for adult PTSD,[47,48] and reduced FKBP5 expression has also been specifically linked with peri-traumatic dissociation, which is associated with PTSD risk.[49]

GC CIRCADIAN RHYTHMS

Cortisol's circadian rhythm, which is critically influenced by GR function,[50] is altered with the progression of PTSD. Intraindividual changes in cortisol circadian parameters are associated with the development of PTSD symptoms. PTSD subjects show a lower cortisol mesor and an overall higher circadian signal-to-noise ratio than controls and depressed patients.[51] A study in offspring of Holocaust survivors, who are at greater risk for PTSD based on having a parent with PTSD, demonstrated that circadian rhythm alterations are actually associated with PTSD but not with PTSD risk, because offspring displayed a lower cortisol mesor but not the rest of the chronobiological alterations found in PTSD.[52]

GC METABOLISM

Early urinary cortisol results of PTSD were highly correlated with total cortisol levels (free cortisol + metabolites) obtained using more sensitive methods of chromatography.[53,54] However, in PTSD, there is some evidence that cortisol metabolites, not just free cortisol, are altered. One of the inactive cortisol metabolites that can be examined is cortisone. Cortisone levels in relation to cortisol levels provide the basis for estimating the activity of 11β-HSD-2, which is the enzyme that degrades cortisol into cortisone, primarily in the kidney (the renal activity of this enzyme is inferred from the urinary-free cortisol to cortisone ratio). Other metabolites include 5α-tetrahydroxycortisol and 5β-tetrahydrocortisol, because cortisol is also degraded by 5α- and 5β-reductases into these inactive metabolites. Cortisone is similarly degraded into

5β-tetrahydrocortisone. 5α- and 5β-reductase activity can be inferred from the ratios of the respective GC metabolites to cortisol or cortisone. Elderly Holocaust survivors, many of whom had PTSD, showed lower activity of 5α-reductase and 11β-HSD-2 activity than comparison subjects.[54]

Cortisol metabolic enzymes have been demonstrated to be subject to developmental programming—just like the GR—and may be important progenitors of physical risk factors (eg, metabolic syndrome) that are often present in combat veterans. An increased risk for hypertension and metabolic disease has been demonstrated in association with early adversity via epigenetic mechanisms.[55] Thus, targeting GC-related enzymes is of interest.[56]

RECALIBRATING HPA AXIS IN PTSD WITH GC TREATMENT

Clearly there is a unique neuroendocrine signature associated with PTSD or exposure to trauma. The question has become whether these neuroendocrine signs represent potential treatment targets. There are no clear answers to this question, because it is still not known which aspects of PTSD-related neuroendocrinology reflect pretraumatic risk factors, and which associate with pathology. Although the associations between PTSD and lower cortisol levels/GR alterations have been relatively robust (as robust as for any biologic marker in mental health or psychiatry), it is not clear whether these changes reflect an attempt at adaptation or homeostasis. The traditional endocrine view that sustained high cortisol levels are damaging would urge caution in attempting to restore low cortisol with simple GC supplementation. Furthermore, as has long been known in endocrinology, such supplementation in the face of a relatively intact HPA axis would induce either suppression of the endogenous HPA-axis and/or exogenous Cushing syndrome. On the other hand, the robust evidence for enhanced GC sensitization cannot be ignored for its potential as a treatment target, particularly because models of PTSD development following trauma exposure are based on the idea that low cortisol does not promote the adaptive mechanisms required to decrease the sympathetic nervous system response. Thus, initial attempts with GC-based treatments in chronic PTSD have begun in several directions, none of which involves attempts to simply provide chronic cortisol treatment over a sustained period of time. Some attempts have been made to use hydrocortisone (Hcort) administration for brief periods of time,[57] or to augment psychotherapy.[58,59] The augmentation strategy is currently being tested in a double-blind, placebo-controlled study in which patients ingest either Hcort or placebo prior to prolonged exposure therapy sessions in which they will engage in an extended imaginal exposure of their trauma.[59] It is hypothesized that supplementing psychotherapy with Hcort will facilitate learning and habituation based on the known effects of GCs on memory and learning.[23] A pilot study (that has led to a multicenter trial, currently ongoing) suggested that the GR-antagonist mifepristone might also be efficacious in PTSD.[60] This treatment would have the net effect of increasing endogenous GCs and is thought to recalibrate the HPA axis by altering GR/MR balance. It can be hypothesized that use of novel GR modulators (partials agonists/antagonists) could fine tune this HPA axis with more tissue-specific precision to get a desired therapeutic effect.[61,62]

GCS IN THE PREVENTION OF PTSD

Given the proposed mechanism for the development of PTSD, it has been suggested that administration of a single high dose of GCs in the acute aftermath of trauma may prevent PTSD, and such studies are ongoing. A successful pilot study has demonstrated that PTSD prophylaxis is possible with a single high dose of Hcort. In a double blind, placebo-controlled, random assignment pilot study, patients were randomized to receive, within 6 hours of a traumatic event, 1 shot of double-blind intravenous Hcort (100–140 mg) and were followed up for 3 months. At the 3-month follow-up assessment, no subjects in the Hcort group were diagnosed with PTSD.[63] A single dose of Hcort (17.5 mg) also improved working memory in combat veterans with chronic PTSD in another study.[59] A recently developed unique animal model of PTSD that captures individual differences in the behavioral response to traumatic stress provided evidence for the effectiveness of early GC administration.[60,62,64] It involves the exposure of a large group of rats to predator scent stress (PSS), and classifies the animals according to their behavior. PSS exposure results in 25% of rats displaying extreme behavioral response (PTSD-like), 25% minimal response (resilient), and 50% an intermediate response.[64] When rats are treated with a high-dose of corticosterone (25 mg/kg), shortly after stress-exposure, the extreme behavioral response disappears.[62]

The use of a single high dose of GC is hypothesized to accomplish a recalibration of GR responsiveness and GC signaling. A single GC boost might reduce GR receptors by homologous down-regulation,[65] and at the same time overcome the lower tonic GC signal by transiently activating the available GRs. A single low dose of DEX (0.5 mg) could significantly down-regulate the number of GR receptors in lymphocytes of PTSD patients and not of controls.[36] A high dose of Hcort might also enhance the stress response by changing the expression of genes that will lead to a reduction of GR sensitivity, which in turn lead to a restoration of basal cortisol, allowing cortisol-induced adaptive changes. The genes that would directly respond to Hcort may not be only those that are involved in GR desensitization, but also those that are necessary for the behavioral adaptation. These stress-sensitive genes are sensitive to GR only at high concentrations of occupied GR in the nucleus, since those DNA-sites are by definition less sensitive than other sites (eg, circadian-responsive sites). In PTSD, these lower-affinity sites may be tonically underactivated and could be reactivated by the Hcort injection.

Investigations of GC-based interventions are ongoing and promising, but what is even more promising is the potential for addressing neuroendocrine alterations at a molecular level. There has been an increased interest in molecular, and particularly epigenetic, mechanisms in PTSD. It should be emphasized that GC-based treatments in PTSD are not mainstream, and they reflect a revolutionary new direction that has not yet been proven effective. The standard of care for PTSD treatment is a combination of psychotherapy and medications, generally selective serotonin reuptake inhibitors (SSRIs), which are the only US Food and Drug Administration (FDA)-approved pharmacotherapy for PTSD. Although both psychotherapy and medications, and certainly their combination, are recognized as first-line treatments in PTSD,[66] they are not always successful. Indeed, the Institute of Medicine Committee on Treatment of Posttraumatic Stress Disorder found inadequate evidence of efficacy for all classes of medications tested in randomized-controlled trials.[67] And although cognitive behavior therapies (emphasizing exposure and cognitive restructuring) have been found to induce improvement or recovery, some of those who enter treatment either do not complete or continue to experience significant symptoms.[68] Thus, there is a continued need to develop and evaluate new interventions for PTSD.

As knowledge about PTSD biology grows, it may be possible in the near future to match treatments for PTSD to more specific clinical and biological presentations. Although the endocrine aspects of PTSD are generally well recognized, biological alterations have been noted in many systems, and in clinical practice there has been a fairly substantial abyss between biological findings and treatment practices. In part, this may reflect the need for comprehensive individualized care of trauma survivors based on unique clinical presentations.

SUMMARY

The normal neuroendocrine response to an acute stressor involves the engagement of complementary biological systems that both prepare the organism for fight or flight and also down-regulate this response and reestablish homeostasis after the threat is removed. Although initial research on the neuroendocrine characteristics of PTSD was premised on the expectation that the biology of PTSD would mirror the biology of the normal stress response, instead, findings of lower cortisol suggested a reconceptualization of PTSD as reflecting a failure of the stress response system. Rather than a heightened cortisol profile, individuals with PTSD show reduced GC signaling. This has been shown to be associated with increased GC responsiveness or sensitivity. GC alterations in PTSD may reflect complex influences and interactions that extend beyond the HPA axis. HPA axis dysregulation may be a result of pretraumatic factors, including early environmental traumas or stressors, and genetic or epigenetic influences.

Future studies will need to take into account the longitudinal trajectory of the disorder and include biological approaches to analyzing a wide range of cellular and molecular markers that may represent more stable upstream indicators (eg, epigenetic markers) than downstream hormonal markers, which are more temporally variable. A better understanding of the mechanisms and networks involved in the failure to recover from traumatic stress will contribute to the development of new treatment targets and the identification of biomarkers of risk, resilience, and recovery.

REFERENCES

1. Yehuda R. Post-traumatic stress disorder. N Engl J Med 2002;346(2):108–14.
2. American Psychiatric Association. Diagnostic and statistical manual of mental disorders: DSM-IV-TR. American Psychiatric Publishing; 2000.
3. Kessler RC, Sonnega A, Bromet E, et al. Posttraumatic stress disorder in the National Comorbidity Survey. Arch Gen Psychiatry 1995;52(12):1048–60.
4. Creamer M, Burgess P, McFarlane AC. Post-traumatic stress disorder: findings from the Australian National Survey of Mental Health and Well-being. Psychol Med 2001;31(7):1237–47.
5. Perkonigg A, Kessler RC, Storz S, et al. Traumatic events and post-traumatic stress disorder in the community: prevalence, risk factors and comorbidity. Acta Psychiatr Scand 2000;101(1):46–59.
6. Kessler RC, Chiu WT, Demler O, et al. Prevalence, severity, and comorbidity of 12-month DSM-IV disorders in the National Comorbidity Survey Replication. Arch Gen Psychiatry 2005;62(6):617–27.
7. Breslau N, Kessler RC, Chilcoat HD, et al. Trauma and posttraumatic stress disorder in the community: the 1996 Detroit Area Survey of Trauma. Arch Gen Psychiatry 1998;55(7):626–32.
8. Greenberg PE, Sisitsky T, Kessler RC, et al. The economic burden of anxiety disorders in the 1990s. J Clin Psychiatry 1999;60(7):427–35.
9. Solomon SD, Davidson JR. Trauma: prevalence, impairment, service use, and cost. J Clin Psychiatry 1997;58(Suppl 9):5–11.
10. Marciniak MD, Lage MJ, Dunayevich E, et al. The cost of treating anxiety: the medical and demographic correlates that impact total medical costs. Depress Anxiety 2005;21(4):178–84.

11. Ouimette P, Cronkite R, Henson BR, et al. Posttraumatic stress disorder and health status among female and male medical patients. J Trauma Stress 2004;17(1):1–9.

12. Schnurr PP, Spiro A III, Paris AH. Physician-diagnosed medical disorders in relation to PTSD symptoms in older male military veterans. Health Psychol 2000; 19(1):91–7.

13. Sareen J, Cox BJ, Stein MB, et al. Physical and mental comorbidity, disability, and suicidal behavior associated with posttraumatic stress disorder in a large community sample. Psychosom Med 2007;69(3):242–8.

14. Heppner PS, Crawford EF, Haji UA, et al. The association of posttraumatic stress disorder and metabolic syndrome: a study of increased health risk in veterans. BMC Med 2009;7:1.

15. Boscarino JA. Posttraumatic stress disorder and physical illness: results from clinical and epidemiologic studies. Ann N Y Acad Sci 2004;1032:141–53.

16. Ahmadi N, Hajsadeghi F, Mirshkarlo HB, et al. Post-traumatic stress disorder, coronary atherosclerosis, and mortality. Am J Cardiol 2011;108(1): 29–33.

17. McEwen BS. Protective and damaging effects of stress mediators. N Engl J Med 1998;338(3):171–9.

18. Cannon WB. Organization for physiological homeostasis. Physiol Rev 1929;9(3): 399–431.

19. de Kloet ER, Joels M, Holsboer F. Stress and the brain: from adaptation to disease. Nat Rev Neurosci 2005;6(6):463–75.

20. Joels M, Sarabdjitsingh RA, Karst H. Unraveling the time domains of corticosteroid hormone influences on brain activity: rapid, slow, and chronic modes. Pharmacol Rev 2012;64(4):901–38.

21. de Kloet ER, Fitzsimons CP, Datson NA, et al. Glucocorticoid signaling and stress-related limbic susceptibility pathway: about receptors, transcription machinery and microRNA. Brain Res 2009;1293:129–41.

22. Mayer EA. The neurobiology of stress and gastrointestinal disease. Gut 2000; 47(6):861–9.

23. Roozendaal B, McEwen BS, Chattarji S. Stress, memory and the amygdala. Nat Rev Neurosci 2009;10(6):423–33.

24. Mason JW, Giller EL, Kosten TR, et al. Urinary free-cortisol levels in posttraumatic stress disorder patients. J Nerv Ment Dis 1986;174(3):145–9.

25. Gill J, Vythilingam M, Page GG. Low cortisol, high DHEA, and high levels of stimulated TNF-alpha, and IL-6 in women with PTSD. J Trauma Stress 2008; 21(6):530–9.

26. Thaller V, Vrkljan M, Hotujac L, et al. The potential role of hypocortisolism in the pathophysiology of PTSD and psoriasis. Coll Antropol 1999;23(2):611–9.

27. Bremner D, Vermetten E, Kelley ME. Cortisol, dehydroepiandrosterone, and estradiol measured over 24 hours in women with childhood sexual abuse-related posttraumatic stress disorder. J Nerv Ment Dis 2007;195(11):919–27.

28. Yehuda R, Southwick SM, Nussbaum G, et al. Low urinary cortisol excretion in patients with posttraumatic stress disorder. J Nerv Ment Dis 1990;178(6): 366–9.

29. Baker DG, West SA, Nicholson WE, et al. Serial CSF corticotropin-releasing hormone levels and adrenocortical activity in combat veterans with posttraumatic stress disorder. Am J Psychiatry 1999;156(4):585–8.

30. Geracioti TD Jr, Baker DG, Ekhator NN, et al. CSF norepinephrine concentrations in posttraumatic stress disorder. Am J Psychiatry 2001;158(8):1227–30.

31. Baker DG, Ekhator NN, Kasckow JW, et al. Plasma and cerebrospinal fluid interleukin-6 concentrations in posttraumatic stress disorder. Neuroimmunomodulation 2001;9(4):209–17.
32. de Kloet CS, Vermetten E, Geuze E, et al. Elevated plasma corticotrophin-releasing hormone levels in veterans with posttraumatic stress disorder. Prog Brain Res 2008;167:287–91.
33. Spivak B, Shohat B, Mester R, et al. Elevated levels of serum interleukin-1 beta in combat-related posttraumatic stress disorder. Biol Psychiatry 1997;42(5): 345–8.
34. Morris MC, Compas BE, Garber J. Relations among posttraumatic stress disorder, comorbid major depression, and HPA function: a systematic review and meta-analysis. Clin Psychol Rev 2012;32(4):301–15.
35. Meewisse ML, Reitsma JB, de Vries GJ, et al. Cortisol and post-traumatic stress disorder in adults: systematic review and meta-analysis. Br J Psychiatry 2007; 191:387–92.
36. Yehuda R, Halligan SL, Grossman R, et al. The cortisol and glucocorticoid receptor response to low dose dexamethasone administration in aging combat veterans and holocaust survivors with and without posttraumatic stress disorder. Biol Psychiatry 2002;52(5):393–403.
37. McFarlane AC. Posttraumatic stress disorder: a model of the longitudinal course and the role of risk factors. J Clin Psychiatry 2000;61(Suppl 5):15–20 [discussion: 21–23].
38. Brewin CR, Andrews B, Valentine JD. Meta-analysis of risk factors for posttraumatic stress disorder in trauma-exposed adults. J Consult Clin Psychol 2000; 68(5):748–66.
39. van Zuiden M, Kavelaars A, Geuze E, et al. Predicting PTSD: Pre-existing vulnerabilities in glucocorticoid-signaling and implications for preventive interventions. Brain Behav Immun 2013;30:12–21.
40. Raison CL, Miller AH. When not enough is too much: the role of insufficient glucocorticoid signaling in the pathophysiology of stress-related disorders. Am J Psychiatry 2003;160(9):1554–65.
41. Yehuda R, Boisoneau D, Lowy MT, et al. Dose-response changes in plasma cortisol and lymphocyte glucocorticoid receptors following dexamethasone administration in combat veterans with and without posttraumatic stress disorder. Arch Gen Psychiatry 1995;52(7):583–93.
42. Yehuda R, Halligan SL, Golier JA, et al. Effects of trauma exposure on the cortisol response to dexamethasone administration in PTSD and major depressive disorder. Psychoneuroendocrinology 2004;29(3):389–404.
43. Yehuda R, Golier JA, Yang RK, et al. Enhanced sensitivity to glucocorticoids in peripheral mononuclear leukocytes in posttraumatic stress disorder. Biol Psychiatry 2004;55(11):1110–6.
44. Sarapas C, Cai G, Bierer LM, et al. Genetic markers for PTSD risk and resilience among survivors of the World Trade Center attacks. Dis Markers 2011;30(2–3): 101–10.
45. Matic G, Milutinovic DV, Nestorov J, et al. Lymphocyte glucocorticoid receptor expression level and hormone-binding properties differ between war trauma-exposed men with and without PTSD. Prog Neuropsychopharmacol Biol Psychiatry 2013;43:238–45.
46. Yehuda R, Cai G, Golier JA, et al. Gene expression patterns associated with posttraumatic stress disorder following exposure to the World Trade Center attacks. Biol Psychiatry 2009;66(7):708–11.

47. Binder EB, Bradley RG, Liu W, et al. Association of FKBP5 polymorphisms and childhood abuse with risk of posttraumatic stress disorder symptoms in adults. JAMA 2008;299(11):1291–305.
48. Klengel T, Mehta D, Anacker C, et al. Allele-specific FKBP5 DNA demethylation mediates gene-childhood trauma interactions. Nat Neurosci 2013;16(1):33–41.
49. Koenen KC, Saxe G, Purcell S, et al. Polymorphisms in FKBP5 are associated with peritraumatic dissociation in medically injured children. Mol Psychiatry 2005;10(12):1058–9.
50. Lightman SL, Conway-Campbell BL. The crucial role of pulsatile activity of the HPA axis for continuous dynamic equilibration. Nat Rev Neurosci 2010;11(10): 710–8.
51. Yehuda R, Teicher MH, Trestman RL, et al. Cortisol regulation in posttraumatic stress disorder and major depression: a chronobiological analysis. Biol Psychiatry 1996;40(2):79–88.
52. Yehuda R, Teicher MH, Seckl JR, et al. Parental posttraumatic stress disorder as a vulnerability factor for low cortisol trait in offspring of holocaust survivors. Arch Gen Psychiatry 2007;64(9):1040–8.
53. Yehuda R, Bierer LM, Sarapas C, et al. Cortisol metabolic predictors of response to psychotherapy for symptoms of PTSD in survivors of the World Trade Center attacks on September 11, 2001. Psychoneuroendocrinology 2009;34(9): 1304–13.
54. Yehuda R, Bierer LM, Andrew R, et al. Enduring effects of severe developmental adversity, including nutritional deprivation, on cortisol metabolism in aging Holocaust survivors. J Psychiatr Res 2009;43(9):877–83.
55. Vickers MH, Sloboda DM. Strategies for reversing the effects of metabolic disorders induced as a consequence of developmental programming. Front Physiol 2012;3:242.
56. Yehuda R, Seckl J. Minireview: stress-related psychiatric disorders with low cortisol levels: a metabolic hypothesis. Endocrinology 2011;152(12):4496–503.
57. Aerni A, Traber R, Hock C, et al. Low-dose cortisol for symptoms of posttraumatic stress disorder. Am J Psychiatry 2004;161(8):1488–90.
58. Pratchett LC, Daly K, Bierer LM, et al. New approaches to combining pharmacotherapy and psychotherapy for posttraumatic stress disorder. Expert Opin Pharmacother 2011;12(15):2339–54.
59. Yehuda R, Golier JA, Bierer LM, et al. Hydrocortisone responsiveness in Gulf War veterans with PTSD: effects on ACTH, declarative memory hippocampal [$_{18}$F] FDG uptake on PET. Psychiatry Res 2010;184(2):117–27.
60. Cohen H, Zohar J, Gidron Y, et al. Blunted HPA axis response to stress influences susceptibility to posttraumatic stress response in rats. Biol Psychiatry 2006;59(12):1208–18.
61. Zalachoras I, Houtman R, Atucha E, et al. Differential targeting of brain stress circuits with a selective glucocorticoid receptor modulator. Proc Natl Acad Sci U S A 2013;110(19):7910–5.
62. Cohen H, Matar MA, Buskila D, et al. Early post-stressor intervention with high-dose corticosterone attenuates posttraumatic stress response in an animal model of posttraumatic stress disorder. Biol Psychiatry 2008;64(8):708–17.
63. Zohar J, Yahalom H, Kozlovsky N, et al. High dose hydrocortisone immediately after trauma may alter the trajectory of PTSD: interplay between clinical and animal studies. Eur Neuropsychopharmacol 2011;21(11):796–809.
64. Cohen H, Zohar J. An animal model of posttraumatic stress disorder: the use of cut-off behavioral criteria. Ann N Y Acad Sci 2004;1032:167–78.

65. Dong Y, Poellinger L, Gustafsson JA, et al. Regulation of glucocorticoid receptor expression: evidence for transcriptional and posttranslational mechanisms. Mol Endocrinol 1988;2(12):1256–64.
66. Foa EB, Keane TM, Friedman MJ, et al. Effective treatments for PTSD: practice guidelines from the International Society for Traumatic Stress Studies. Guilford Press; 2009.
67. National Research Council. Treatment of posttraumatic stress disorder: an assessment of the evidence. Washington, DC: The National Academies Press; 2008.
68. Bradley R, Greene J, Russ E, et al. A multidimensional meta-analysis of psychotherapy for PTSD. Am J Psychiatry 2005;162(2):214–27.

Endocrine Effects of Anorexia Nervosa

Karen Klahr Miller, MD

KEYWORDS

- Anorexia nervosa • Hypogonadism • Hypercortisolemia • Growth hormone
- Osteoporosis

KEY POINTS

- Anorexia nervosa is a disease of psychiatric origin and is characterized by chronic starvation, with resultant neuroendocrine dysregulation.
- Endocrine complications of anorexia nervosa include hypothalamic amenorrhea, growth hormone resistance, and hypercortisolemia.
- Appetite hormone dysregulation has also been shown in girls and women with anorexia nervosa.
- Bone loss is prevalent and severe and a consequence of neuroendocrine hormone dysregulation in anorexia nervosa.
- The standard-of-care treatment of anorexia nervosa is multidisciplinary care aimed at psychological and nutritional recovery.
- Most, but not all, endocrine abnormalities, improve with psychological and nutritional recovery of anorexia nervosa.

EPIDEMIOLOGY

In 1874, Sir William Gull, one of Queen Victoria's physicians, coined the term anorexia nervosa to name a syndrome he had described in 1868 in an address to the Annual Meeting of the British Medical Association in Oxford, United Kingdom.[1] He reported having treated several girls and women between the ages of 16 and 23 years with severe emaciation for which he could discern no organic cause (including tuberculosis, a common causes of weight loss at the time). He noted the cardinal features of the disease to be bradycardia, hypothermia, and an endocrine complication, amenorrhea, that tended to reverse with refeeding. He also noted that the disease could on

Disclosure: Dr Miller has no relevant conflicts to disclose. This work was completed with the support of the following NIH grants: R01 DK052625 and R01 MH083657.
Harvard Medical School and Neuroendocrine Unit, BUL 457B, Massachusetts General Hospital, 55 Fruit Street, Boston, MA 02114, USA
E-mail address: kkmiller@partners.org

occasion be fatal. Although he reported that anorexia nervosa occurred primarily in women, he noted that it also occurred in men. He concluded that the syndrome was of psychiatric origin and although, in retrospect, the disease had likely existed for centuries (for example, Mary Queen of Scots' teenage illness has been attributed by some to anorexia nervosa), Gull's disease construct forms the basis of the current conception of the disease. The definition and understanding of anorexia nervosa have evolved, and continue to do so, with the most recent changes to the diagnostic criteria (Diagnostic and Statistical Manual of Mental Disorders V [DSM V]) published in May of 2013. The DSM V criteria no longer include amenorrhea as a necessary condition of the diagnosis, recognizing that vulnerability to neuroendocrine dysregulation is highly variable, and many women with all of the psychiatric features of anorexia nervosa and very low weight continue to have regular menstrual cycles. The DSM V are similar to those of the previous DSM diagnostic criteria, but broader, and require low body weight, restrictive eating behavior, fear of gaining weight, and body image disturbance. Anorexia nervosa is further subclassified into 2 types: restricting and binge-eating/purging, the latter characterized by recurrent episodes of binge eating or purging behaviors. There is significant crossover between the two types,[2] and the anorexia nervosa binge-eating/purging type differs from bulimia nervosa in that the former requires low weight for the diagnostic criteria to be met.

Anorexia nervosa is the third most common chronic disorder in adolescent girls[3] and has a reported prevalence of 0.3% to 3% in women.[4–6] The syndrome rarely affects boys and men, and less is known about the effects of anorexia nervosa in men that in women, though they seem to suffer from many of the same neuroendocrine complications as in girls and women. This article focuses on endocrine effects of anorexia nervosa in women.

Anorexia nervosa is commonly a chronic disease, particularly in adults. Between 20% and 30% of women with anorexia nervosa are afflicted chronically; 30% achieve partial recovery and 50% sustain a full recovery.[7] Anorexia nervosa carries a high risk of death, with a standardized mortality ratio of 11 to 12 times that expected,[8,9] and a particularly high risk of suicide of 56 times that expected for age and sex.[9] Alcoholism, advanced age, history of suicide attempt, severity and length of time of disease, and diuretic use all increase the risk of death from the disease.[9] Medical and endocrine complications of the disease include electrolyte disturbances, primarily hyponatremia, and hypokalemia, both of which occur in 20% of patients, and hypokalemia is observed in patients with binge-eating/purging type anorexia nervosa.[10] Hyponatremia can be severe enough to cause seizures, and may be caused by syndrome of inappropriate anti-diuretic hormone or primary polydipsia. Hypernatremia from diabetes insipidus has been reported but is rarely observed. Decreased T4 to T3 conversion is common.[11] Mild transaminitis (in 12%), anemia of chronic disease (in 39%), and leukocytopenia (in 34%) are commonly seen. With severely low weight, pancytopenia can occur.[12] Congestive heart failure secondary to ipecac, used to self-induce vomiting, is usually reversible with discontinuation of the offending agent. The endocrine complications about which most is known include hypothalamic amenorrhea, growth hormone (GH) resistance, hypercortisolemia, appetite hormone dysregulation, and bone loss (**Table 1**), and these are discussed in detail later.

HYPOTHALAMIC AMENORRHEA

The most widely recognized endocrine complication of anorexia nervosa is amenorrhea, which occurs in many, but not all, girls and women with anorexia nervosa. The early seminal characterization of minimum weight for height necessary for

Table 1 Endocrine dysfunction in women and adolescent girls with anorexia nervosa		
	Women and Adolescent Girls with Anorexia Nervosa	Implicated in Bone Loss
Hypothalamic Amenorrhea	✓	✓
GH Resistance	✓	
↑GH	✓	
↓IGF-I	✓	✓
Hypercortisolemia	✓	✓
Appetite Hormone Dysregulation	✓	
↑PYY	✓	✓
↓Leptin	✓	
↑Ghrelin	✓	

Abbreviations: IGF-I, insulinlike growth factor I; PYY, peptide YY.

menarche and normal reproductive function, as described by Frisch and McArthur[13] in the 1970s, is a concept that formed the basis for understanding the cause of amenorrhea that has evolved over the subsequent decades. It is now understood that many, but not all, women with anorexia nervosa develop hypothalamic amenorrhea, which may, in part, be regulated by adipocyte adipokine secretion. The physiology underlying hypothalamic amenorrhea was first described in a detailed manner in an article by Boyar and colleagues,[14] published in the New England Journal of Medicine in 1974. In that paper and subsequent work, Boyar and colleagues[14] carefully delineated several patterns of dysregulated luteinizing hormone (LH) pulsatility in amenorrheic women with anorexia nervosa. LH pulses reflect gonadotrophin-releasing hormone (GnRH) pulsatility and are readily measurable in the periphery by frequent blood sampling, in contrast with GnRH. Boyar and colleagues[14] described altered LH, and therefore GnRH pulsatility, in women with anorexia nervosa, including an absence of pulsations and pubertal patterns in which pulsatility occurs only during the night. They also showed reversal to normal of LH pulsatility in women who regained weight and recovered menses. They also showed that the degree of immaturity of LH pattern did not correlate reliably with duration of illness, degree of fatness, or extent of deficit from ideal weight, and that regaining of menses did not show a simple relationship to weight.[15] These observations reflect 2 important concepts observed in clinical practice that are still not well understood, namely: (1) that although many women with very low weight develop hypothalamic amenorrhea, others of comparable low weight remain eumenorrheic; and (2) although many women with anorexia nervosa recover normal reproductive function with weight restoration, approximately 15% remain amenorrheic.[16] A partial understanding of the mechanisms underlying these phenomena has occurred with the recognition of adipose tissue as an endocrine organ that secretes peptides that regulate energy balance, appetite, and other functions, including reproduction. Most of this work has focused on leptin, a 16-kDa peptide, primarily expressed in adipocytes and secreted in response to short-term caloric intake. It is thought that leptin's primary role is to signal inadequate energy stores, and leptin has been shown in both humans and animals to directly regulate reproductive function. Leptin receptors are present in the hypothalamus, and congenital leptin deficiency is characterized by hypogonadotropic hypogonadism in addition to obesity.[17] Particularly relevant to identifying the cause of hypothalamic amenorrhea in anorexia nervosa, leptin has been shown to play an important causal role in starvation-associated hypothalamic amenorrhea. In an important study by Ahima and colleagues,[18] leptin replacement prevented the delay of estrous in mice caused by 48 hours of fasting, suggesting that the acute decrease in leptin observed with fasting is responsible for the impairment in reproduction function observed with starvation. Similarly, mean serum leptin levels are lower in association with lower body fat mass in women with anorexia nervosa who experience amenorrhea than in women with anorexia nervosa of comparable mean low weight but without amenorrhea.[19] However, there is considerable overlap between leptin levels in the two groups, and there is no threshold below which amenorrhea is a certainty or above which eumenorrhea can be predicted to resume.[19] The implications of these findings include that leptin levels cannot be used clinically to set recovery goals and that hypoleptinemia is only one factor of many that likely are implicated in the pathophysiology of the hypothalamic amenorrhea in women with anorexia nervosa. Other factors that may be involved include kisspeptin, cortisol, and/or appetite-regulating peptides, but none has been specifically implicated as a factor in the pathophysiology of hypothalamic amenorrhea in anorexia nervosa. Kisspeptin, the endogenous ligand for the hypothalamic kisspeptin receptor, inactivating mutations of which result in pubertal failure,[20,21] is one candidate. Acute, but not chronic, administration of kisspeptin has been shown to result in gonadotropin release in a group of women with hypothalamic amenorrhea,[22] but women with anorexia nervosa specifically have not been studied. Leptin administration to 8 healthy-weight women with functional hypothalamic amenorrhea (body mass index [BMI] 18.8–24.4 kg/m^2) resulted in ovulatory cycles in 3 but also resulted in weight loss.[23] Therefore, leptin administration, should it become more widely available, is not an appropriate therapeutic option for women with anorexia nervosa.

The mechanisms underlying lack of recovery of hypothalamic amenorrhea in some women with anorexia nervosa despite weight recovery are incompletely understood. One study showed lower leptin levels compared with healthy women of similar mean BMI and persistence of disordered eating–related psychological symptoms in a group of such women, possibly reflecting incomplete recovery of fat mass and psychological symptoms in some of the women.[24]

Hypothalamic amenorrhea in women with anorexia nervosa results in hypoandrogenemia in addition to hypoestrogenemia, with a further reduction in free testosterone levels in women with anorexia nervosa receiving oral contraceptives. This finding has been shown in a group of 169 women with anorexia nervosa compared with 21 healthy controls[25] and follows logically because, in women of reproductive age, approximately 60% of serum testosterone is secreted from the ovaries, whereas 40% is of adrenal origin, as shown in bilateral oophorectomy studies.[26] Studies in adults have shown no decrement in the adrenally derived prohormone dehydroepiandrosterone sulfate (DHEAS) compared with lean controls,[25] and dehydroepiandrosterone (DHEA) levels stimulate normally with cosyntropin.[27] In contrast, a study in adolescent girls showed low DHEAS levels in relation to a laboratory-generated normal range.[28] The consequences, if any, of relative androgen deficiency in women with anorexia nervosa are not known, but may include a reduction in muscle mass or bone mass, and or negative effects on mood, as observed in hypogonadal men, although testosterone levels are 10 to 20 times greater in men than in healthy women and therefore the relevance of relatively low androgen levels in women cannot be extrapolated from data in men. With regard to muscle mass, a small, 1-year, randomized, placebo-controlled study of low-dose transdermal testosterone (300 μg daily) showed increases in lean body mass,[29] suggesting a possible effect of hypogonadism to cause a relative reduction in muscle mass. In contrast, the same study showed no effect on bone mass, despite an acute increase in a marker of bone formation.[29] A cross-sectional study showed an inverse relationship between serum androgen levels and severity of depression and anxiety symptoms in women with anorexia nervosa such that, in general, women with the lowest androgen levels experienced the most severe depression and anxiety symptoms.[30] Whether relative androgen deficiency contributes to affective comorbidities and whether androgen replacement therapy would be effective therapeutically is unknown. In addition, although the data regarding androgen effects on libido and sexual function in postmenopausal women show effectiveness on these end points, whether low libido or sexual dysfunction are prevalent and affected by relative androgen deficiency in women with anorexia nervosa and/or responds to low-dose androgen therapy has not been studied.

GH RESISTANCE

Roth and colleagues[31] reported an increase in GH with fasting in healthy subjects in 1963 in *Science*, and, in contrast with what was expected given the known effects of GH to stimulate insulinlike growth factor I (IGF-I) release from the liver, subsequent studies showed low IGF-I levels, a phenomenon termed GH resistance because the liver is resistant to the usual effects of GH. Studies in the 1990s established that both basal and pulsatile GH release are increased in women with anorexia nervosa, the former 4 times and the latter 20 times the levels observed in healthy-weight women of comparable age.[32] GH secretion is also higher in adolescent girls with anorexia nervosa than in healthy adolescent girls, including during the time of their physiologic peak in GH.[33] However, despite the increase in GH secretion, IGF-I levels are low in anorexia nervosa, and this cannot be attributed to decreases in binding globulins. This was shown by Stoving and colleagues,[34] who reported reduced IGF-I bioactivity using a kinase receptor activation assay. The low serum IGF-I levels are thought to cause the increase in GH through a feedback mechanism. Even high doses of GH are ineffective in overcoming GH resistance in women with anorexia nervosa, as was shown by Fazeli and colleagues,[35] who administered GH at a mean maximum daily dose of 1.4 mg/d for 12 weeks to a group of women with anorexia nervosa and observed no significant resultant increase in serum IGF-I levels. These doses of GH resulted in a reduction in fat mass and leptin levels, likely from the IGF-I–independent effects of GH, with no benefit to lean body mass or bone, likely because GH effects are mediated primarily by IGF-I.

Studies suggest that GH resistance reverses with weight gain in women with anorexia nervosa. IGF-I levels seem to increase in a stepwise fashion with weight gain, resulting in a reduction of GH levels to normal through intact feedback mechanisms.[32,34,36]

HYPERCORTISOLEMIA

In 1977, Boyar and colleagues[11] were also the first to establish that anorexia nervosa can be accompanied by hypercortisolemia. They reported that 24-hour mean plasma cortisol concentrations were nearly double in women with anorexia nervosa compared with healthy controls because of an increased half-life and decreased clearance rate rather than an increased cortisol production rate. In addition, 24-hour urinary cortisol was increased in 2 of 5 patients in whom the data were available. A subsequent study by Doerr and colleagues[37] in 1980 established lack of dexamethasone suppressibility of cortisol and the reversibility of the hypercortisolemia with a modest amount of weight gain, although subsequent studies have identified a subgroup of patients with anorexia nervosa in whom hypercortisolemia persists despite weight recovery.[38–40] Subsequent studies have also established an increased serum cortisol response to cortrosyn[27] and increased midnight salivary cortisol levels[41] in anorexia nervosa. Although women with hypercortisolemia secondary to anorexia nervosa are underweight in contrast with the characteristic central adiposity of Cushing syndrome, there are consequences of hypercortisolemia in anorexia nervosa that mirror those observed in Cushing syndrome. For example, women with anorexia nervosa and higher urine free cortisol levels tend to accumulate proportionally more trunk, than extremity, fat during recovery.[42] Higher serum cortisol levels similarly predict future weight gain and return of menses in adolescent girls with anorexia nervosa,[43] the latter likely being a consequence, at least partially, of the former. Another impactful consequence of hypercortisolemia that mirrors that observed in Cushing syndrome is bone loss, which is discussed later. In addition, degree of hypercortisolemia is associated with severity of depression, anxiety, and reduced bone mineral density in anorexia nervosa.[44]

APPETITE HORMONE DYSREGULATION

A recent area of investigation has been appetite regulation in anorexia nervosa, which is characterized by restrictive eating behavior despite low weight, leading to speculation about the presence of appetite hormone dysregulation in this syndrome. Although increased serum levels of anorexigenic hormones and suppressed serum levels of orexigenic hormones would be predicted in this state of chronic starvation, this has proved only partially to be the case. Serum levels of the anorexigenic hormone leptin are suppressed, as predicted based on lower fat mass, the source of leptin secretion.[45,46] However, the anorexigenic hormone peptide YY (PYY), which is secreted by intestinal L cells in response to food intake, is increased in both girls and women with anorexia nervosa compared with normal controls,[47,48] leading to speculation that dysregulation of the neuropeptide Y (NPY)-PYY appetite regulatory system may play a causal role in the development of anorexia nervosa in some patients. However, this hypothesis is difficult to test, and it is unclear whether it is the case. PYY levels are positively associated with degree of eating disorder thinking and behavior as determined by self-administered questionnaires, independently of weight,[49] suggesting a possible relationship between the psychological features of anorexia nervosa and PYY. Mean serum levels of the orexigenic hormone ghrelin, which is released by oxyntic cells of the stomach, seems to be higher in girls and women with anorexia nervosa than controls,[50–52] as would be predicted in a nutritionally deprived population. However, one study reported low ghrelin levels in women with anorexia nervosa and binge-eating/purging type[53] and another showed an amplified reduction in ghrelin levels during a euglycemic hyperinsulinemic clamp,[54] raising the question of whether the normal ghrelin suppressive secretory response to food is exaggerated in anorexia nervosa and might lead to an increased sensation of satiety in such patients.

NEUROENDOCRINE DYSREGULATION AND BONE LOSS

Hypogonadism, GH resistance, hypercortisolemia, and appetite hormone dysregulation contribute to the severe bone loss observed in girls and women with anorexia nervosa. Despite a mean age in the mid-20s in most studies, more than 90% of women with anorexia nervosa have osteopenia and 40% have osteoporosis,[55] with fewer than 15% of such women having normal bone density at all skeletal sites.[10] Bone mineral density decreases at a mean rate of 2.5% per year in women with anorexia nervosa,[56] and adolescent girls with anorexia nervosa do not experience the sharp increase in bone mineral density that normally occurs during puberty,[57] which results in lower bone mineral density in girls with anorexia nervosa compared with appropriate controls at a critical time for accrual of bone toward peak bone mass.[58] The consequence is an increased fracture risk in adolescent girls as well as women with anorexia nervosa.[10] Studies have reported a 30% prevalence of history of fracture in women with anorexia nervosa[10] and a fracture rate 7 times that expected for sex and age.[59] Newer imaging modalities have shown abnormalities in bone microarchitecture, both the trabecular and cortical components, in both women[60] and girls[61,62] with anorexia nervosa. Moreover, bone strength, as determined by finite element analysis modeling, is reduced in anorexia nervosa.[63] Bredella and colleagues[62] showed abnormalities in bone microarchitecture in girls with recent-onset anorexia nervosa, before decrements in bone mineral density are evident. This finding suggests that anorexia nervosa exerts deleterious effects on bone early in the disease, and, that early intervention may be necessary to prevent bone loss. Although bone mass generally increases with weight recovery, residual bone loss is common,[64] and weight recovery may take years to achieve. Therefore, early intervention with the goal of weight and neuroendocrine function restoration is important, and research into therapeutic strategies aimed at treating low bone mineral density is important.

The pathophysiology of bone loss is complex, and several neuroendocrine systems have been implicated (see **Table 1**). Bone formation is reduced, and bone resorption is increased in women with anorexia nervosa,[65] resulting in particularly severe bone loss in this disease. In contrast, both bone formation and resorption are suppressed in adolescent girls with anorexia nervosa,[66] reflecting important differences in skeletal physiology during adolescence versus adulthood. Adolescence is a period of heightened bone turnover (reflected by an increase in markers of bone metabolism, both formation and resorption) leading to rapid accrual of bone mass in the attainment of peak bone mass. Bone metabolism overall is suppressed in adolescent girls with anorexia nervosa, preventing the normal rapid bone mass accrual seen in this age group. Because of these differences in underlying skeletal physiology between these two age groups, caution is advised in extrapolating research results from one age group to the other. Studies in both adults and adolescents implicate hypogonadism, hypercortisolemia, relative IGF-I deficiency, and appetite hormone dysregulation in the pathogenesis of bone loss; however, significant differences in response to therapies in the two groups of women have been observed.

The importance of hypogonadism as a contributing factor has been highlighted in several studies. The regaining of menses has been shown as critical to skeletal recovery, independent of weight gain.[56] In 1 study, weight gain without reproductive function recovery did not result in skeletal recovery.[56] In another study, bone mineral density in 74 women with anorexia nervosa and amenorrhea was compared with that of 42 women with anorexia nervosa and eumenorrhea.[19] Both groups showed low mean bone mineral density, particularly at the spine. However, although the mean posteroanterior spine T score in the amenorrheic group was −1.9 (1.9 standard deviations less than the mean for a healthy young woman), that of the eumenorrheic group was −0.9. Bone mineral density is similarly lower in women with anorexia nervosa than in normal-weight women with hypothalamic amenorrhea.[67] These studies suggest that gonadal steroid deficiency is a significant contributor to bone loss in women with anorexia nervosa; roughly as important a factor as nutritional state (ie, weight).

However, amenorrhea may simply be a marker of degree of undernutrition and/or degree of neuroendocrine dysregulation. Undernutrition, as reflected in body mass index, is an important determinant of weight, with lean body mass the most predictive body composition component.[57] The only fat depot that studies have shown to be strongly associated with bone mineral density in anorexia nervosa is bone marrow fat, which is increased in anorexia nervosa and negatively correlates with bone mineral density.[68] Whether this observation holds clues to the pathogenesis of bone loss in anorexia nervosa is unknown. Because osteoblasts and adipocytes share a common mesenchymal stem cell precursor, the increased bone marrow fat in anorexia nervosa may provide a key to understanding the mechanisms underlying reduced bone formation or simply reflect a default into the fat lineage caused by impaired osteoblastogenesis. No specific macronutrient or micronutrient component of the diet has been identified as an important determinant of bone mineral density. The cause and development of bone loss in this population does not seem to involve calcium and vitamin D deficiency, because both women and girls with anorexia nervosa ingest comparable amounts to those of healthy counterparts (largely in the form of supplements[69,70]) but have lower bone mineral density.

Direct effects of hypogonadism on bone, if present, may be secondary to relative estrogen or androgen deficiency. Data in support of estrogen mediation are stronger than those for androgen mediation, mostly in the form of small, prospective controlled studies of gonadal hormone administration. Oral estrogens at doses used routinely to treat postmenopausal osteoporosis do not seem to increase bone mineral density in women with anorexia nervosa,[71] although at the higher oral contraceptive doses they may help prevent further bone loss,[72] but the data in this regard are not conclusive. The most important role of estrogen, which may have a significant impact, is in older adolescents, in whom peak bone mass attainment is inhibited by the effects of starvation. Misra and colleagues[73] showed that estrogen administration in low doses designed to mimic estrogen levels observed in puberty (100 μg of 17-beta estradiol with cyclic progesterone transdermally in girls with a bone age $\geq$15 years and oral ethinyl estradiol 3.75 μg daily from 0 to 6 months, 7.5 μg from 6 to 12 months, and 11.25 μg from 12 to 18 months in girls with bone age <15 years) increased bone mineral density significantly, although these interventions resulted in less than normal bone accrual rates during an 18-month period. Although low-dose estrogen is the most promising therapy for adolescent bone loss in anorexia nervosa so far investigated, further studies are needed to optimize therapy to achieve normalization of bone mineral density and attainment of optimal peak bone mass. Although low-dose testosterone administration stimulates bone formation over a period of weeks to months,[29,74] it does not result in significant increases in bone mineral density in women with anorexia nervosa.[29] Neither DHEA nor ethinyl estradiol 20 μg/levonorgesterol 0.1 mg daily administered to a group of young adults and adolescents improved bone mineral density after controlling for increases in weight,[28] but a subsequent study combining the two hormonal strategies resulted in preservation of spine and total-body bone mineral density compared with placebo, which was associated with decreases in bone mineral density at these sites.[75] A small, randomized, controlled study of DHEA 100 mg daily (double the dose administered in the two previous studies) showed no effects on bone mass but did show an increase BMI.[76] These findings have not been replicated.

The importance of GH as a bone anabolic agent cannot be overstated, as shown by numerous studies establishing it as one of the primary factors responsible for linear growth in children and maintenance of normal bone mass in adults. The actions of GH are largely mediated through its stimulation of IGF-I secretion. IGF-I is anabolic to bone, stimulates osteoblast differentiation, and also exerts antiresorptive effects. Therefore, GH resistance, and the accompanying absence of normal IGF-I levels in women with anorexia nervosa, are of central importance in the development of bone loss in this population. Low serum IGF-I levels are associated with low markers of bone formation, suggesting that a lack of normal anabolic action accompanies relative IGF-I deficiency in anorexia nervosa.[57] Moreover, Lawson and colleagues[60] showed an association between serum IGF-I levels and bone microarchitectural parameters. Recombinant IGF-I (rhIGF-I) replacement therapy has been shown to increase bone mineral density in women with anorexia nervosa compared with placebo (2.8% when combined with oral contraceptives and 1.4% when administered alone) over 9 months.[72] However, this increase is not large enough to result in normal bone mineral density, and rhIGF-I is not approved by the US Food and Drug Administration for this indication. In addition, it is not known whether IGF-I replacement therapy is effective at increasing bone density in adolescents with anorexia nervosa.

Consistent with the deleterious effects of hypercortisolemia on the skeletal system observed in patients with Cushing syndrome, hypercortisolemia may be a factor contributing to bone loss in women with anorexia nervosa. Bone mineral density is inversely associated with pooled frequently sampled serum cortisol levels in both women and girls with anorexia nervosa.[44,77] At this time, it is unknown how to translate the known relationship between hypercortisolemia and low bone mineral density into a clinical strategy, because lowering of cortisol levels is predicted to result in weight loss and may cause adrenal insufficiency.

The interplay between appetite hormone dysregulation and bone mineral density has been investigated, with resultant data mostly suggesting indirect effects. The exception is that of PYY, levels of which are paradoxically high in women and girls with anorexia nervosa and strongly inversely correlated with bone mineral density, even after controlling for weight.[78] In contrast, no direct relationship between ghrelin or leptin and bone mineral density in anorexia nervosa has been shown. However, leptin may mediate bone loss through its effects on reproduction, and further studies on the effects of appetite hormones on skeletal physiology are warranted and ongoing.

Nonhormonal treatments for low bone density have also been investigated, particularly bisphosphonates. Risedronate has been shown to be effective at increasing bone mineral density in women with anorexia nervosa, although, as in other cited therapeutic studies, bone mineral density did not normalize with a 1-year course of therapy.[29] In contrast, Golden and colleagues[79] studied the effects of alendronate administration on bone mineral density in adolescent girls with anorexia nervosa, and showed no increase in bone mineral density at any skeletal site after accounting for increases caused by weight gain over time. Whether the differences in effects are attributable to specific age-based or endocrine-based differences between adults and adolescents, differences in recovery rates, or other factors is unknown. In addition, the effects of bisphosphonates on fetal development are unknown and therefore these medications should not be used in women or adolescent girls who are pregnant or at risk of becoming pregnant during or shortly after their use.

A question that is often raised is whether weight-bearing exercise is beneficial to skeletal health in patients with anorexia nervosa, as it has shown to be for postmenopausal women. Health care providers routinely restrict exercise in women with anorexia nervosa in order to aid in the restoration of energy balance and promote weight gain. A recent study confirmed that exercise exerts deleterious effects on bone mineral density in underweight women with anorexia nervosa.[80] However, a beneficial effect was shown in women who were weight-recovered from anorexia nervosa.[80] Further research is warranted to more fully understand the mechanisms responsible for bone loss in anorexia nervosa and to determine the most effective and safest therapies.

IMPLICATIONS

Neuroendocrine hormone dysregulation, including hypothalamic amenorrhea, GH resistance, and hypercortisolemia, has serious implications for the health of girls and women with anorexia nervosa. In most patients with anorexia nervosa, this results in severe bone loss, which increases the risk for fractures. The pathophysiology of bone loss in anorexia nervosa is incompletely understood, and further studies are warranted to determine an optimal treatment strategy that results in normalization of bone mass. It is important when evaluating research results and considering therapeutic options to bear in mind that, because adolescent skeletal physiology differs in fundamental ways from that of adult skeletal physiology, results from investigations in one age group cannot be extrapolated to the other.

Neuroendocrine dysfunction largely reverses with weight gain and psychiatric recovery, including reproductive dysfunction, which usually recovers with weight gain but can be permanent. In such cases, assisted-reproductive technologies may be successful. Bone loss tends to reverse also, especially in those who regain menses with weight gain, but residual deficits often persist. The mainstay of therapy for anorexia nervosa remains a treatment team approach, usually consisting of a psychologist and/or psychologist, nutritionist, and primary care physician, with the therapeutic goal of restoration of psychological health and weight restoration.

REFERENCES

1. Gull WW. Address in medicine delivered before the Annual Meeting of the British Medical Association at Oxford. Lancet 1868;2:171–6.
2. Eddy KT, Keel PK, Dorer DJ, et al. Longitudinal comparison of anorexia nervosa subtypes. Int J Eat Disord 2002;31(2):191–201.
3. Lucas AR, Beard CM, O'Fallon WM, et al. 50-year trends in the incidence of anorexia nervosa in Rochester, Minn.: a population-based study. Am J Psychiatry 1991;148(7):917–22.
4. Garfinkel PE, Lin E, Goering P, et al. Should amenorrhoea be necessary for the diagnosis of anorexia nervosa? Evidence from a Canadian community sample. Br J Psychiatry 1996;168(4):500–6.
5. Hoek HW, van Hoeken D. Review of the prevalence and incidence of eating disorders. Int J Eat Disord 2003;34(4):383–96.
6. Walters EE, Kendler KS. Anorexia nervosa and anorexic-like syndromes in a population-based female twin sample. Am J Psychiatry 1995;152(1):64–71.
7. Fairburn CG, Harrison PJ. Eating disorders. Lancet 2003;361(9355):407–16.
8. Huas C, Caille A, Godart N, et al. Factors predictive of ten-year mortality in severe anorexia nervosa patients. Acta Psychiatr Scand 2011;123(1):62–70.
9. Keel PK, Dorer DJ, Eddy KT, et al. Predictors of mortality in eating disorders. Arch Gen Psychiatry 2003;60(2):179–83.
10. Miller KK, Grinspoon SK, Ciampa J, et al. Medical findings in outpatients with anorexia nervosa. Arch Intern Med 2005;165(5):561–6.
11. Boyar RM, Hellman LD, Roffwarg H, et al. Cortisol secretion and metabolism in anorexia nervosa. N Engl J Med 1977;296(4):190–3.
12. Sabel AL, Gaudiani JL, Statland B, et al. Hematological abnormalities in severe anorexia nervosa. Ann Hematol 2013;92(5):605–13.
13. Frisch RE, McArthur JW. Menstrual cycles: fatness as a determinant of minimum weight for height necessary for their maintenance or onset. Science 1974; 185(4155):949–51.

14. Boyar RM, Katz J, Finkelstein JW, et al. Anorexia nervosa. Immaturity of the 24-hour luteinizing hormone secretory pattern. N Engl J Med 1974;291(17):861–5.

15. Katz JL, Boyar R, Roffwarg H, et al. Weight and circadian luteinizing hormone secretory pattern in anorexia nervosa. Psychosom Med 1978;40(7):549–67.

16. Jocoangeli F, Masala S, Staar Mezzasalma F, et al. Amenorrhea after weight recovery in anorexia nervosa: role of body composition and endocrine abnormalities. Eat Weight Disord 2006;11:e20–6.

17. Strobel A, Issad T, Camoin L, et al. A leptin missense mutation associated with hypogonadism and morbid obesity. Nat Genet 1998;18(3):213–5.

18. Ahima RS, Prabakaran D, Mantzoros C, et al. Role of leptin in the neuroendocrine response to fasting. Nature 1996;382(6588):250–2.

19. Miller KK, Grinspoon S, Gleysteen S, et al. Preservation of neuroendocrine control of reproductive function despite severe undernutrition. J Clin Endocrinol Metab 2004;89(9):4434–8.

20. de Roux N, Genin E, Carel JC, et al. Hypogonadotropic hypogonadism due to loss of function of the KiSS1-derived peptide receptor GPR54. Proc Natl Acad Sci U S A 2003;100(19):10972–6.

21. Seminara SB, Messager S, Chatzidaki EE, et al. The GPR54 gene as a regulator of puberty. N Engl J Med 2003;349(17):1614–27.

22. Jayasena CN, Nijher GM, Chaudhri OB, et al. Subcutaneous injection of kisspeptin-54 acutely stimulates gonadotropin secretion in women with hypothalamic amenorrhea, but chronic administration causes tachyphylaxis. J Clin Endocrinol Metab 2009;94(11):4315–23.

23. Wolt CK, Chan JL, Bullen J, et al. Recombinant human leptin in women with hypothalamic amenorrhea. N Engl J Med 2004;351(10):987–97.

24. Brambilla F, Monteleone P, Bortolotti F, et al. Persistent amenorrhoea in weight-recovered anorexics: psychological and biological aspects. Psychiatry Res 2003;118(3):249–57.

25. Miller KK, Lawson EA, Mathur V, et al. Androgens in women with anorexia nervosa and normal-weight women with hypothalamic amenorrhea. J Clin Endocrinol Metab 2007;92(4):1334–9.

26. Judd HL, Lucas WE, Yen SS. Effect of oophorectomy on circulating testosterone and androstenedione levels in patients with endometrial cancer. Am J Obstet Gynecol 1974;118(6):793–8.

27. Lawson EA, Misra M, Meenaghan E, et al. Adrenal glucocorticoid and androgen precursor dissociation in anorexia nervosa. J Clin Endocrinol Metab 2009;94(4):1367–71.

28. Gordon CM, Grace E, Emans SJ, et al. Effects of oral dehydroepiandrosterone on bone density in young women with anorexia nervosa: a randomized trial. J Clin Endocrinol Metab 2002;87(11):4935–41.

29. Miller KK, Meenaghan E, Lawson EA, et al. Effects of risedronate and low-dose transdermal testosterone on bone mineral density in women with anorexia nervosa: a randomized, placebo-controlled study. J Clin Endocrinol Metab 2011;96(7):2081–8.

30. Miller KK, Wexler TL, Zha AM, et al. Androgen deficiency: association with increased anxiety and depression symptom severity in anorexia nervosa. J Clin Psychiatry 2007;68(6):959–65.

31. Roth J, Glick SM, Yalow RS, et al. Hypoglycemia: a potent stimulus to secretion of growth hormone. Science 1963;140:987–8.

32. Stoving RK, Veldhuis JD, Flyvbjerg A, et al. Jointly amplified basal and pulsatile growth hormone (GH) secretion and increased process irregularity in women

with anorexia nervosa: indirect evidence for disruption of feedback regulation within the GH-insulin-like growth factor I axis. J Clin Endocrinol Metab 1999; 84(6):2056–63.

33. Misra M, Miller KK, Bjornson J, et al. Alterations in growth hormone secretory dynamics in adolescent girls with anorexia nervosa and effects on bone metabolism. J Clin Endocrinol Metab 2003;88(12):5615–23.

34. Stoving RK, Chen JW, Glintborg D, et al. Bioactive insulin-like growth factor (IGF) I and IGF-binding protein-1 in anorexia nervosa. J Clin Endocrinol Metab 2007;92(6):2323–9.

35. Fazeli PK, Lawson EA, Prabhakaran R, et al. Effects of recombinant human growth hormone in anorexia nervosa: a randomized, placebo-controlled study. J Clin Endocrinol Metab 2010;95(11):4889–97.

36. Hill KK, Hill DB, McClain MP, et al. Serum insulin-like growth factor-I concentrations in the recovery of patients with anorexia nervosa. J Am Coll Nutr 1993; 12(4):475–8.

37. Doerr P, Fichter M, Pirke KM, et al. Relationship between weight gain and hypothalamic pituitary adrenal function in patients with anorexia nervosa. J Steroid Biochem 1980;13(5):529–37.

38. Gwirtsman HE, Kaye WH, Curtis SR, et al. Energy intake and dietary macronutrient content in women with anorexia nervosa and volunteers. J Am Diet Assoc 1989;89(1):54–7.

39. Schweitzer I, Szmukler GI, Maguire KP, et al. The dexamethasone suppression test in anorexia nervosa. The influence of weight, depression, adrenocorticotrophic hormone and dexamethasone. Br J Psychiatry 1990;157:713–7.

40. Walsh BT, Katz JL, Levin J, et al. The production rate of cortisol declines during recovery from anorexia nervosa. J Clin Endocrinol Metab 1981;53(1): 203–5.

41. Putignano P, Dubini A, Toja P, et al. Salivary cortisol measurement in normal-weight, obese and anorexic women: comparison with plasma cortisol. Eur J Endocrinol 2001;145(2):165–71.

42. Grinspoon S, Thomas L, Miller K, et al. Changes in regional fat redistribution and the effects of estrogen during spontaneous weight gain in women with anorexia nervosa. Am J Clin Nutr 2001;73(5):865–9.

43. Misra M, Prabhakaran R, Miller KK, et al. Role of cortisol in menstrual recovery in adolescent girls with anorexia nervosa. Pediatr Res 2006;59(4 Pt 1):598–603.

44. Lawson EA, Donoho D, Miller KK, et al. Hypercortisolemia is associated with severity of bone loss and depression in hypothalamic amenorrhea and anorexia nervosa. J Clin Endocrinol Metab 2009;94(12):4710–6.

45. Grinspoon S, Gulick T, Askari H, et al. Serum leptin levels in women with anorexia nervosa. J Clin Endocrinol Metab 1996;81(11):3861–3.

46. Hebebrand J, Blum WF, Barth N, et al. Leptin levels in patients with anorexia nervosa are reduced in the acute stage and elevated upon short-term weight restoration. Mol Psychiatry 1997;2(4):330–4.

47. Misra M, Miller KK, Tsai P, et al. Elevated peptide YY levels in adolescent girls with anorexia nervosa. J Clin Endocrinol Metab 2006;91(3):1027–33.

48. Pfluger PT, Kampe J, Castaneda TR, et al. Effect of human body weight changes on circulating levels of peptide YY and peptide YY3-36. J Clin Endocrinol Metab 2007;92(2):583–8.

49. Lawson EA, Eddy KT, Donoho D, et al. Appetite-regulating hormones cortisol and peptide YY are associated with disordered eating psychopathology, independent of body mass index. Eur J Endocrinol 2011;164(2):253–61.

50. Misra M, Miller KK, Kuo K, et al. Secretory dynamics of ghrelin in adolescent girls with anorexia nervosa and healthy adolescents. Am J Physiol Endocrinol Metab 2005;289(2):E347–56.
51. Monteleone P, Serritella C, Martiadis V, et al. Plasma obestatin, ghrelin, and ghrelin/obestatin ratio are increased in underweight patients with anorexia nervosa but not in symptomatic patients with bulimia nervosa. J Clin Endocrinol Metab 2008;93(11):4418–21.
52. Usdan LS, Khaodhiar L, Apovian CM. The endocrinopathies of anorexia nervosa. Endocr Pract 2008;14(8):1055–63.
53. Germain N, Galusca B, Grouselle D, et al. Ghrelin and obestatin circadian levels differentiate bingeing-purging from restrictive anorexia nervosa. J Clin Endocrinol Metab 2010;95(6):3057–62.
54. Karczewska-Kupczewska M, Straczkowski M, Adamska A, et al. Increased suppression of serum ghrelin concentration by hyperinsulinemia in women with anorexia nervosa. Eur J Endocrinol 2010;162(2):235–9.
55. Grinspoon S, Thomas E, Pitts S, et al. Prevalence and predictive factors for regional osteopenia in women with anorexia nervosa. Ann Intern Med 2000; 133(10):790–4.
56. Miller KK, Lee EE, Lawson EA, et al. Determinants of skeletal loss and recovery in anorexia nervosa. J Clin Endocrinol Metab 2006;91(8):2931–7.
57. Soyka LA, Misra M, Frenchman A, et al. Abnormal bone mineral accrual in adolescent girls with anorexia nervosa. J Clin Endocrinol Metab 2002;87(9): 4177–85.
58. Misra M, Aggarwal A, Miller KK, et al. Effects of anorexia nervosa on clinical, hematologic, biochemical, and bone density parameters in community-dwelling adolescent girls. Pediatrics 2004;114(6):1574–83.
59. Rigotti NA, Neer RM, Skates SJ, et al. The clinical course of osteoporosis in anorexia nervosa. A longitudinal study of cortical bone mass. JAMA 1991; 265(9):1133–8.
60. Lawson EA, Miller KK, Bredella MA, et al. Hormone predictors of abnormal bone microarchitecture in women with anorexia nervosa. Bone 2010;46(2):458–63.
61. Faje AT, Karim L, Taylor A, et al. Adolescent girls with anorexia nervosa have impaired cortical and trabecular microarchitecture and lower estimated bone strength at the distal radius. J Clin Endocrinol Metab 2013;98(5):1923–9.
62. Bredella MA, Misra M, Miller KK, et al. Distal radius in adolescent girls with anorexia nervosa: trabecular structure analysis with high-resolution flat-panel volume CT. Radiology 2008;249(3):938–46.
63. Walsh CJ, Phan CM, Misra M, et al. Women with anorexia nervosa: finite element and trabecular structure analysis by using flat-panel volume CT. Radiology 2010;257(1):167–74.
64. Herzog W, Minne H, Deter C, et al. Outcome of bone mineral density in anorexia nervosa patients 11.7 years after first admission. J Bone Miner Res 1993;8(5): 597–605.
65. Grinspoon S, Baum H, Lee K, et al. Effects of short-term recombinant human insulin-like growth factor I administration on bone turnover in osteopenic women with anorexia nervosa. J Clin Endocrinol Metab 1996;81(11):3864–70.
66. Misra M, Soyka LA, Miller KK, et al. Serum osteoprotegerin in adolescent girls with anorexia nervosa. J Clin Endocrinol Metab 2003;88(8):3816–22.
67. Grinspoon S, Miller K, Coyle C, et al. Severity of osteopenia in estrogen-deficient women with anorexia nervosa and hypothalamic amenorrhea. J Clin Endocrinol Metab 1999;84(6):2049–55.

68. Bredella MA, Fazeli PK, Miller KK, et al. Increased bone marrow fat in anorexia nervosa. J Clin Endocrinol Metab 2009;94(6):2129–36.
69. Hadigan CM, Anderson EJ, Miller KK, et al. Assessment of macronutrient and micronutrient intake in women with anorexia nervosa. Int J Eat Disord 2000; 28(3):284–92.
70. Misra M, Tsai P, Anderson EJ, et al. Nutrient intake in community-dwelling adolescent girls with anorexia nervosa and in healthy adolescents. Am J Clin Nutr 2006;84(4):698–706.
71. Klibanski A, Biller BM, Schoenfeld DA, et al. The effects of estrogen administration on trabecular bone loss in young women with anorexia nervosa. J Clin Endocrinol Metab 1995;80(3):898–904.
72. Grinspoon S, Thomas L, Miller K, et al. Effects of recombinant human IGF-I and oral contraceptive administration on bone density in anorexia nervosa. J Clin Endocrinol Metab 2002;87(6):2883–91.
73. Misra M, Katzman D, Miller KK, et al. Physiologic estrogen replacement increases bone density in adolescent girls with anorexia nervosa. J Bone Miner Res 2011;26(10):2430–8.
74. Miller KK, Grieco KA, Klibanski A. Testosterone administration in women with anorexia nervosa. J Clin Endocrinol Metab 2005;90(3):1428–33.
75. Divasta AD, Feldman HA, Giancaterino C, et al. The effect of gonadal and adrenal steroid therapy on skeletal health in adolescents and young women with anorexia nervosa. Metabolism 2012;61(7):1010–20.
76. Bloch M, Ish-Shalom S, Greenman Y, et al. Dehydroepiandrosterone treatment effects on weight, bone density, bone metabolism and mood in women suffering from anorexia nervosa-a pilot study. Psychiatry Res 2012;200(2–3):544–9.
77. Misra M, Miller KK, Almazan C, et al. Alterations in cortisol secretory dynamics in adolescent girls with anorexia nervosa and effects on bone metabolism. J Clin Endocrinol Metab 2004;89(10):4972–80.
78. Utz AL, Lawson EA, Misra M, et al. Peptide YY (PYY) levels and bone mineral density (BMD) in women with anorexia nervosa. Bone 2008;43(1):135–9.
79. Golden NH, Iglesias EA, Jacobson MS, et al. Alendronate for the treatment of osteopenia in anorexia nervosa: a randomized, double-blind, placebo-controlled trial. J Clin Endocrinol Metab 2005;90(6):3179–85.
80. Waugh EJ, Woodside DB, Beaton DE, et al. Effects of exercise on bone mass in young women with anorexia nervosa. Med Sci Sports Exerc 2011;43(5): 755–63.

Adverse Effects of Depression on Glycemic Control and Health Outcomes in People with Diabetes

A Review

François Pouwer, PhD[a,*], Giesje Nefs, PhD[a], Arie Nouwen, PhD[b]

KEYWORDS

- Type 1 diabetes • Type 2 diabetes • Depression • Mortality
- Cardiovascular disease • Microvascular disease • Review

KEY POINTS

- Depression is common in people with diabetes, affecting 10% to 30%.
- Depression in diabetes is associated with suboptimal self-care behaviors.
- Depressed people with diabetes are more often in suboptimal glycemic control.
- Depression is associated with an increased risk of having/developing complications.
- Depression is associated with an increased risk of mortality in people with diabetes.

INTRODUCTION

Diabetes mellitus is an increasingly common metabolic disorder. The World Health Organization (WHO) recently estimated the number of persons with diabetes at more than 347 million (WHO fact sheet 312).[1] These figures are expected to increase to 366 million by 2030.[2] Diabetes is a serious disease. It is well known that people with diabetes mellitus have a 2-fold to 4-fold increased risk of coronary heart disease and also an increased risk for microvascular diseases such as retinopathy, nephropathy, and neuropathy.[3–5] In recent years, important advances have been achieved in the psychosocial aspects of diabetes. A considerable part of these studies have focused on depression. The present article provides an update on the prevalence of depression in people with type 1 or type 2 diabetes. It also describes the temporal associations between depression, diabetes, and the adverse health consequences that are associated with depression in people with diabetes, focusing on the onset or

[a] Department of Medical and Clinical Psychology, Center of Research on Psychology in Somatic Diseases (CoRPS), Tilburg University, Warandelaan 2, PO Box 90153, Tilburg 5000 LE, The Netherlands; [b] School of Health and Social Sciences, Middlesex University, The Town Hall, The Burroughs, Hendon, London NW4 4BT, UK
* Corresponding author.
E-mail address: f.pouwer@tilburguniversity.edu

Endocrinol Metab Clin N Am 42 (2013) 529–544
http://dx.doi.org/10.1016/j.ecl.2013.05.002
0889-8529/13/$ – see front matter © 2013 Elsevier Inc. All rights reserved.

progression of microvascular and macrovascular complications of diabetes and mortality. Potential mechanisms that could link depression with adverse health outcomes are also be discussed, with a focus on the role of impaired diabetes self-care behaviors and suboptimal glycemic control.

Depression in People with Type 1 Diabetes

A review in 2006, including 4 controlled and 10 uncontrolled studies, found that the prevalence of clinical depression in controlled studies was 12% for people with diabetes compared with 3% for control subjects.[6] In uncontrolled studies the prevalence of clinical depression in people with diabetes was 13%.[6] However, this review included only 1 controlled study using a psychiatric diagnostic interview to determine the prevalence of depression. All other studies relied on self-report questionnaires assessing depressive symptoms.[6]

A subsequent study confirmed the increased prevalence of depressive symptoms in people with type 1 diabetes.[7] Based on data that had been collected within the framework of the Coronary Artery Calcification in Type 1 Diabetes Study,[7] 458 participants with type 1 diabetes and 546 participants without diabetes completed the Beck Depression Inventory II (BDI-II). Depressive symptoms (defined as a high BDI-II score) were more common in people with type 1 diabetes compared with controls (18% vs 6%, P<.0001). Those who reported having diabetes complications had higher mean BDI-II scores than those without complications (11 vs 6, P<.0001). Moreover, people with type 1 diabetes reported using more antidepressant medications (21% vs 12%, P = .0003).[7]

Since 2006, only 1 additional study examined the prevalence of depression in type 1 diabetes using both diagnostic criteria and self-report questionnaires. In a study from 3 Dutch outpatient hospitals, approximately one-third of people with type 1 diabetes reported low mood when data from the WHO-5 questionnaire were used.[8] When using the Center for Epidemiologic Studies Depression Scale (CES-D) questionnaire, the prevalence of depressive affect was 25% and 30% for men and women with type 1 diabetes, respectively.[8] Using the WHO Composite International Diagnostic Interview (CIDI), 8% of the people with type 1 diabetes were diagnosed with a major depressive disorder. In that study, depression was associated with suboptimal glycemic control and the presence of proliferative retinopathy.[8]

As in the general population, the prevalence of depression is higher in women with type 1 diabetes than in men.[9] A recent systematic review examined the prevalence of depression in young people (aged up to 25 years) with diabetes.[10] The review included 23 articles, but only 8 studies used a control group (healthy controls or another chronic condition) or norm populations. Of the 5 studies that made comparisons with a control group, 2 reported that young people with type 1 diabetes were more often depressed.[10] The results regarding the prevalence of depression in young people with type 1 diabetes therefore remain inconclusive.

In summary, there is some evidence that the prevalence of depression is increased in people with type 1 diabetes. However, the number of controlled studies is limited and most relied on self-report questionnaires to assess depression. Controlled studies using diagnostic criteria are needed. Most studies of the associations between type 1 diabetes and depression that have been conducted so far were cross sectional, limiting any conclusions about the causal nature and direction of the relationship between type 1 diabetes and depression.[6,9]

Depression in People with Type 2 Diabetes

In a systematic review with meta-analysis, Ali and colleagues[11] (2006) estimated the prevalence and odds of depression in adults with type 2 diabetes, compared with those without diabetes. The researchers included 10 controlled studies that were published between 1980 and 2005. The prevalence of depression seemed to be increased in people with type 2 diabetes compared with those without (18% vs 10%, odds ratio [OR] 1.6, 95% confidence interval [CI] 1.2–2.0). Depression was particularly common in women with diabetes (24%) compared with men (13%).[11]

The increased prevalence of depression in diabetes seems to be a global phenomenon. In a survey that has been carried out in 60 countries across the globe, the self-reported 1-year prevalence of depressive symptoms in diabetes was 9.3% (95% CI 7.3–11.3) compared with 3.2% in people without a comorbid condition. However, diabetes was not the only condition in which increased levels of depression were found, and the prevalence of depression was greater in people with arthritis (10.7%, 95% CI 9.1–12.3), angina (15.0%, 95% CI 12.9–17.2), and asthma (18.1%, 95% CI 15.9–20.3).[12]

In a large cross-sectional study that included more than 200,000 adults from 47 countries from almost all continents, the associations between diabetes and an episode of depressive symptoms were investigated.[13] In that study, both diabetes and presence of an episode of depressive symptoms were determined by self-report. Results showed that, on a global level, individuals with diabetes had increased odds of an episode of depressive symptoms compared with those without diabetes (adjusted OR 2.36, 95% CI 1.91–2.92).[13] Comparable associations were found in South American, Asian, and European countries (ORs>1.97), but not in the African continent (OR 0.86, 95% CI 0.54–1.37).[13]

A recent systematic review and meta-analysis showed that the prevalence of depression is increased in people with known type 2 diabetes but not in people with undiagnosed diabetes or impaired glucose metabolism (prediabetes) compared with controls.[14] This finding could be regarded as support for the hypothesis of a psychological burden of diabetes, which states that particularly the burden of the knowledge of having diabetes, and having to manage a chronic disease and its complications, explain the high prevalence of depression in people with diabetes. The prevalence of depression was not increased in people with prediabetes or undiagnosed diabetes, which suggests that a disturbed glucose metabolism in the early phase of the disease is not associated with depression.[14] An important limitation of that systematic review is that data on diabetes complications were not available. Data from the Longitudinal Aging Study Amsterdam (LASA) showed that, compared with controls who did not report having a chronic disease, the prevalence of depression was not higher in people with type 2 diabetes only who did not have diabetes complications.[15] However, in people with both type 2 diabetes and complications of diabetes and/or comorbid disease, the prevalence of depression was more than doubled, compared with healthy controls.[15]

Temporal Associations Between Depression and Type 2 Diabetes

The association between diabetes and depression is likely to be bidirectional in nature, with depression increasing the risk of developing diabetes and diabetes increasing the risk of depression. Since the seventeenth century, it has been suggested that depression plays a role in the cause of (type 2) diabetes.[16] Four meta-analyses have tested whether depression is associated with a higher risk for the onset of type 2 diabetes.[17–20] Any prospective association between depression and the onset of type 1 diabetes is yet to be established. Based on 9 longitudinal epidemiologic studies, Knol and colleagues[17] (2006) were the first to conclude that depression increases the risk for type 2 diabetes by 37%. In 2008, Mezuk and colleagues[19] (2008) published an update of this review, and included a total of 13 studies that investigated depression as a risk factor for diabetes. In this meta-analytical review, the risk for incident diabetes was 60% higher in depressed participants, compared with nondepressed controls (rate ratio [RR] 1.60, 95% CI 1.37–1.88).[19] The most recent meta-analysis included 23 prospective studies and confirmed that people with depressive symptoms are at increased risk to develop diabetes (unadjusted risk 1.57, 95% CI 1.37–1.77, and adjusted risk 1.38, 95% CI 1.23–1.55).[20] This study also reported a new, additional meta-analysis of 5 prospective studies that tested use of antidepressant medication as a risk factor for type 2 diabetes. The use of antidepressant drugs was associated with increased risk to develop diabetes (hazard ratio [HR] 1.68, 95% CI 1.17–2.40). Rotella and Mannucci[20] concluded that depression should be included in the list of risk factors that are being described by the American Diabetes Association as a reason to initiate early diabetes screening (physical inactivity, family history of diabetes, previous gestational diabetes, hypertension, hypertriglyceridemia, polycystic ovary syndrome). However, the practical value of this recommendation is unclear. It has not been tested yet whether the use of early diabetes screening in depressed individuals enables earlier recognition of diabetes and results in better health outcomes.

Another systematic review with meta-analysis that has focused on the temporal associations between type 2 diabetes and depression has studied the incidence of depression in people with type 2 diabetes.[21] This meta-analysis included 11 prospective studies that investigated whether people with type 2 diabetes are at increased risk to develop depression, showing that the incidence of depression is also 24% increased in people with type 2 diabetes compared with healthy controls.[21]

Depression and Incident Type 2 Diabetes: a Role for Emotional Stress?

Four meta-analyses have all concluded that depression is an (established) risk factor for the development of type 2 diabetes. However, chronic emotional stress is an established risk factor for the development of depression.[22] In 2 recent reviews it was concluded that the results of several prospective studies on the potential role of stress suggest that a high level of emotional stress or anxiety in general, sleeping problems, anger, and hostility are associated with an increased risk for the development of type 2 diabetes.[23,24] Conflicting results were found regarding other potential sources of chronic stress, such as childhood neglect, life events, and work stress.[23] The investigators emphasized that publication bias may have occurred in this research area, as a result from so-called fishing, in which investigators search their datasets for significant associations.[23] Publication bias may also have occurred because of the tendency of reviewers and editors to reject manuscripts with negative results for publication. Using prospective data from 9514 participants of the British Household Panel Survey, Mommersteeg and colleagues[25] (2012) showed that participants with a high level of psychological distress at the baseline assessment had a 33% higher hazard of developing diabetes during follow-up (HR 1.33, 95% CI 1.10–1.61) relative to those with a low level of psychological distress, adjusted for age, sex, education level, and household income. However, when the investigators adjusted the analyses for level of energy, health status, health problems, and activity level, higher psychological distress was no longer associated with incident diabetes (HR 1.10, 95% CI 0.91–1.34). This finding could indicate that the association between psychological stress and diabetes risk is mediated or confounded by low energy level and impaired health status.[25]

Prenatal stress factors may also play a role in programming offspring and accelerate the development of both type 1 and type 2 diabetes.[26,27] A large Danish study used data from the Danish Civil Registration System to identify almost 2 million singleton births in Denmark born in a period of 30 years and linked them to their parents, grandparents, and siblings. The researchers categorized these children as being exposed to serious prenatal stress (bereavement) during prenatal life if "their mothers lost an elder child, husband or parent during the period from 1 year before conception to the child's birth."[26,27] Children exposed to prenatal stress because their mothers experienced traumatic father or sibling deaths had a doubled risk to develop type 1 diabetes (adjusted incidence RRs [aIRRs] 2.03, 95% CI 1.22–3.38). Using data from the same database, the investigators also found that children exposed to bereavement during their prenatal life were also more likely to have a type 2 diabetes diagnosis later in their lives (aIRR 1.31, 95% CI 1.01–1.69). The results were most pronounced when death of an elder child occurred (aIRR 1.51, 95% CI 0.94–2.44) or when the bereavement took place in the second trimester of pregnancy (aIRR 2.08, 95% CI 1.15–3.76).[27] In a large Swedish study of 7251 men, aged 47 to 56 years at the start of the study, it was tested whether self-perceived stress at baseline predicted newly diagnosed diabetes over a period of 35 years of follow-up.[28] It was reported that, in an age-adjusted Cox regression analysis, men with permanent stress had a higher risk of diabetes (HR 1.52, 95% CI 1.26–1.82) compared with men with no (referent) or periodic stress (HR 1.09; 95% CI 0.94–1.27). This association was attenuated but remained significant after adjustment for age, socioeconomic status, physical inactivity, body mass index (BMI), systolic blood pressure, and use of antihypertensive medication (HR 1.45, 95% CI 1.20–1.75).[28]

Depression and Poor Health Outcomes

People with diabetes mellitus have a 2-fold to 4-fold increased risk of coronary heart disease and also an increased risk for microvascular complications such as retinopathy, nephropathy, and neuropathy, and cognitive decline and dysfunction including Alzheimer disease.[29] In the past 2 decades, mounting evidence has shown that these complications are compounded by depression. Further, depression in diabetes can lead to suboptimal glycemic control and increased mortality.

In their early systematic review published in 2001, de Groot and colleagues[30] searched the literature for articles examining the associations between depression and diabetes complications. The investigators found 27 cross-sectional studies that met their inclusion criteria. Depression was significantly associated with a variety of diabetes complications, including retinopathy, nephropathy, neuropathy, macrovascular complications, and sexual dysfunction. The effect sizes ranged from small to moderate ($r = 0.17$–0.32). However, as the investigators noted, all studies were cross-sectional in nature and thus there was a need for prospective, longitudinal studies.[30]

In 2003, Black and colleagues[31] published the results of a longitudinal study that examined the effect of depression and diabetes on the incidence of adverse health outcomes among older Mexican Americans. They used longitudinal data from the Hispanic Established Population for the Epidemiologic Study of the Elderly (EPESE) survey. Both main effects and interaction effects of diabetes and depressive symptoms were studied. The investigators reported a synergistic effect of diabetes and depression, associated with a higher incidence of both macrovascular and microvascular complications, and greater incidence of disability in activities of daily living, after adjustment for sociodemographic characteristics such as sex, age, education, acculturation, and marital status.[31]

Katon and colleagues[32] investigated whether comorbid depression in patients with diabetes was associated with an increased risk for dementia. Data from a prospective cohort study were used, comprising 3837 people with diabetes from primary care settings.[32] Participants without International Classification of Diseases Ninth Revision (ICD-9) diagnosis of dementia before baseline were followed for a period of 5-years.

Cox proportional hazard regression models showed that people with diabetes and co-morbid major depression (as indicated by the PHQ-9) had an increased risk of dementia (fully adjusted HR 2.69, 95% CI 1.77, 4.07) compared to people without depression.[32] Another study conducted by the same group was designed to test the same hypothesis with a different dataset.[33] The investigators analyzed data from a sample of 19,239 people with diabetes aged 30 to 75 years; all participants were members of a diabetes registry. Cox proportional hazard regression models showed that 80 of 3766 patients (2.1%) with comorbid depression and diabetes (incidence rate of 5.5 per 1000 person-years) versus 158 of 15,473 patients (1.0%) with diabetes alone (incidence rate of 2.6 per 1000 person-years) had 1 or more ICD-9 Clinical Modification diagnoses of dementia. Patients with comorbid depression had a doubled risk of dementia during this 3-year to 5-year period (adjusted HR 2.02, 95% confidence interval 1.73–2.35).[33] Sieu and colleagues[34] examined whether depression is associated with a higher incidence of retinopathy among adults with type 2 diabetes after controlling for sociodemographic factors, health risk behaviors, and clinical characteristics. To test this hypothesis, data from the Pathways Epidemiologic Follow-Up Study were used. The Pathways Study is a prospective cohort study investigating the impact of depression in people with type 2 diabetes in primary care. Cox proportional hazard models showed that severity of depression was associated with an increased risk of incident retinopathy (OR 1.03, 95% CI 1.002–1.051) as well as time to incident retinopathy (HR 1.025, 95% CI 1.009–1.041) over a 5-year follow-up period.[34] Williams and colleagues[35] also used data from The Pathways Study, this time to test the hypothesis that depression is associated with an increased risk of incident diabetic foot ulcers. That analysis was conducted using a sample of 3474 adults with type 2 diabetes who had no prior diabetic foot ulcers or amputations. Mean follow-up was 4.1 years. Patients with a high score on the 9-item Patient Health Questionnaire, which indicates major depression, had a 2-fold increased risk of incident diabetic foot ulcers (adjusted HR 2.00, 95% CI 1.24–3.25). Minor depression was not significantly associated with incident diabetic foot ulcers (adjusted HR 1.37, 95% CI 0.77–2.44).[35]

Lin and colleagues[36] focused on the associations between baseline depression and the risks for the development of advanced macrovascular and microvascular complications among a group of 4623 people with type 2 diabetes in primary care. Advanced microvascular complications were assessed, including blindness, end-stage renal disease, amputations, and renal failure deaths. Advanced macrovascular complications comprised myocardial infarction, stroke, cardiovascular risk procedures, and deaths. Medical record review, ICD-9 diagnostic and procedural codes, and death certificate data were used to ascertain outcomes in the 5-year follow-up. Major depression was associated with a significantly higher risk of both microvascular complications (HR 1.36, 95% CI 1.05–1.75) and macrovascular complications (1.24, 95% CI 1.0–1.54), after adjustment for prior complications and demographic, clinical, and diabetes self-care variables.[36]

In a small study (n = 76) among women with type 1 or type 2 diabetes, the women who were diagnosed with a major depressive disorder at baseline (n = 16) were at increased risk to develop coronary heart disease (HR 5.2, 95% CI 1.4–18.9) during a 10-year follow-up period, after adjustment for BMI.[37] In that study, depression did not predict the development of clinically apparent peripheral or cerebrovascular disease.[37]

In another large cohort study from the United States, data from the Veterans Administration electronic medical records were analyzed. Scherrer and colleagues[38] studied a cohort of 345,949 persons who had not been diagnosed with cardiovascular disease in fiscal years 1999 and 2000. Results showed that persons with type 2 diabetes alone and persons diagnosed with major depression had a 30% increased risk for myocardial infarction. Persons with a double diagnosis (both type 2 diabetes and major depressive disorder) were at 82% increased risk for myocardial infarction (HR 1.82, 95% CI 1.69–1.97) compared with those without either condition.[38]

Gonzalez and colleagues[39] investigated longitudinal data in a group of 333 persons (73% with type 2 diabetes) who were diagnosed after clinical examination with diabetic peripheral neuropathy, but did not have peripheral vascular disease. Depression and other diabetes complications were assessed by self-report. Cox regression showed that baseline depression was an independent predictor of a first foot ulceration over 18 months (HR 1.68, 95% CI 1.20–2.35). Further analyses showed that foot self-care did not mediate the positive association between depression and foot ulceration.[39]

Williams and colleagues[40] investigated the association between diagnosed depression and incident nontraumatic lower limb amputations in 531,973 veterans with diabetes. The investigators used data from the Diabetes Epidemiology Cohorts.[40] Depression was defined by diagnostic codes or antidepressant prescriptions. Persons with a diagnosed depression had a higher risk of major amputation(s) (HR 1.33, 95% CI 1.15–1.55). There was no statistically significant association between depression and minor amputations (adjusted HR 1.01, 95% CI 0.90–1.13).[40]

A recent systematic review and meta-analysis tested whether depression in diabetes is associated with a higher all-cause mortality and/or higher cardiovascular mortality.[41] This systematic review included 16 prospective studies and concluded that baseline depression was associated with an almost 50% higher risk of all-cause mortality during follow-up (HR 1.46, 95% CI 1.29–1.66). Meta-analysis of the results of 5 studies showed that depression was associated with a 39% higher cardiovascular mortality at follow-up (HR 1.39, 95% CI 1.11–1.73).[41]

In sum, a large number of prospective studies have shown that depressed persons with diabetes are at increased risk for adverse health outcomes, namely microvascular and macrovascular complications and higher mortality. Results in this area might have been biased, because the studies were mainly conducted in the United States. Moreover, publication bias may also have occurred, resulting from fishing expeditions in which investigators search existing datasets for significant associations. Such a publication bias may also have resulted from the tendency of reviewers and editors to reject manuscripts with negative results for publication. It is therefore important that research groups that intend to conduct a new epidemiologic cohort study prospectively describe and publish the design of their study.

Why is Depression Linked with Poor Health Outcomes?

There is abundant evidence showing that depression in people with diabetes is associated with poor health outcomes in the long term. However, the behavioral and pathophysiologic mechanisms that explain this association are probably complex and still only partly understood. One mechanism that has received considerable attention from researchers is suboptimal glycemic control. In a landmark study, Lustman and colleagues[42] (2000) summarized the literature regarding the associations between depression and glycemic control. A total of 24 cross-sectional studies were included, and a small to moderate standardized effect size was found, with higher levels of depression being associated with suboptimal glycemic control.[42] This association was evident in both type 1 diabetes and type 2 diabetes, and greater in studies that had investigated interview-diagnosed depression (effect size 0.28), compared with studies that had used self-report measures for depression (effect size 0.15). However, in a small longitudinal study that included people with type 1 (n = 28) or type 2 diabetes (n = 62), Georgiades and colleagues[43] (2007) found that changes in depressive symptoms were not associated with changes in glycemic control (hemoglobin A1c [HbA$_{1c}$]) or fasting blood glucose levels over a period of 1 year. In a larger subsequent study with 2 assessments, with a 6-month interval, depressive symptoms and glycemic control were measured in 253 adults with type 2 diabetes.[44] Baseline depressive symptom severity predicted suboptimal glycemic control 6 months later, but not after the analysis was adjusted for baseline glycemic control. In contrast, baseline glycemic control predicted depressive symptoms at follow-up among participants who used insulin (beta = 0.31, P = .002), but not in people using oral medication alone (beta = −0.10, P = .210).[44] Recent prospective studies suggest that diabetes-specific emotional distress may be a more consistent predictor of suboptimal glycemic control than either major depressive disorder or depressive symptoms.[45,46]

Depressed individuals often lack energy, may find it difficult to concentrate, frequently have low self-esteem, and are often inactive; moreover, eating problems are also a common symptom of depression.[47] These depression symptoms may all affect glycemic control via suboptimal self-care behaviors. In a large cohort study among 4117 people with diabetes, baseline depression was associated with suboptimal use of diabetes control medications among people with diabetes and poor disease control over a 5-year follow-up period.[48] In the same study, depression was not associated with delayed intensification of treatment.[48] Treatment intensification was defined as an increased medication dosage in a class, an increase in the number of medication classes, or a switch to a different class within 3-month periods before and after notation of the target levels.[48]

Gonzalez and colleagues[49] conducted a systematic review with meta-analysis examining the association between depression and treatment nonadherence in people with type 1 and type 2 diabetes. They included 47 studies, showing that depression was significantly associated with nonadherence to the diabetes treatment regimen (z = 9.97, P<.0001). Effect sizes were largest for missed medical appointments and composite measures of self-care.[49] It is also of clinical relevance that eating problems are particularly common in people with depression. A recent study showed that, in teenage girls with diabetes, depression is strongly associated with disturbed eating behaviors; 75% of the girls with a high depression score also reported disturbed eating behaviors.[50] However, metabolic control was not significantly associated with either depression or disturbed eating behaviors in that study.[50] In a recent systematic review of 13 controlled studies, the prevalence of eating problems in young adults with type 1 diabetes was compared with peers without type 1 diabetes.[51] Eating problems were particularly common in young people with type 1 diabetes, with disordered eating behavior affecting 39% of the participants with diabetes and eating disorders affecting 7% (vs 3% in controls).[51] People with diabetes and disturbed eating behaviors were often in suboptimal glycemic control.[51]

Another potential mechanism that could link depression with poor health outcomes is delay of insulin therapy.[52] Results of the United Kingdom Prospective Diabetes Study have shown that beta-cell function deteriorates gradually.[53] As a result, for many people with type 2 diabetes, insulin therapy is unavoidable in the long term, but a considerable percentage are reluctant to start insulin therapy and would blame themselves when they had to start with insulin therapy.[53,54] Again, many people with depression lack energy, have poor self-esteem, find it difficult to make decisions, and have problems concentrating. These symptoms could contribute to a further delay in insulin therapy. A cross-sectional study in insulin-naive outpatients with type 2 diabetes confirmed that depression was associated with more negative appraisals of insulin therapy.[52] Whether depression is associated with negative appraisals of insulin therapy or a delay of insulin therapy should now be investigated in prospective studies. Negative appraisals of insulin are common not only among patients with diabetes. In the Diabetes Attitudes Wishes and Needs (DAWN) Study, a considerable percentage of nurses and general practitioners (50%–55%) responded that they would delay insulin therapy until necessary, but specialists and opinion leaders were less likely to do so.[54] At present, there is a need for longitudinal studies that test the hypothesis that depression is associated with timing of insulin therapy, or that test the hypothesis that depression leads to poor health outcomes via delay of insulin therapy.

Depression could also contribute to poor health outcomes via decreased levels of physical activity. Koopmans and colleagues[55] found in a large primary care sample of people with type 2 diabetes that depression was associated with lower levels of physical activity. In the Heart and Soul Study, a cohort with people with stable coronary heart disease, depressive symptoms were associated with a 31% higher rate of cardiovascular events (HR 1.31, 95% CI 1.00–1.71, $P = .04$) after adjustment for comorbid conditions and disease severity.[56] Statistical adjustment for potential biologic mediators that were also measured at baseline (heart-rate variability, serotonin, cortisol, 24-hour excretion of norepinephrine, omega-3 polyunsaturated fatty acids, and C-reactive protein) attenuated this association slightly (HR 1.24, 95% CI 0.94–1.63, $P = .12$). After further adjustment for potential behavioral mediators, including physical inactivity, there was no significant association (HR 1.05, 95% CI 0.79–1.40, $P = .75$).[56] Thus, in the Heart and Soul Study, decreased levels of physical activity mediated the association between depression and cardiovascular events; this may also be the case with depression and poor health outcomes in people with diabetes. Again, several physiologic mechanisms have been described that may link depression with poor health outcomes in diabetes, but these mechanisms are currently understudied. In psychiatric research, depression was associated with several biologic changes, such as increased inflammation, disturbed platelet function and serotonin metabolism, heart-rate variability, dysfunction of the autonomic nervous system, altered polyunsaturated fatty acid metabolism, and disturbed functioning of the hypothalamus-pituitary-adrenal (HPA) axis, which in turn have been related to increased (cardiovascular) mortality.[57–63] Hood and colleagues[64] analyzed data from SEARCH for Diabetes in Youth (SEARCH), an observational study of 2359 children diagnosed with diabetes at less than 20 years of age. Six of 8 markers of inflammation were significantly associated with depression in youth with diabetes in bivariate analyses. Adiponectin, leptin, C-reactive protein, serum amyloid A, apolipoprotein B, and low-density lipoprotein levels differed by depression category. With the exception of serum amyloid A, all were in the expected direction (ie, increased depression was associated with greater metabolic abnormalities or systemic inflammation).[64] In a group of 215 postmenopausal women (48% had type 2 diabetes), Wagner and colleagues[65] investigated whether acute stress and lifetime history of major depressive disorder were associated with functional and biochemical markers of endothelial function and whether this relationship varied by diabetes status. Women with a lifetime history of depression had lower nitric oxide generation and lower flow-mediated dilatation of the brachial artery compared with never-depressed controls.[65] Diabetes moderated the effect of mental stress on nitric oxide.[65]

Depression and Suboptimal Glycemic Control: a Role for Individual Depression Symptoms?

Depression is a heterogenous condition. According to the Diagnostic and Statistical Manual, fourth edition (DSM-IV), major depressive disorder consists of 9 symptoms of which at least 5 should be present for at least 2 weeks, including 1 of the 2 core symptoms (anhedonia and dysphoria).[47] Therefore the cluster of symptoms that is present can vary widely between people who are diagnosed with a major depressive disorder. Moreover, some symptoms of depression, as mentioned in the DSM-IV, are so-called double-barreled items. One of these features involves change in appetite. This can mean increased appetite nearly every day with subsequent weight gain (eg, a change of more than 5% of body weight in a month), but it can also mean a decreased appetite, resulting in significant weight loss when not dieting, or decrease or increase in appetite nearly every day. Other complex criteria are, for example, insomnia or hypersomnia nearly every day or psychomotor agitation or retardation nearly every day. However, a few studies have investigated the association between these individual symptoms of depression or symptom cluster and glycemic control. For example, Bot and colleagues[66] showed that particularly the symptoms of depressed mood, sleeping difficulties, and appetite problems were significantly related to higher baseline and 1-year follow-up HbA_{1c} values. Suicidal ideation (beta = 0.14, P = .001) was significantly related to higher baseline HbA_{1c} levels. Associations were more pronounced in type 1 diabetes than in type 2 diabetes.[66] Another recent study examined whether different depression symptom clusters were differentially associated with suboptimal glycemic control.[67] Cross-sectional baseline data from a cohort study of 5772 people with type 2 diabetes in primary care were used. Symptoms of depressed mood, anhedonia, and anxiety were measured using the Edinburgh Depression Scale. Anhedonia in particular was associated with suboptimal glycemic control (OR 1.29, 95% CI 1.09–1.52), whereas both depressed mood (OR 1.04, 95% CI 0.88–1.22) and anxiety (OR 0.99, 95% CI 0.83–1.19) were not. This association was not attenuated by alcohol consumption or physical activity.[67]

Psychosocial Interventions and Glycemic Control

Thus, depression seems to be an important risk factor for poor health outcomes in people with diabetes. An important clinical question is whether psychotherapeutic or pharmacologic interventions that reduce depression also have a beneficial effect on health outcomes. A meta-analysis of 14 randomized controlled trials with a total of 1724 people with diabetes showed that depression can be effectively treated in this group, with large effects for psychotherapeutic interventions (often combined with diabetes self-management), and moderate effects for pharmacologic treatments.[68] The same review concluded that both pharmacotherapy and collaborative care reduced depressive symptoms but had no effect on glycemic control, except for sertraline.[68]

In their recent Cochrane systematic review, Baumeister and colleagues[69] included randomized controlled trials that tested psychological and pharmacologic interventions for depression in adults with diabetes and depression. Primary outcomes were depression and glycemic control, and secondary outcomes were adherence to diabetes treatment regimens, diabetes complications, and all-cause mortality. In total, 19 trials were included, with 1592 participants. Eight psychological intervention studies had beneficial effects on short-term (end of treatment), medium-term (1 to 6 months after treatment), and long-term (more than 6 months after treatment) depression severity.[69] Evidence with regard to the effect of psychological intervention on glycemic control was heterogeneous and inconclusive. Eight trials compared pharmacologic interventions versus a placebo treatment, showing a moderate beneficial effect of antidepressant medication on short-term depression severity. Moreover, in 5 trials, glycemic control slightly improved in the short term (HbA_{1c} −0.4%, 95% CI −0.6 to −0.1, P = .002). The investigators concluded that medium-term and long-term depression and glycemic control outcomes as well as health care costs, diabetes complications, and mortality have not been examined in pharmacologic intervention trials.[69]

At present, there is no evidence that successful treatment of depression can decrease the risk for adverse health outcomes. Bogner and colleagues[70] tested the hypothesis that implementing a depression management program would decrease the risk of mortality compared with depressed people with diabetes in usual-care practices. The investigators conducted a multisite, practice-randomized, controlled trial, the Prevention of Suicide in Primary Care Elderly: Collaborative Trial (PROSPECT). Depressed people with diabetes who were assigned to the intervention group were less likely to have died during the 5-year follow-up interval than depressed people with diabetes in usual care, after accounting for baseline differences among participants (adjusted HR 0.49, 95% CI 0.24–0.98).[70] However, in a letter to the Editor, Thombs and Ziegelstein[71] argued that the PROSPECT care intervention was not originally designed specifically to improve survival. They also expressed concerns that the statistical methods used by Bogner and colleagues[70] could result in model overfitting. Models that have been overfitted generally have poor predictive value, because they generally exaggerate minor fluctuations in the data.

New, innovative interventions have been developed in order to treat depression in people with diabetes. For example, Van Bastelaar and colleagues[72] conducted a randomized controlled trial showing that depression in people with diabetes can be effectively treated with a Web-based intervention. In that study, Web-based treatment also reduced diabetes-specific emotional distress but did not affect HbA_{1c} levels.[72,73]

Another randomized controlled trial by Van Son and colleagues[74,75] showed that mindfulness-based cognitive behavior therapy reduced emotional distress and increased health-related quality of life in people with diabetes who had low levels of emotional well-being at baseline. Future research is needed to test whether these interventions have long-term effects on mental health, self-care behaviors, and health outcomes.

SUMMARY

Research in the past decades has shown that depression is common in people with type 1 or type 2 diabetes, affecting 10% to 30% of cases. A considerable number of prospective studies have shown that depressed persons with diabetes are at increased risk for microvascular and macrovascular complications of diabetes and have higher mortality. The biologic and behavioral mechanisms that link depression with these adverse health outcomes are still unclear. One plausible mechanism is that depression contributes to suboptimal glycemic control via less adequate self-care behaviors, because several studies have shown that depressed persons with diabetes more frequently have lower levels of physical activity, are more frequently nonadherent to treatment recommendations, and have disturbed eating behaviors. Depression may also be associated with delayed treatment intensification; for example, delayed initiation of insulin therapy. However, most of the studies that have been conducted in this area had a cross-sectional design and relied on self-report measures of depression only, not using the psychiatric diagnostic interview to assess depression. Moreover, these studies were mostly conducted in people with type 2 diabetes. Prospective studies that investigate the mechanisms that link depression with adverse health outcomes are now urgently needed. In addition, more research is needed to find more effective and efficient ways to treat depression in people with diabetes, and to develop and test new interventions that can not only treat depression but also help to reduce the associated health risks of depressed people with diabetes.

REFERENCES

1. WHO Fact sheet No 312, Available at: www.who.int/mediacentre/factsheets/fs312/en. Accessed June 25, 2013.
2. Wild S, Roglic G, Green A, et al. Global prevalence of diabetes: estimates for the year 2000 and projections for 2030. Diabetes Care 2004;27:1047–53.
3. Williams R, Van Gaal L, Lucioni C. Assessing the impact of complications on the costs of type II diabetes. Diabetologia 2002;45:S13–7.
4. Gregg EW, Beckles GL, Williamson DF, et al. Diabetes and physical disability among older U.S. adults. Diabetes Care 2000;23:1272–7.
5. Roglic G, Unwin N, Bennett PH, et al. The burden of mortality attributable to diabetes: realistic estimates for the year 2000. Diabetes Care 2005;28:2130–5.
6. Barnard KD, Skinner TC, Peveler R. The prevalence of co-morbid depression in adults with type 1 diabetes: systematic literature review. Diabet Med 2006;23(4):445–8.
7. Gendelman N, Snell-Bergeon JK, McFann K, et al. Prevalence and correlates of depression in individuals with and without type 1 diabetes. Diabetes Care 2009;32(4):575–9.
8. Pouwer F, Geelhoed-Duijvestijn PH, Tack CJ, et al. Prevalence of comorbid depression is high in out-patients with type 1 or type 2 diabetes mellitus. Results from three out-patient clinics in the Netherlands. Diabet Med 2010;27(2):217–24.
9. Roy T, Lloyd CE. Epidemiology of depression and diabetes: a systematic review. J Affect Disord 2012;142(Suppl):S8–21.
10. Johnson B, Eiser C, Young V, et al. Prevalence of depression among young people with type 1 diabetes: a systematic review. Diabet Med 2013;30(2):199–208.
11. Ali S, Stone MA, Peters JL, et al. The prevalence of co-morbid depression in adults with type 2 diabetes: a systematic review and meta-analysis. Diabet Med 2006;23(11):1165–73.
12. Moussavi S, Chatterji S, Verdes E, et al. Depression, chronic diseases, and decrements in health: results from the World Health Surveys. Lancet 2007;370(9590):851–8.
13. Mommersteeg PM, Herr R, Pouwer F, et al. The association between diabetes and an episode of depressive symptoms in the 2002 World Health Survey: an analysis of 231,797 individuals from 47 countries. Diabet Med 2013;30(6):e208–14.
14. Nouwen A, Nefs G, Caramlau I, et al. Prevalence of depression in individuals with impaired glucose metabolism or undiagnosed diabetes: a systematic review and meta-analysis of the European Depression in Diabetes (EDID) Research Consortium. Diabetes Care 2011;34(3):752–62.
15. Pouwer F, Beekman AT, Nijpels G, et al. Rates and risks for co-morbid depression in patients with type 2 diabetes mellitus: results from a community-based study. Diabetologia 2003;46(7):892–8.
16. Willis T. Pharmaceutice rationalis sive diatriba de medicamentorum operationibus in humano corpore. [Oxford]: E Theatro Sheldoniano, M.DC.LXXV.
17. Knol M, Twisk J, Beekman A, et al. Depression as a risk factor for the onset of type 2 diabetes: a meta-analysis. Diabetologia 2006;49:837–45.
18. Cosgrove MP, Sargeant LA, Griffin SJ. Does depression increase the risk of developing type 2 diabetes? Occup Med (Lond) 2008;58(1):7–14.
19. Mezuk B, Eaton WW, Albrecht S, et al. Depression and type 2 diabetes over the lifespan. Diabetes Care 2008;31:2383–90.

20. Rotella F, Mannucci E. Depression as a risk factor for diabetes: a meta-analysis of longitudinal studies. J Clin Psychiatry 2013;74(1):31–7.
21. Nouwen A, Winkley K, Twisk J, et al. European Depression in Diabetes (EDID) Research Consortium. Type 2 diabetes mellitus as a risk factor for the onset of depression: a systematic review and meta-analysis. Diabetologia 2010; 53(12):2480–6.
22. MacQueen G, Frodl T. The hippocampus in major depression: evidence for the convergence of the bench and bedside in psychiatric research? Mol Psychiatry 2011;16(3):252–64.
23. Pouwer F, Kupper N, Adriaanse MC. Does emotional stress cause type 2 diabetes mellitus? A review from the European Depression in Diabetes (EDID) Research Consortium. Discov Med 2010;9(45):112–8.
24. Cappuccio FP, D'Elia LD, Strazzullo P, et al. Quantity and quality of sleep and incidence of type 2 diabetes: a systematic review and meta-analysis. Diabetes Care 2010;33:414–20.
25. Mommersteeg PM, Herr R, Zijlstra WP, et al. Higher levels of psychological distress are associated with a higher risk of incident diabetes during 18 year follow-up: results from the British Household Panel Survey. BMC Public Health 2012;12:1109.
26. Virk J, Li J, Vestergaard M, et al. Early life disease programming during the preconception and prenatal period: making the link between stressful life events and type-1 diabetes. PLoS One 2010;5(7):e11523.
27. Li J, Olsen J, Vestergaard M, et al. Prenatal exposure to bereavement and type-2 diabetes: a Danish longitudinal population based study. PLoS One 2012;7(8): e43508.
28. Novak M, Björck L, Giang KW, et al. Perceived stress and incidence of type 2 diabetes: a 35-year follow-up study of middle-aged Swedish men. Diabet Med 2013;30(1):e8–16.
29. Lu FP, Lin KP, Kuo HK. Diabetes and the risk of multi-system aging phenotypes: a systematic review and meta-analysis. PLoS One 2009;4(1):e4144.
30. de Groot M, Anderson R, Freedland KE, et al. Association of depression and diabetes complications: a meta-analysis. Psychosom Med 2001;63(4):619–30.
31. Black SA, Markides KS, Ray LA. Depression predicts increased incidence of adverse health outcomes in older Mexican Americans with type 2 diabetes. Diabetes Care 2003;26(10):2822–8.
32. Katon WJ, Lin EH, Williams LH, et al. Comorbid depression is associated with an increased risk of dementia diagnosis in patients with diabetes: a prospective cohort study. J Gen Intern Med 2010;25(5):423–9.
33. Katon W, Lyles CR, Parker MM, et al. Association of depression with increased risk of dementia in patients with type 2 diabetes: the Diabetes and Aging Study. Arch Gen Psychiatry 2012;69(4):410–7.
34. Sieu N, Katon W, Lin EH, et al. Depression and incident diabetic retinopathy: a prospective cohort study. Gen Hosp Psychiatry 2011;33(5):429–35.
35. Williams LH, Rutter CM, Katon WJ, et al. Depression and incident diabetic foot ulcers: a prospective cohort study. Am J Med 2010;123(8):748–54.e3.
36. Lin EH, Rutter CM, Katon W, et al. Depression and advanced complications of diabetes: a prospective cohort study. Diabetes Care 2010;33(2):264–9.
37. Clouse RE, Lustman PJ, Freedland KE, et al. Depression and coronary heart disease in women with diabetes. Psychosom Med 2003;65:376–83.
38. Scherrer JF, Garfield LD, Chrusciel T, et al. Increased risk of myocardial infarction in depressed patients with type 2 diabetes. Diabetes Care 2011;34(8):1729–34.

39. Gonzalez JS, Vileikyte L, Ulbrecht JS, et al. Depression predicts first but not recurrent diabetic foot ulcers. Diabetologia 2010;53(10):2241–8.
40. Williams LH, Miller DR, Fincke G, et al. Depression and incident lower limb amputations in veterans with diabetes. J Diabet Complications 2011;25(3):175–82.
41. Van Dooren FE, Nefs G, Schram MT, et al. Depression and risk of mortality in people with diabetes mellitus: a systematic review and meta-analysis. PLoS One 2013;8(3):e57058.
42. Lustman PJ, Anderson RJ, Freedland KE, et al. Depression and poor glycemic control: a meta-analytic review of the literature. Diabetes Care 2000;23(7):934–42.
43. Georgiades A, Zucker N, Friedman KE, et al. Changes in depressive symptoms and glycemic control in diabetes mellitus. Psychosom Med 2007;69(3):235–41.
44. Aikens JE, Perkins DW, Lipton B, et al. Longitudinal analysis of depressive symptoms and glycemic control in type 2 diabetes. Diabetes Care 2009; 32(7):1177–81.
45. Aikens JE. Prospective associations between emotional distress and poor outcomes in type 2 diabetes. Diabetes Care 2012;35:2472–8.
46. Fisher L, Mullan JT, Arean P, et al. Diabetes distress but not clinical depression or depressive symptoms is associated with glycemic control in both cross-sectional and longitudinal analyses. Diabetes Care 2010;33:23–8.
47. American Psychiatric Association. Diagnostic and statistical manual of mental disorders. 4th edition. Text revision. Washington, DC: American Psychiatric Publishing; 2000.
48. Katon W, Russo J, Lin EH, et al. Diabetes and poor disease control: is comorbid depression associated with poor medication adherence or lack of treatment intensification? Psychosom Med 2009;71(9):965–72.
49. Gonzalez JS, Peyrot M, McCarl LA, et al. Depression and diabetes treatment nonadherence: a meta-analysis. Diabetes Care 2008;31(12):2398–403.
50. Colton PA, Olmsted MP, Daneman D, et al. Depression, disturbed eating behavior, and metabolic control in teenage girls with type 1 diabetes. Pediatr Diabetes 2013;14(5):372–6.
51. Young V, Eiser C, Johnson B, et al. Eating problems in adolescents with type 1 diabetes: a systematic review with meta-analysis. Diabet Med 2013;30(2):189–98.
52. Makine C, Karşidağ C, Kadioğlu P, et al. Symptoms of depression and diabetes-specific emotional distress are associated with a negative appraisal of insulin therapy in insulin-naïve patients with type 2 diabetes mellitus. A study from the European Depression in Diabetes [EDID] Research Consortium. Diabet Med 2009;26(1):28–33.
53. Turner RC, Cull CA, Frighi V, et al. Glycemic control with d1. diet, sulfonylurea, metformin, or insulin in patients with type 2 diabetes mellitus: progressive requirement for multiple therapies (UKPDS 49). UK Prospective Diabetes Study (UKPDS) Group. JAMA 1999;281(21):2005–12.
54. Peyrot M, Rubin RR, Lauritzen T, et al, International DAWN Advisory Panel. Resistance to insulin therapy among patients and providers: results of the cross-national Diabetes Attitudes, Wishes, and Needs (DAWN) study. Diabetes Care 2005;28(11):2673–9.
55. Koopmans B, Pouwer F, de Bie RA, et al. Depressive symptoms are associated with physical inactivity in patients with type 2 diabetes. The DIAZOB Primary Care Diabetes study. Fam Pract 2009;26(3):171–3.
56. Whooley MA, de Jonge P, Vittinghoff E, et al. Depressive symptoms, health behaviors, and risk of cardiovascular events in patients with coronary heart disease. JAMA 2008;300(20):2379–88.

57. de Jonge P, Rosmalen JG, Kema IP, et al. Psychophysiological biomarkers explaining the association between depression and prognosis in coronary artery patients: a critical review of the literature. Neurosci Biobehav Rev 2010;35(1): 84–90.

58. Howren MB, Lamkin DM, Suls J. Associations of depression with C-reactive protein, IL-1, and IL-6: a meta-analysis. Psychosom Med 2009;71(2):171–86.

59. Kop WJ, Stein PK, Tracy RP, et al. Autonomic nervous system dysfunction and inflammation contribute to the increased cardiovascular mortality risk associated with depression. Psychosom Med 2010;72(7):626–35.

60. Stuart MJ, Baune BT. Depression and type 2 diabetes: inflammatory mechanisms of a psychoneuroendocrine co-morbidity. Neurosci Biobehav Rev 2012; 36(1):658–76.

61. Korczak DJ, Pereira S, Koulajian K, et al. Type 1 diabetes mellitus and major depressive disorder: evidence for a biological link. Diabetologia 2011;54(10): 2483–93.

62. Champaneri S, Wand GS, Malhotra SS, et al. Biological basis of depression in adults with diabetes. Curr Diab Rep 2010;10(6):396–405.

63. Pouwer F, Nijpels G, Beekman AT, et al. Fat food for a bad mood. Could we treat and prevent depression in type 2 diabetes by means of omega-3 polyunsaturated fatty acids? A review of the evidence. Diabet Med 2005;22(11):1465–75.

64. Hood KK, Lawrence JM, Anderson A, et al, SEARCH for Diabetes in Youth Study Group. Metabolic and inflammatory links to depression in youth with diabetes. Diabetes Care 2012;35(12):2443–6.

65. Wagner JA, Tennen H, Finan PH, et al. Lifetime history of depression, type 2 diabetes, and endothelial reactivity to acute stress in postmenopausal women. Int J Behav Med 2012;19(4):503–11.

66. Bot M, Pouwer F, de Jonge P, et al. Differential associations between depressive symptoms and glycaemic control in outpatients with diabetes. Diabet Med 2013;30(3):e115–22.

67. Nefs G, Pouwer F, Denollet J, et al. Suboptimal glycemic control in type 2 diabetes: a key role for anhedonia? J Psychiatr Res 2012;46(4):549–54.

68. Van der Feltz-Cornelis CM, Nuyen J, Stoop C, et al. Effect of interventions for major depressive disorder and significant depressive symptoms in patients with diabetes mellitus: a systematic review and meta-analysis. Gen Hosp Psychiatry 2010;32(4):380–95.

69. Baumeister H, Hutter N, Bengel J. Psychological and pharmacological interventions for depression in patients with diabetes mellitus and depression. Cochrane Database Syst Rev 2012;(12):CD008381.

70. Bogner HR, Morales KH, Post EP, et al. Diabetes, depression, and death: a randomized controlled trial of a depression treatment program for older adults based in primary care (PROSPECT). Diabetes Care 2007;30(12):3005–10.

71. Thombs BD, Ziegelstein RC. Diabetes, depression, and death: a randomized controlled trial of a depression treatment program for older adults based in primary care (PROSPECT): response to Bogner et al. Diabetes Care 2008; 31(6):e54.

72. van Bastelaar KM, Pouwer F, Cuijpers P, et al. Web-based cognitive behavioral therapy (W-CBT) for diabetes patients with co-morbid depression: design of a randomised controlled trial. BMC Psychiatry 2008;19(8):9.

73. van Bastelaar KM, Pouwer F, Cuijpers P, et al. Web-based depression treatment for type 1 and type 2 diabetic patients: a randomized, controlled trial. Diabetes Care 2011;34(2):320–5.

74. van Son J, Nyklíček I, Pop VJ, et al. Testing the effectiveness of a mindfulness-based intervention to reduce emotional distress in outpatients with diabetes (DiaMind): design of a randomized controlled trial. BMC Public Health 2011; 11:131.

75. van Son J, Nyklíček I, Pop VJ, et al. The effects of a mindfulness-based intervention on emotional distress, quality of life, and HbA1c in outpatients with diabetes (DiaMind): a randomized controlled trial. Diabetes Care 2013;36(4):823–30.

Effects of Antipsychotic Medications on Appetite, Weight, and Insulin Resistance

Chao Deng, PhD

KEYWORDS

- Antipsychotic • Appetite • Obesity • Weight gain • Insulin resistance
- Glucose dysregulation

KEY POINTS

- Although some atypical antipsychotic drugs, particularly olanzapine and clozapine, have more severe weight-gain side effects, all antipsychotics, including typical antipsychotics currently used clinically, may cause some degree of weight gain.
- There are time-dependent changes in weight gain associated with antipsychotic medication, with development of a 3-stage time course; in particular, rapid weight gain in the initial stage is a good indicator for a long-term outcome of weight gain and obesity.
- Accumulated data suggest that increasing appetite and food intake, as well as delayed satiety signaling, are key behavioral changes related to weight gain/obesity induced by antipsychotics.
- Antipsychotics may induce insulin resistance, glucose dysregulation, and even type 2 diabetes mellitus independent of weight gain and adiposity.
- There are also time-dependent changes for insulin and glucose dysregulation associated with antipsychotic medication.
- Current evidence from clinical trials in first-episode psychotic patients shows that typical antipsychotics such as haloperidol have a relatively high risk for weight gain/obesity and glucometabolic side effects.
- Monitoring weight gain is important but insufficient. Periodic monitoring of blood sugar may also be required during antipsychotic therapy, particularly for drugs with high diabetic liabilities such as olanzapine and clozapine.
- There are marked individual variations in weight gain and other metabolic side effects associated with antipsychotics. For example, irrespective of the antipsychotic drug some patients lose weight, some maintain weight, and some gain weight.

Continued

Funding Sources: This study was supported by a Project grant (APP1044624) from the National Health and Medical Research Council (NHMRC), Australia.
Conflicts of Interest: None.
Antipsychotic Research Laboratory, School of Health Sciences, Illawarra Health and Medical Research Institute, University of Wollongong, Northfields Avenue, Wollongong, New South Wales 2522, Australia
E-mail address: chao@uow.edu.au

Endocrinol Metab Clin N Am 42 (2013) 545–563
http://dx.doi.org/10.1016/j.ecl.2013.05.006
0889-8529/13/$ – see front matter © 2013 Elsevier Inc. All rights reserved.

endo.theclinics.com

Continued

- Mechanisms for antipsychotic-related weight gain, insulin resistance, and glucose dysregulation have yet to be elucidated. Current results suggest that antagonistic effects of atypical antipsychotics on serotonin 5-HT_{2C} and histamine H_1 receptors play an important role in weight-gain/obesity side effects, whereas muscarinic M_3 receptors have been identified as most closely linked with diabetic side effects. However, blockade of dopamine D_2 receptors may be a common mechanism for these metabolic side effects in both atypical and typical antipsychotics.

INTRODUCTION

Mental disorders are the greatest overall cause of disability.[1] Antipsychotic drugs (APDs) are the most widely prescribed medications and are used frequently to control various mental disorders such as schizophrenia, bipolar disorder, dementia, major depression, Tourette syndrome, eating disorders, and even substance abuse.[2,3] Unfortunately, APDs may cause some serious side effects, including extrapyramidal and metabolic side effects. Since typical APDs were introduced into clinics in the 1950s their side effects of increasing body weight have been reported, but have gained less attention because these drugs often have worse and problematic extrapyramidal side effects.[4] In the 1980s and 1990s, clozapine, olanzapine, and other atypical APDs with reduced extrapyramidal side effects were widely introduced into psychiatric clinics, and currently form the first line of APD treatment.[5,6] Unfortunately, atypical APDs, particularly clozapine and olanzapine, cause serious metabolic side effects, such as substantial weight gain, intra-abdominal obesity, hyperlipidemia, insulin resistance, hyperglycemia, and type 2 diabetes mellitus (T2DM).[7–10] These adverse effects are a major risk for cardiovascular disease, stroke, and premature death (by 20–30 years).[7,11] In addition to medical consequences, weight gain and obesity can lead to noncompliance with medication, which is a primary problem for the treatment of schizophrenia because cessation of APD treatment dramatically (up to 5-fold) increases the relapse rate for these patients.[12,13] Given that the majority of patients with psychiatric disorders face chronic, even life-long, treatment with APDs, the risks of weight gain, obesity, and other metabolic symptoms are major considerations for individual APD maintenance treatment. This review focuses on the effects of APDs on weight gain, appetite, insulin resistance, and glucose dysregulation, as well as relevant underlying mechanisms that may be help to prevent and treat weight gain/obesity and other metabolic side effects caused by APD therapy.

WEIGHT GAIN AND OBESITY INDUCED BY ANTIPSYCHOTICS
Weight-Gain/Obesity Side Effects: Typical Versus Atypical APDs

It had been reported since the 1950s that treatment with some typical APDs (such as chlorpromazine) is associated with weight gain; however, many psychiatrists still hold believe that atypical APDs are associated with significant weight gain and obesity side effects, whereas typical APDs are not.[14] For example, the commonly used typical APD, haloperidol, was once believed to have a minimal weight-gain side effect.[14] However, a recent report on the European First-Episode Schizophrenia Trial (EUFEST) has clearly shown that 1 year of treatment with haloperidol caused clinically significant weight gain (≥7% from baseline) in 53% of patients, with an average weight gain of 7.3 kg.[15] A dramatic weight gain (9.56 kg) was also observed in another study of first-episode patients after 1 year treatment with haloperidol.[16] Therefore, while certain atypical APDs (such as olanzapine and clozapine) might lead to greater weight gain, typical APDs could also lead to significant weight and other metabolic changes in patients.

Underestimation of weight-gain and obesity side effects has also been the case for atypical APDs. In 2005, the National Institutes of Health–funded CATIE (The Clinical Antipsychotic Trials of Intervention Effectiveness) study reported the effects of the atypical APDs olanzapine, quetiapine, risperidone, and ziprasidone on body weight over an 18-months period in chronic schizophrenia patients who had an average of more than 14 years' APD medication history.[17] The CATIE study found that olanzapine treatment caused significant weight gain ($\geq$7% from baseline) in a higher proportion of patients (30%) than quetiapine (16%), risperidone (14%), and ziprasidone (7%). Patients treated with olanzapine also gained more weight (average addition 0.9 kg [2 lb] per month) than patients treated with quetiapine (average addition 0.23 kg [0.5 lb] per month) and risperidone (average addition 0.18 kg [0.4 lb] per month), whereas ziprasidone-treated patients lost body weight (average loss 0.14 kg [−0.3 lb] per month).[17] However, the subsequent EUFEST and CAFE (Comparison of Atypical Antipsychotics for First Episode) studies showed that these atypical APDs caused more severe weight gain in first-episode schizophrenia patients.[15,18] The CAFE study reported that after a 12-week treatment, significant weight gain ($\geq$7% body weight) occurred in a large number of first-episode schizophrenia patients treated with olanzapine (59.8%), compared with risperidone (32.5%) and quetiapine (29.2%). Furthermore, after 52 weeks' treatment, 80% of olanzapine-treated patients gained at least 7% body weight (with an average 1.76 kg [3.88 lb] per month), compared with 57.6% of risperidone treated (with an average 1.28 kg [2.81 lb] per month) and 50% of quetiapine-treated (with an average 1.29 kg [2.85 lb] per month) patients.[18] The EUFEST study confirmed that after 12 months of treatment, olanzapine caused the most significant weight gain in first-episode schizophrenia (in 86% of patients with an average 1.16 kg [2.56 lb] per month) compared with quetiapine (in 65% of patients with an average 0.88 kg [1.94 lb] per month), amisulpride (in 63% of patients with an average [1.78 lb] per month), and ziprasidone (in 37% of patients with an average 0.4 kg [0.88 lb] per month).[15] In another study of first-episode patients, dramatic weight gain was observed in olanzapine (average 12.02 kg), risperidone (8.99 kg), and haloperidol (9.56 kg) treatment after 1 year.[16] It is interesting that ziprasidone and amisulpride have been widely regarded as atypical APDs with low weight gain risk in previous studies[10]; ziprasidone was even found to cause weight loss in the CATIE study.[17] Therefore, it is worth exploring why a lesser weight-gain side effect was observed in the CATIE study. The main difference between these studies was that subjects in the CATIE study had a chronic APD medication history (average >14 years) in comparison with first-episode patients without previous APD medication in the EUFEST and CAFE studies.[15,17,18] These clinical trials indicate that previous studies on patients with chronic schizophrenia may have underestimated the magnitude of weight-gain/obesity side effects associated with APDs. Furthermore, although mean weight gain and the incidence of clinically significant weight gain may vary between APDs, olanzapine and clozapine have the highest risk; accumulated evidence indicates that both typical and atypical APDs have more weight-gain and other metabolic side effects than placebo-level effects.[9,10,15]

Time Course of APD-Induced Weight Gain/Obesity

Although various APDs cause weight gain at different magnitudes, both typical and atypical APDs exhibit a similar temporal course of weight gain that includes

3 stages: stage 1, an early acceleration stage in which APDs induce a rapid increase in body weight within the first few months of treatment (eg, about 3 months for clozapine, olanzapine, risperidone, and haloperidol); stage 2, a middle stage in which body weight continues to increase at a much steadier rate for a period of at least a year or longer; and stage 3, further treatment that leads to a plateau of weight gain, representing a possible "ceiling effect" of APDs, in which patients will maintain the heavier weight with ongoing APD treatment.[19,20] For example, patients with first-episode psychosis treated with olanzapine or haloperidol gained weight rapidly during the first 12 weeks (mean ± standard deviation [SD]: olanzapine, 9.2 ± 5.31 kg; haloperidol, 3.7 ± 4.9 kg), then continued to gain weight until a plateau was reached (olanzapine, 15.5 ± 9.6 kg; haloperidol, 7.1 ± 6.7 kg) at approximately 1 year, after which weight gain remained at this high level (olanzapine, 15.4 ± 10.0 kg; haloperidol, 7.5 ± 9.2 kg) up to the end of 2 years.[20] The changes in body mass index (BMI; calculated as weight in kilograms divided by height in meters squared, ie, kg/m^2) during the 2-year study period followed a pattern similar to that for weight gain; in the olanzapine group the mean BMI increased from 23.6 ± 4.8 (mean ± SD) at baseline to 26.4 ± 4.6 at 12 weeks, 28.8 ± 4.5 at 1 year, and 28.3 ± 4.0 at 2 years, compared with the haloperidol group's increase from 23.9 ± 4.5 at baseline to 24.8 ± 4.1 at 12 weeks, 26.2 ± 4.3 at 1 year, and 26.6 ± 4.4 at 2 years.[20] Several long-term studies indicate that some APDs may take a much longer time to reach the plateau.[19,21,22] This temporal course is well mimicked in an animal model of olanzapine-induced weight gain.[23,24] Although the final weight plateau is often reached after several years, accumulated evidence indicates that rapid weight gain in the first few weeks (Stage 1) of APD treatment is a strong indicator for the long-term outcome of weight gain and obesity.[25–27] Therefore, although the time course of weight gain has been observed to have a similar pattern in various APDs, the exact time course of weight gain induced by a specific APD still remains a topic of further research.

Are Weight-Gain and Obesity Side Effects of APD Dose Dependent?

To date, the possible relationship between APD dosages and associated weight gain has not been systematically investigated. Simon and colleagues[28] reviewed publications between 1975 and 2008, and suggested that olanzapine and clozapine appear to have dose-dependent and serum concentration–dependent weight-gain side effects. For example, Perry and colleagues[29] reported associations of weight gain with both olanzapine dosages and plasma concentrations. More recently, in an 8-week, randomized clinical trial of olanzapine, 10-, 20-, and 40-mg (oral) doses in 634 patients with schizophrenia or schizoaffective disorder, a significant dose-related change in weight gain was found, which suggested that higher than standard doses of olanzapine may be associated with greater weight gain compared with standard doses.[30] This finding was supported by a study into long-acting olanzapine injection, in which clear dose-dependent changes of weight gain were observed; a high dose (300 mg every 2 weeks) had a higher weight gain than medium (405 mg every 4 weeks) and low (150 mg every 2 weeks) doses in schizophrenia patients.[31] Risperidone-induced weight gain could be dose related to some extent but data are contradictory, and no study has assessed risperidone serum concentrations in association with weight gain.[28] Current evidence indicates that other APDs including aripiprazole, amisulpride, quetiapine, sertindole, and ziprasidone have no dose-related metabolic effects; however, no study has assessed serum concentrations of these APDs.[28] Therefore, prescribing the lowest possible effective doses, at least for clozapine, olanzapine, and risperidone, will be helpful in minimizing their weight-gain side effects.

EFFECTS OF ANTIPSYCHOTIC MEDICATION ON APPETITE AND FOOD INTAKE

Theoretically, gain in body weight results from an imbalance between energy intake and energy expenditure, whereby overeating and/or less energy expenditure (such as decreasing resting metabolism and activity) may contribute to overweight and obesity. Over the past 15 years, accumulated data from both clinical and animal studies suggest that increasing appetite and food intake, as well as delayed satiety signaling, are key behavioral changes related to APD-induced weight gain/obesity.[32–34] On the other hand, there is less understanding of to what extent changes of resting metabolism rate and activity/sedation affect weight gain associated with APD medication, although current evidence suggests that they may play an important role in the development of APD-induced weight gain.[19,35,36]

Altered eating behaviors have been reported in several clinical studies with treatment involving various APDs. Gothelf and colleagues[37] first reported that increased food intake, but not resting energy expenditure and physical activity, was associated with olanzapine-induced weight gain in schizophrenia patients. A randomized double-blind study found that both clozapine and olanzapine were associated with food craving and binge eating over the 6-week treatment period.[38] Compared with those taking clozapine, patients receiving olanzapine tended to have higher rates of food craving (olanzapine 48.9% vs clozapine 23.3%) and binge eating (olanzapine 16.7% vs clozapine 8.9%), which also occurred earlier (1 week vs 3 weeks for binge eating).[38] In another study[33] eating behavior in patients treated with atypical APDs (clozapine, olanzapine, risperidone, quetiapine, or ziprasidone) were also compared with healthy controls by recording appetite sensation before and after a standardized breakfast using visual analog scales. The investigators found that: (1) atypical APD-treated patients showed greater adiposity and a higher degree of hunger following the standardized breakfast; and (2) patients had significantly higher cognitive dietary restraint, disinhibition, and susceptibility to hunger than controls. The patients treated with atypical APDs were also more reactive to external eating cues.[34] Furthermore, a recent study reported that, consistent with the significant increase in body weight, food consumption, and disinhibited eating, 1 week of treatment with olanzapine enhanced both the anticipatory and consummatory reward response to food rewards in the brain's reward circuitry, including the inferior frontal cortex, striatum, and anterior cingulate cortex, but decreased activation in the brain region (the lateral orbital frontal cortex) believed to inhibit feeding behavior.[39]

These clinical findings are confirmed in animal studies where APD-induced hyperphagia is repeatedly found in animal models of APD-induced weight gain.[23,40–43] Furthermore, recently olanzapine has been found to selectively increase rats' response to sucrose pellets in an operant conditioning without affecting free-feeding intake of sucrose; by contrast, sibutramine (a noradrenaline/serotonin reuptake inhibitor and a weight-reducing agent) prevented the increase of rats' response to sucrose pellets induced by olanzapine.[44] It has been well established that the hypothalamic arcuate nucleus plays a crucial role in appetite and energy homeostasis through activation of 2 distinct populations of anorexigenic and orexigenic neurons: neurons that express appetite inhibiting cocaine- and amphetamine-related transcript (CART) and pro-opiomelanocortin (POMC), and neurons that express appetite-stimulating agouti-related peptide (AgRP) and neuropeptide Y (NPY).[45] Using the animal model for olanzapine-induced weight gain, it has been revealed that olanzapine elevated the expression of appetite-stimulating AgRP and NPY, and decreased appetite-inhibiting POMC.[46,47] These results suggest that patients treated with APDs may develop abnormal eating behaviors in response to altered appetite sensations and increased susceptibility to hunger, which may lead to a positive energy balance and contribute to gain in body weight.

INSULIN RESISTANCE, GLUCOSE DYSREGULATION, AND DIABETES ASSOCIATED WITH ANTIPSYCHOTIC MEDICATION
Effects of Atypical APDs

Validated evidence over the past 20 years has indicated that APD medication significantly increases the risk of insulin resistance, glucose dysregulation, and the development of T2DM.[5,48,49] Although patients with psychiatric disorders such as schizophrenia have been observed to have an increased risk of developing diabetes regardless of antipsychotics, suggesting that the disease itself may be a predisposing risk factor,[50–52] APD medication has been widely recognized as a main contributor in these metabolic disorders.[7,48,49] An analysis of the US Food and Drug Administration Adverse Event database also showed that adjusted report ratios for T2DM were the following: olanzapine 9.6 (95% confidence interval [CI] 9.2–10.0), risperidone 3.8 (95% CI 3.5–4.1), quetiapine 3.5 (95% CI 3.2–3.9), clozapine 3.1 (95% CI 2.9–3.3), ziprasidone 2.4 (95% CI 2.0–2.9), aripiprazole 2.4 (95% CI 1.9–2.9), and haloperidol 2.0 (95% CI 1.7–2.3), which suggests differential risks of diabetes across various APDs.[53]

Owing to relatively short trial periods, many clinical trials have not been able to capture most new cases of diabetes; however, numerous studies have shown strong relationships between APDs and indicators of insulin resistance and glucose dysregulation.[48,54] In the CATIE study of patients with chronic schizophrenia, compared with baseline the fasting blood glucose (FBG) level was most elevated with olanzapine (15.0 ± 2.8 mg/dL; mean ± standard error), followed by quetiapine (6.8 ± 2.5 mg/dL), risperidone (6.7 ± 2.0 mg/dL), perphenazine (5.2 ± 2.0 mg/dL), and ziprasidone (2.3 ± 3.9 mg/dL).[17] The EUFEST study has reported a similar incidence rate of hyperglycemia among various APDs after 1 year of treatment with haloperidol (18%), amisulpride (21%), olanzapine (30%), quetiapine (22%) and ziprasidone (22%), with a significant increase of fasting insulin level (haloperidol 2.0 ± 1.4 mU/L, amisulpride 8.6 ± 3.1 mU/L, olanzapine 2.5 ± 3.9 mU/L, quetiapine 2.1 ± 1.2 mU/L, and ziprasidone 0.1 ± 2.0 mU/L).[15] Chronically elevated insulin levels and concurrent hyperglycemia are consistent with insulin resistance, and may indicate T2DM.[55] In fact, numerous clinical studies have reported that chronic APD treatment increases insulin resistance. Using the homeostasis model assessment index for insulin resistance (HOMA-IR), chronic (8 weeks to 5 months) treatment with olanzapine, clozapine, and risperidone has been repeatedly reported to significantly increase the HOMA-IR,[56–61] although risperidone was normally observed to have a lesser effect on HOMA-IR.[58,60,61] Furthermore, patients with chronic olanzapine treatment also showed a greater decrease in insulin sensitivity during an oral glucose tolerance test than those treated with risperidone.[61] Using a frequently sampled intravenous glucose tolerance test and minimal model analysis, significant insulin resistance and impairment of glucose effectiveness were reported in nonobese patients chronically treated with clozapine and olanzapine, but with a lesser effect in patients treated with risperidone and quetiapine.[62,63] Recently, a 2-step euglycemic, hyperinsulinemic clamp procedure has been used to assess changes in insulin sensitivity in nondiabetic patients with schizophrenia or schizoaffective disorder treated with olanzapine or risperidone, whereby olanzapine and risperidone treatment caused a decrement in insulin sensitivity.[59] These results were confirmed in numerous animal studies using the HOMA-IR or euglycemic/hyperinsulinemic clamp procedures: chronic treatment with olanzapine and clozapine caused insulin resistance, a reduction in insulin sensitivity, and glucose dysregulation.[64–68]

Effects of Typical APDs Using Haloperidol as an Example

Although over the past 15 years the metabolic side effects of atypical APDs have attracted most attention, there is evidence that treatment with some typical APDs also increases the risk of insulin resistance, glucose dysregulation, and T2DM.[11,49,69,70] Since they were introduced to clinics in the 1950s, chlorpromazine and thioridazine have been repeatedly reported to cause abnormal glucose tolerance, insulin resistance, and even T2DM.[70–76] Although, on the other hand, it was generally believed that haloperidol did not increase the risk of insulin resistance and T2DM,[49] recent evidence from clinical trials in first-episode patients showed that haloperidol may have a higher risk than originally thought. As discussed earlier, the EUFEST study has reported that 1 year of treatment with haloperidol has an incidence rate of hyperglycemia and increased fasting insulin levels similar to that of the atypical APDs olanzapine and quetiapine.[15] Another randomized, double-blind trial in patients with first-episode schizophrenia also found that both FBG and 2-hour postprandial blood glucose (PPBG) levels were significantly increased by a 6-week treatment with haloperidol (FBG, $6.8 \pm 14.1/dL$, mean $\pm$ SD; PPBG, 6.7 ± 12.6 mg/dL), olanzapine, (FBG, 6.6 ± 12.7 mg/dL; PPBG, 21.5 ± 32.2 mg/dl), and risperidone (FBG, 4.3 ± 12.5 mg/dL; PPBG, 21.0 ± 23.4 mg/dL), with a similar incidence rate of diabetes induced by APD treatment (haloperidol 9.7%, olanzapine 11.4%, risperidone 9.1%) by World Health Organization criteria.[69] A 1-year treatment of haloperidol in drug-naïve first-episode patients showed a similarly increased insulin level and HOMA-IR in comparison with olanzapine and risperidone.[77] Analyzing data from the Italian Health Search Database also showed that, In initially nondiabetic and APD-free patients, the diabetic risk ratios were 12.4% (95% CI 6.3–24.5) for haloperidol, 18.7% (95% CI 8.2–42.8) for risperidone, 20.4% (95% CI 6.9–60.3) for olanzapine, and 33.7% (95% CI 9.2–123.6) for quetiapine, with no significant difference between various drug groups.[78] These findings were confirmed by a large population-based study conducted in Denmark, which included 345,937 patients treated with an APD and 1,426,488 unexposed control subjects. A significantly higher relative risk compared with the general population was observed in drug-naïve patients treated with olanzapine (1.35, 95% CI 1.18–1.54), risperidone (1.24, 95% CI 1.09–1.40), sertindole (9.53, 95% CI 1.34–67.63), perphenazine (1.60, 95% CI 1.45–1.77), ziprasidone (3.09, 95% CI 1.54–6.17), and haloperidol (1.32, 95% CI 1.17–1.49), but not in patients treated with aripiprazole, amisulpride, or quetiapine.[79] These results suggest that treatment with haloperidol, like chlorpromazine and thioridazine, is associated an increased risk of glucose and insulin dysregulation.

Indirect Effects of APD-Induced Weight Gain and Obesity Versus Direct Effects of APDs on Insulin Resistance and Glucose Dysregulation

Given the well-established association between obesity and insulin resistance and hyperglycemia, APD-induced dysregulation of glucose homeostasis has been frequently linked to the high propensity of these drugs for weight gain and obesity. For example, many studies have found the increased HOMA-IR induced by chronic treatment of olanzapine, clozapine, or risperidone to be correlated with weight gain and adiposity.[58,77,80] Weight gain and adiposity were also found to be significantly correlated with changes in insulin sensitivity in patients following a 12-week treatment with olanzapine and risperidone.[59] In 2010, Kim and colleagues[81] reported that BMI contributed one-quarter to one-third of the variance in insulin resistance in olanzapine-treated patients. However, growing evidence has demonstrated that treatment with APDs, particularly short-term treatment, can directly affect insulin resistance and glucose homeostasis independent of weight gain.[82] In fact, clinical studies have shown impaired glucose regulation without weight gain in some schizophrenia patients treated with APDs.[83] Insulin resistance has also been reported to be induced by olanzapine treatment within days without any weight gain.[84,85] Diabetic ketoacidosis has been reported in patients in early treatment with various APDs and without weight gain.[86] In APD-naïve schizophrenia patients, 2 weeks' treatment of olanzapine decreased insulin secretory response to a hyperglycemic challenge, which suggests that olanzapine might directly impair pancreatic β-cell function.[87] Data from animal studies also showed that acute treatment, even a single acute dose, of olanzapine, risperidone, or clozapine can cause hyperglycemia and hyperinsulinemia, impair insulin sensitivity, and induce insulin resistance.[66,88–91] An in vitro study also showed that olanzapine and clozapine can directly decrease glucose-stimulated insulin secretion from pancreatic β cells.[92] Furthermore, olanzapine and clozapine can significantly decrease the insulin-stimulated glucose transport rate by about 40% in 3T3-L1 adipocytes, whereas clozapine and risperidone reduced the insulin-stimulated glucose transport rate by about 40% in primary cultured rat adipocytes.[93] Therefore, these typical APDs may directly induce insulin resistance by directly impairing insulin-responsive glucose resistance in adipocytes.[93]

Time Course of APD-Induced Insulin Dysregulation

Although a growing body of evidence has shown that short-term/acute APD treatment decreases fasting plasma insulin levels and attenuates glucose-stimulated insulin response,[87,88,91,92,94] as already discussed, chronic treatment is associated with hyperinsulinemia, insulin resistance, and T2DM.[49,59,95] The apparent conflict in reports between chronic and short-term APD treatment may be reconciled by a hypothesis of time-dependent changes of APD-induced insulin dysregulation. This hypothesis is supported by a recent report that found time-dependent changes of glucose-stimulated insulin response in individuals with schizophrenia: decreased insulin levels during the first 2 weeks of olanzapine treatment compared with their baseline levels, followed by a return to baseline levels after 4 weeks of treatment, and increased insulin response following 8 weeks of olanzapine treatment.[96] In another study in schizophrenia patients who started or switched to a different APD for 3 months, a time-dependent worsening of plasma glucose levels was observed in subjects taking clozapine, olanzapine, and quetiapine.[97] A recent animal study also demonstrated that acute treatment of rats with olanzapine showed both glucose dysregulation and insulin resistance; however, rats treated intermittently with olanzapine (once per week) showed a marked worsening in both glucose dysregulation and insulin resistance over the course of a 10-week treatment.[67] The mechanisms underlying this time-dependent change in APD-induced insulin and glucose dysregulation have not been investigated, however.

NEUROPHARMACOLOGIC MECHANISMS FOR APD-INDUCED WEIGHT GAIN AND GLUCOMETABOLIC SIDE EFFECTS

In contrast to typical APDs (such as haloperidol) that are largely potent and selective D_2 antagonists, atypical APDs have binding affinities for various neurotransmitter receptors, such as dopamine D_2, serotonin 5-HT$_{2A}$ and 5-HT$_{2C}$, adrenergic α_{1-2}, muscarinic M_1 and M_3, and histamine H_1 receptors.[98] Among these receptors, dopamine D_2 and 5-HT$_2$ receptors play critical roles in the therapeutic effects of atypical APDs.[99,100]

Accumulated evidence has revealed that the antagonistic properties of 5-HT_{2C} and H_1 receptors are involved in APD-induced weight gain.[32,101,102] In fact, among APDs, clozapine and olanzapine have the highest affinities for 5-HT_{2C} and H_1 receptors, and have the highest risk of weight-gain/obesity side effects.[36,98,103] Therefore, the neuropharmacologic mechanisms reviewed here are mainly from studies on olanzapine and clozapine. It is worth noting that because of the variations in receptor-binding profiles between different APDs, the mechanisms underlying the weight gain and glucometabolic side effects might not be exactly the same between various APDs.

Over the past 30 years the 5-HT receptor has been revealed to regulate appetite and body weight, mainly through acting at the hypothalamic 5-HT_{2C} receptors.[104] In fact, 5-HTergic neurons project to the hypothalamic POMC neurons that coexpress 5-HT_{2C} receptors, and 5-HT has been found to influence appetite by activating anorexigenic POMC neurons and melanocortin-4 receptors.[104] Considering the finding that olanzapine decreases expression of POMC in animal studies,[46,47] APDs may therefore increase appetite by inhibiting POMC neurons through the 5-HT_{2C} receptors. It is interesting that 5-HT_{2C} agonists reduce food intake by advancing satiety, and these effects are reversed by 5-HT_{2C} antagonists.[105,106] These results suggest that blockade of 5-HT_{2C} receptors could possibly be the mechanism for the clinical findings showing that treatment with both clozapine and olanzapine could induce food craving and binge eating in patients.[38] Furthermore, the role of 5-HT_{2C} in APD-induced weight gain was confirmed by an animal study, which showed that the initial (5 days) increase in weight gain and food intake associated with olanzapine treatment could be mimicked by combining a 5-HT_{2C} antagonist (SB243213) with haloperidol, but not by an H_1 antagonist alone or in combination with haloperidol.[107] However, there is clear evidence that 1-week and 12-week treatment with olanzapine reduces the expression of hypothalamic H_1 receptors, and H_1 receptor changes have been correlated with increased food intake and weight gain in rats.[24] Olanzapine and clozapine have been reported to activate the hypothalamic adenosine monophosphate-activated protein kinase (AMPK) pathway via H_1 receptors to increase food intake and gain in body weight.[108] Olanzapine has also been reported to regulate feeding behavior in rats by modulating histaminergic neurotransmission.[109] The role of the H_1 receptor in APD-induced weight gain has also been supported by findings that cotreatment of betahistine (an H_1 agonist and an H_3 antagonist) can significantly reduce olanzapine-induced weight gain in both schizophrenia patients and animals.[110–112] It has also been postulated that different neural mechanisms are responsible for the 3 stages of weight gain induced by APDs.[19]

APD affinity for the muscarinic M_3 receptor has been identified as most closely linked to its diabetic side effects,[113–115] and can even be used to predict its diabetogenic liability.[113] Consistently, olanzapine and clozapine, 2 of the APDs associated with a high risk of insulin resistance, glucose dysregulation, and diabetic side effects, possess the highest M_3 receptor-binding affinity.[116] M_3 receptors play a crucial role in the regulation of insulin secretion through both the peripheral and central cholinergic pathways.[117] An in vitro study has shown that olanzapine and clozapine can impair cholinergic-stimulated insulin secretion.[92] A recent animal study found that a single subcutaneous injection of darifenacin (a selective M_3 muscarinic antagonist) significantly decreased insulin response to glucose challenge in comparison with controls.[118] M_3 receptors are widely expressed in the hypothalamic arcuate nucleus and ventromedial nucleus, and the dorsal vagal complex of the brainstem, brain regions well documented for their role in insulin and glucagon secretion and glucose homeostasis.[119,120] Recently, Weston-Green[121] found that a 2-week treatment with olanzapine decreased fasting insulin levels and correlated with an increase in

M_3 receptor-binding density in the arcuate nucleus, ventromedial nucleus, and dorsal vagal complex. In addition, acute central treatment with olanzapine via intracerebroventricular infusion induced hepatic insulin resistance and increased hypothalamic AMPK expression.[122] Results from the 2 studies suggest that olanzapine may block M_3 receptor signaling pathways in the brain, thus affecting insulin production and insulin resistance. Therefore, APDs may act through both peripheral and central M_3 antagonism to impair compensatory insulin response, resulting in diabetes.

Since the introduction of APDs in the 1950s, binding at dopamine D_2 receptors (antagonism or partial agonism) remains the only mechanism common to the therapeutic efficacy of all APDs.[100] There is evidence that both atypical and typical APDs can cause weight gain and other metabolic side effects. In particular, recent clinical data from studies in first-episode patients demonstrated haloperidol (a potent and selective D_2 antagonist) to be associated with weight gain, insulin resistance, and glucose dysregulation, as already discussed; it is therefore reasonable to propose D_2 receptors as a possible common mechanism underlying these side effects. Although it has been the subject of fewer investigations, there is some evidence supporting the involvement of D_2 receptors in APD-induced weight gain, insulin resistance, and glucose dysregulation. As discussed earlier, only treatment using a 5-HT_{2C} antagonist combined with haloperidol can mimic olanzapine-induced weight gain.[107] A relationship between a functional promoter region polymorphism in *DRD2* and weight gain induced by olanzapine and risperidone has been reported in first-episode schizophrenia.[123] Dopamine and D_2 receptors are key components of the reward system controlling the desire for food and, hence, regulation of body weight.[124] A previous study by the author's group[125] found that D_2 receptor density in the rostral part of the caudate putamen in obese mice was significantly lower compared with that in lean mice. It is well established that blockade of dopamine D_2 receptor activity in the mesolimbic and nigrostriatal pathways is the common mechanism of APD action,[100,126] and that these are also key pathways for food reward.[127] In fact, reduced striatal activation was detected by functional magnetic resonance imaging during reward anticipation, owing to appetite-provoking cues in chronic schizophrenia under APD treatment.[128] Therefore, APDs may increase appetite and food intake by acting on dopamine D_2–mediated reward.[127] It is interesting that D_2-like receptors are also expressed in pancreatic β cells, which function to inhibit glucose-stimulated insulin secretion,[129] and permanent lack of D_2 receptor–mediated inhibition (such as in D_2 knockout mice *Drd2$^{-/-}$*) eventually results in glucose intolerance.[130] It has been reported that a single subcutaneous injection of raclopride (a D_2/D_3 selective antagonist) can enhance insulin secretion and marginally decrease insulin sensitivity.[118] Therefore, this may provide a mechanism to explain why chronic treatment of some typical APDs (such as haloperidol) leads to glucose dysregulation, hyperinsulinemia, and, eventually, diabetes.

SUMMARY

Over the past 20 years it has been established that treatment with atypical APDs is associated with serious weight gain, obesity, and other metabolic side effects such as insulin resistance, glucose dysregulation, and T2DM; however, the metabolic side effects associated with some typical APDs are possibly underestimated. Emerging evidence over the past 5 to 6 years from the studies in first-episode psychotic and drug-naïve patients show that some commonly used typical APDs (such as haloperidol) may also cause significant weight gain, insulin resistance, glucose dysregulation, and even T2DM, particularly under chronic treatment. In fact, although some atypical APDs, particularly clozapine and olanzapine, have a higher liability than others in inducing metabolic side effects, current evidence indicates that all APDs have more weight gain and other metabolic side effects than placebo-level effects.

It is worth noting that variations in weight gain and other metabolic side effects are observed not only among APDs; marked individual variations have also been observed in all reported clinical studies and, irrespective of the APD, some subjects lose weight, some maintain weight, and some gain weight.[15,17] It is also noteworthy that not all weight gain is detrimental. For those patients who are underweight before APD treatment, possibly reflecting that their psychotic illness has caused them to neglect themselves, weight gain associated with APD is beneficial if the medication results in these individuals returning to a premorbid and healthy weight.[131] This individual variation could be related to both genetic and nongenetic factors (such as gender, age, and initial body weight/BMI).[132,133] Although there is no reliable biomarker for the prediction of weight gain, several studies have identified female gender, younger age, and a low BMI before the first APD treatment as risk factors for APD-induced weight gain and obesity.[133–136] A diagnosis of undifferentiated schizophrenia or schizophrenia spectrum disorder was also identified as a possible predictor for APD-induced weight gain.[133,136] As APD-induced weight gain has a time-dependent development, and particularly because rapid weight gain in the first few weeks of APD treatment is a good indicator for a long-term outcome of weight gain and obesity,[19,27] weight monitoring during the early phase of APD therapy is crucial for prevention of this serious side effect. Because insulin resistance and glucose dysregulation may develop independently of weight gain, monitoring only weight gain is not sufficient, and periodic monitoring of blood sugar may also be required during APD therapy, particularly for drugs with high diabetic liabilities such as olanzapine and clozapine. Although current evidence suggests that multiple neurotransmitter receptors such as $5-HT_{2C}$, histamine H_1, and muscarinic M_3 (and possibly also dopamine D_2 receptors) are involved in weight gain/obesity and insulin and glucose dysregulation associated with APDs, one important issue that needs to be investigated is how these neurotransmitter systems interact during the time-dependent development of these side effects. An improved understanding of the mechanisms underlying the time-dependent development of these metabolic side effects could help in designing better strategies to prevent and treat these devastating side effects and their associated cardiovascular disease, stroke, and premature death.

REFERENCES

1. Murray CJ, Lopez AD. The Global Burden of Disease: a comprehensive assessment of mortality and disability from diseases, injuries and risk factors in 1990 and projected to 2020. Cambridge (MA): Harvard School of Public Health; 1996.
2. Lambert T. Managing the metabolic adverse effects of antipsychotic drugs in patients with psychosis. Australian Prescriber 2011;34(4):97–9.
3. Newcomer J. Second-generation atypical antipsychotics and metabolic effects. a comprehensive literature review. CNS Drugs 2005;19:1–93.
4. Hasan A, Wobrock T, Reich-Erkelenz D, et al. Treatment of first-episode schizophrenia: pharmacological and neurobiological aspects. Drug Discov Today 2011;8(1–2):31–5.
5. Vohora D. Atypical antipsychotic drugs: current issues of safety and efficacy in the management of schizophrenia. Curr Opin Investig Drugs 2007;8(7): 531–8.

6. Asenjo Lobos C, Komossa K, Rummel-Kluge C, et al. Clozapine versus other atypical antipsychotics for schizophrenia. Cochrane Database Syst Rev 2010;(11):CD006633.

7. Stahl SM, Mignon L, Meyer JM. Which comes first: atypical antipsychotic treatment or cardiometabolic risk? Acta Psychiatr Scand 2009;119(3):171–9.

8. Lambert MT, Copeland LA, Sampson N, et al. New-onset type-2 diabetes associated with atypical antipsychotic medications. Prog Neuropsychopharmacol Biol Psychiatry 2006;30(5):919–23.

9. Allison D, Mentore J, Heo M, et al. Antipsychotic-induced weight gain: a comprehensive research synthesis. Am J Psychiatry 1999;156(11):1686–96.

10. Correll CU, Lencz T, Malhotra AK. Antipsychotic drugs and obesity. Trends Mol Med 2011;17(2):97–107.

11. Newcomer JW. Metabolic considerations in the use of antipsychotic medications: a review of recent evidence. J Clin Psychiatry 2007;68(Suppl 1):20–7.

12. Robinson D, Woerner MG, Alvir JMJ, et al. Predictors of relapse following response from a first episode of schizophrenia or schizoaffective disorder. Arch Gen Psychiatry 1999;56(3):241–7.

13. Weiden PJ, Mackell JA, McDonnell DD. Obesity as a risk factor for antipsychotic noncompliance. Schizophr Res 2004;66(1):51–7.

14. Nasrallah HA. Folie en masse! It's so tempting to drink the Kool-Aid. Curr Psychiatr 2011;10(3):12–6.

15. Kahn RS, Fleischhacker WW, Boter H, et al. Effectiveness of antipsychotic drugs in first-episode schizophrenia and schizophreniform disorder: an open randomised clinical trial. Lancet 2008;371(9618):1085–97.

16. Perez-Iglesias R, Vazquez-Barquero JL, Amado JA, et al. Effect of antipsychotics on peptides involved in energy balance in drug-naive psychotic patients after 1 year of treatment. J Clin Psychopharmacol 2008;28(3):289–95.

17. Lieberman JA, Stroup TS, McEvoy JP, et al. Effectiveness of antipsychotic drugs in patients with chronic schizophrenia. N Engl J Med 2005;353(12):1209–23.

18. Patel JK, Buckley PF, Woolson S, et al. Metabolic profiles of second-generation antipsychotics in early psychosis: findings from the CAFE study. Schizophr Res 2009;111(1–3):9–16.

19. Pai N, Deng C, Vella S-L, et al. Are there different neural mechanisms responsible for three stages of weight gain development in anti-psychotic therapy: temporally based hypothesis. Asian J Psychiatr 2012;5(4):315–8.

20. Zipursky RB, Gu H, Green AI, et al. Course and predictors of weight gain in people with first-episode psychosis treated with olanzapine or haloperidol. Br J Psychiatry 2005;187:537–43.

21. Henderson DC, Cagliero E, Gray C, et al. Clozapine, diabetes mellitus, weight gain, and lipid abnormalities: a five-year naturalistic study. Am J Psychiatry 2000;157(6):975–81.

22. Gentile S. Long-term treatment with atypical antipsychotics and the risk of weight gain: a literature analysis. Drug Saf 2006;29(4):303–19.

23. Huang X-F, Han M, Huang X, et al. Olanzapine differentially affects 5-HT2A and 2C receptor mRNA expression in the rat brain. Behav Brain Res 2006;171(2):355–62.

24. Han M, Deng C, Burne TH, et al. Short- and long-term effects of antipsychotic drug treatment on weight gain and H1 receptor expression. Psychoneuroendocrinology 2008;33(5):569–80.

25. Bai YM, Lin C-C, Chen J-Y, et al. Association of initial antipsychotic response to clozapine and long-term weight gain. Am J Psychiatry 2006;163(7):1276–9.

26. Kinon BJ, Kaiser CJ, Ahmed S, et al. Association between early and rapid weight gain and change in weight over one year of olanzapine therapy in patients with schizophrenia and related disorders. J Clin Psychopharmacol 2005;25(3):255–8.

27. Case M, Treuer T, Karagianis J, et al. The potential role of appetite in predicting weight changes during treatment with olanzapine. BMC Psychiatry 2010; 10:72.

28. Simon V, van Winkel R, De Hert M. Are weight gain and metabolic side effects of atypical antipsychotics dose dependent? A literature review. J Clin Psychiatry 2009;70(7):1041–50.

29. Perry PJ, Argo TR, Carnahan RM, et al. The association of weight gain and olanzapine plasma concentrations. J Clin Psychopharmacol 2005;25(3): 250–4.

30. Citrome L, Stauffer VL, Chen L, et al. Olanzapine plasma concentrations after treatment with 10, 20, and 40 mg/d in patients with schizophrenia: an analysis of correlations with efficacy, weight gain, and prolactin concentration. J Clin Psychopharmacol 2009;29(3):278–83.

31. Kane JM, Detke HC, Naber D, et al. Olanzapine long-acting injection: a 24-week, randomized, double-blind trial of maintenance treatment in patients with schizophrenia. Am J Psychiatry 2010;167(2):181–9.

32. Deng C, Weston-Green K, Huang XF. The role of histaminergic H1 and H3 receptors in food intake: a mechanism for atypical antipsychotic-induced weight gain? Prog Neuropsychopharmacol Biol Psychiatry 2010;34(1):1–4.

33. Blouin M, Tremblay A, Jalbert M-E, et al. Adiposity and eating behaviors in patients under second generation antipsychotics. Obesity 2008;16(8):1780–7.

34. Sentissi O, Viala A, Bourdel MC, et al. Impact of antipsychotic treatments on the motivation to eat: preliminary results in 153 schizophrenic patients. Int Clin Psychopharmacol 2009;24(5):257–64.

35. Cuerda C, Merchan-Naranjo J, Velasco C, et al. Influence of resting energy expenditure on weight gain in adolescents taking second-generation antipsychotics. Clin Nutr 2011;30(5):616–23.

36. Coccurello R, Moles A. Potential mechanisms of atypical antipsychotic-induced metabolic derangement: clues for understanding obesity and novel drug design. Pharmacol Ther 2010;127(3):210–51.

37. Gothelf D, Falk B, Singer P, et al. Weight gain associated with increased food intake and low habitual activity levels in male adolescent schizophrenic inpatients treated with olanzapine. Am J Psychiatry 2002;159(6):1055–7.

38. Kluge M, Schuld A, Himmerich H, et al. Clozapine and olanzapine are associated with food craving and binge eating: results from a randomized double-blind study. J Clin Psychopharmacol 2007;27(6):662–6.

39. Mathews J, Newcomer JW, Mathews JR, et al. Neural correlates of weight gain with olanzapine. Arch Gen Psychiatry 2012;69(12):1226–37.

40. Cooper GD, Goudie AJ, Halford JC. Acute effects of olanzapine on behavioural expression including the behavioural satiety sequence in female rats. J Psychopharmacol 2010;24(7):1069–78.

41. Thornton-Jones Z, Neill JC, Reynolds GP. The atypical antipsychotic olanzapine enhances ingestive behaviour in the rat: a preliminary study. J Psychopharmacol 2002;16(1):35–7.

42. Minet-Ringuet J, Even PC, Guesdon B, et al. Effects of chronic neuroleptic treatments on nutrient selection, body weight, and body composition in the male rat under dietary self-selection. Behav Brain Res 2005;163(2):204–11.

43. Weston-Green K, Huang X-F, Deng C. Olanzapine treatment and metabolic dysfunction: a dose response study in female Sprague Dawley rats. Behav Brain Res 2011;217(2):337–46.
44. van der Zwaal EM, Janhunen SK, Luijendijk MC, et al. Olanzapine and sibutramine have opposing effects on the motivation for palatable food. Behav Pharmacol 2012;23(2):198–204.
45. Schwartz MW, Woods SC, Porte D, et al. Central nervous system control of food intake. Nature 2000;404(6778):661–71.
46. Ferno J, Varela L, Skrede S, et al. Olanzapine-induced hyperphagia and weight gain associate with orexigenic hypothalamic neuropeptide signaling without concomitant AMPK phosphorylation. PLoS One 2011;6(6):e20571.
47. Weston-Green K, Huang X-F, Deng C. Alterations to melanocortinergic, GABAergic and cannabinoid neurotransmission associated with olanzapine-induced weight gain. PLoS One 2012;7(3):e33548.
48. Allison DB, Newcomer JW, Dunn AL, et al. Obesity among those with mental disorders: a National Institute of Mental Health meeting report. Am J Prev Med 2009;36(4):341–50.
49. De Hert M, Detraux J, van Winkel R, et al. Metabolic and cardiovascular adverse effects associated with antipsychotic drugs. Nat Rev Endocrinol 2012;8(2):114–26.
50. Henderson DC. Atypical antipsychotic-induced diabetes mellitus: how strong is the evidence? CNS Drugs 2002;16(2):77–89.
51. Meyer JM, Stahl SM. The metabolic syndrome and schizophrenia. Acta Psychiatr Scand 2009;119(1):4–14.
52. Davoodi N, Kalinichev M, Korneev SA, et al. Hyperphagia and increased meal size are responsible for weight gain in rats treated sub-chronically with olanzapine. Psychopharmacology (Berl) 2009;203(4):693–702.
53. Baker RA, Pikalov A, Tran Q-V, et al. Atypical antipsychotic drugs and diabetes mellitus in the US Food and Drug Administration Adverse Event database: a systematic Bayesian signal detection analysis. Psychopharmacol Bull 2009; 42(1):11–31.
54. Simpson GM, Weiden P, Pigott T, et al. Six-month, blinded, multicenter continuation study of ziprasidone versus olanzapine in schizophrenia. Am J Psychiatry 2005;162(8):1535–8.
55. Ahrén B. Autonomic regulation of islet hormone secretion—Implications for health and disease. Diabetologia 2000;43(4):393–410.
56. Rettenbacher MA, Hummer M, Hofer A, et al. Alterations of glucose metabolism during treatment with clozapine or amisulpride: results from a prospective 16-week study. J Psychopharmacol 2007;21(4):400–4.
57. Ebenbichler CF, Laimer M, Eder U, et al. Olanzapine induces insulin resistance: results from a prospective study. J Clin Psychiatry 2003;64(12):1436–9.
58. Wu R-R, Zhao J-P, Zhai J-G, et al. Sex difference in effects of typical and atypical antipsychotics on glucose-insulin homeostasis and lipid metabolism in first-episode schizophrenia. J Clin Psychopharmacol 2007;27(4):374–9.
59. Hardy TA, Henry RR, Forrester TD, et al. Impact of olanzapine or risperidone treatment on insulin sensitivity in schizophrenia or schizoaffective disorder. Diabetes Obes Metab 2011;13(8):726–35.
60. Sato Y, Yasui-Furukori N, Furukori H, et al. A crossover study on the glucose metabolism between treatment with olanzapine and risperidone in schizophrenic patients. Exp Clin Psychopharmacol 2010;18(5):445–50.

61. Smith RC, Lindenmayer J-P, Davis JM, et al. Effects of olanzapine and risperidone on glucose metabolism and insulin sensitivity in chronic schizophrenic patients with long-term antipsychotic treatment: a randomized 5-month study. J Clin Psychiatry 2009;70(11):1501–13.

62. Henderson DC, Cagliero E, Copeland PM, et al. Glucose metabolism in patients with schizophrenia treated with atypical antipsychotic agents: a frequently sampled intravenous glucose tolerance test and minimal model analysis. Arch Gen Psychiatry 2005;62(1):19–28.

63. Henderson DC, Copeland PM, Borba CP, et al. Glucose metabolism in patients with schizophrenia treated with olanzapine or quetiapine: a frequently sampled intravenous glucose tolerance test and minimal model analysis. J Clin Psychiatry 2006;67(5):789–97.

64. Coccurello R, Brina D, Caprioli A, et al. 30 days of continuous olanzapine infusion determines energy imbalance, glucose intolerance, insulin resistance, and dyslipidemia in mice. J Clin Psychopharmacol 2009;29(6):576–83.

65. Chintoh AF, Mann SW, Lam TK, et al. Insulin resistance following continuous, chronic olanzapine treatment: an animal model. Schizophr Res 2008;104(1–3): 23–30.

66. Albaugh VL, Henry CR, Bello NT, et al. Hormonal and metabolic effects of olanzapine and clozapine related to body weight in rodents. Obesity 2006;14(1): 36–51.

67. Boyda HN, Procyshyn RM, Tse L, et al. Intermittent treatment with olanzapine causes sensitization of the metabolic side-effects in rats. Neuropharmacology 2012;62(3):1391–400.

68. Boyda HN, Tse L, Procyshyn RM, et al. Preclinical models of antipsychotic drug-induced metabolic side effects. Trends Pharmacol Sci 2010;31(10):484–97.

69. Saddichha S, Manjunatha N, Ameen S, et al. Diabetes and schizophrenia—effect of disease or drug? Results from a randomized, double-blind, controlled prospective study in first-episode schizophrenia. Acta Psychiatr Scand 2008; 117(5):342–7.

70. Park S, Hong SM, Lee JE, et al. Chlorpromazine exacerbates hepatic insulin sensitivity via attenuating insulin and leptin signaling pathway, while exercise partially reverses the adverse effects. Life Sci 2007;80(26):2428–35.

71. Amamoto T, Kumai T, Nakaya S, et al. The elucidation of the mechanism of weight gain and glucose tolerance abnormalities induced by chlorpromazine. J Pharm Sci 2006;102(2):213–9.

72. Lorenzen J, Remvig J. Diabetes mellitus in a psychotic patient with recovery during chlorpromazine therapy. Dan Med Bull 1957;4(4):134–6.

73. Schwarz L, Munoz R. Blood sugar levels in patients treated with chlorpromazine. Am J Psychiatry 1968;125(2):253–5.

74. Meltzer HY, Perry E, Jayathilake K. Clozapine-induced weight gain predicts improvement in psychopathology. Schizophr Res 2003;59(1):19–27.

75. Amdisen A. Diabetes mellitus as a side effect of treatment with tricyclic neuroleptics. Acta Psychiatr Scand 1964;40(Suppl 180):411–4.

76. Price WA, Giannini AJ. Thioridazine and diabetes. J Clin Psychiatry 1983;44(12): 469.

77. Perez-Iglesias R, Mata I, Pelayo-Teran JM, et al. Glucose and lipid disturbances after 1 year of antipsychotic treatment in a drug-naive population. Schizophr Res 2009;107(2–3):115–21.

78. Sacchetti E, Turrina C, Parrinello G, et al. Incidence of diabetes in a general practice population: a database cohort study on the relationship with

    haloperidol, olanzapine, risperidone or quetiapine exposure. Int Clin Psycho-
    pharmacol 2005;20(1):33–7.
79. Kessing LV, Thomsen AF, Mogensen UB, et al. Treatment with antipsychotics
    and the risk of diabetes in clinical practice. Br J Psychiatry 2010;197(4):
    266–71.
80. Tschoner A, Engl J, Rettenbacher M, et al. Effects of six second generation
    antipsychotics on body weight and metabolism—risk assessment and results
    from a prospective study. Pharmacopsychiatry 2009;42(1):29–34.
81. Kim SH, Nikolics L, Abbasi F, et al. Relationship between body mass index and
    insulin resistance in patients treated with second generation antipsychotic
    agents. J Psychiatr Res 2010;44(8):493–8.
82. Guenette MD, Giacca A, Hahn M, et al. Atypical antipsychotics and effects of
    adrenergic and serotonergic receptor binding on insulin secretion in-vivo: an
    animal model. Schizophr Res 2013;146(1–3):162–9.
83. Newcomer JW, Haupt DW, Fucetola R, et al. Abnormalities in glucose regulation
    during antipsychotic treatment of schizophrenia. Arch Gen Psychiatry 2002;
    59(4):337–45.
84. Koller EA, Doraiswamy PM. Olanzapine-associated diabetes mellitus. Pharma-
    cotherapy 2002;22(7):841–52.
85. Laimer M, Ebenbichler CF, Kranebitter M, et al. Olanzapine-induced hypergly-
    cemia: role of humoral insulin resistance-inducing factors. J Clin Psychophar-
    macol 2005;25(2):183–5.
86. Guenette M, Hahn M, Cohn T, et al. Atypical antipsychotics and diabetic ketoa-
    cidosis: a review. Psychopharmacology (Berl) 2013;226(1):1–12.
87. Chiu CC, Chen KP, Liu HC, et al. The early effect of olanzapine and risperidone
    on insulin secretion in atypical-naive schizophrenic patients. J Clin Psychophar-
    macol 2006;26(5):504–7.
88. Houseknecht KL, Robertson AS, Zavadoski W, et al. Acute effects of atypical
    antipsychotics on whole-body insulin resistance in rats: implications for adverse
    metabolic effects. Neuropsychopharmacology 2007;32(2):289–97.
89. Chintoh AF, Mann SW, Lam L, et al. Insulin resistance and secretion in vivo:
    effects of different antipsychotics in an animal model. Schizophr Res 2009;
    108(1–3):127–33.
90. Boyda HN, Tse L, Procyshyn RM, et al. A parametric study of the acute effects of
    antipsychotic drugs on glucose sensitivity in an animal model. Prog Neuropsy-
    chopharmacol Biol Psychiatry 2010;34(6):945–54.
91. Girault EM, Alkemade A, Foppen E, et al. Acute peripheral but not central
    administration of olanzapine induces hyperglycemia associated with hepatic
    and extra-hepatic insulin resistance. PLoS One 2012;7(8):e43244.
92. Johnson DE, Yamazaki H, Ward KM, et al. Inhibitory effects of antipsychotics on
    carbachol-enhanced insulin secretion from perfused rat islets: role of musca-
    rinic antagonism in antipsychotic-induced diabetes and hyperglycemia.
    Diabetes 2005;54(5):1552–8.
93. Vestri HS, Maianu L, Moellering DR, et al. Atypical antipsychotic drugs directly
    impair insulin action in adipocytes: effects on glucose transport, lipogenesis,
    and antilipolysis. Neuropsychopharmacology 2007;32(4):765–72.
94. Chintoh AF, Mann SW, Lam L, et al. Insulin resistance and decreased glucose-
    stimulated insulin secretion after acute olanzapine administration. J Clin Psycho-
    pharmacol 2008;28(5):494–9.
95. Lambert TJ, Chapman LH. Diabetes, psychotic disorders and antipsychotic
    therapy: a consensus statement. Med J Aust 2005;182(6):310.

96. Chiu C-C, Chen C-H, Chen B-Y, et al. The time-dependent change of insulin secretion in schizophrenic patients treated with olanzapine. Prog Neuropsychopharmacol Biol Psychiatry 2010;34(6):866–70.

97. van Winkel R, De Hert M, Wampers M, et al. Major changes in glucose metabolism, including new-onset diabetes, within 3 months after initiation of or switch to atypical antipsychotic medication in patients with schizophrenia and schizoaffective disorder. J Clin Psychiatry 2008;69(3):472–9.

98. Nasrallah HA. Atypical antipsychotic-induced metabolic side effects: insights from receptor-binding profiles. Mol Psychiatry 2008;13:27–35.

99. Meltzer H, Massey B. The role of serotonin receptors in the action of atypical antipsychotic drugs. Curr Opin Pharmacol 2011;11:59–67.

100. Kapur S, Mamo D. Half a century of antipsychotics and still a central role for dopamine D2 receptors. Prog Neuropsychopharmacol Biol Psychiatry 2003; 27(7):1081–90.

101. Kroeze WK, Hufeisen SJ, Popadak BA, et al. H1-histamine receptor affinity predicts short-term weight gain for typical and atypical antipsychotic drugs. Neuropsychopharmacology 2003;28(3):519–26.

102. Matsui-Sakata A, Ohtani H, Sawada Y. Receptor occupancy-based analysis of the contributions of various receptors to antipsychotics-induced weight gain and diabetes mellitus. Drug Metab Pharmacokinet 2005;20(5):368–78.

103. Correll CU, Kane JM, Manu P. Obesity and coronary risk in patients treated with second-generation antipsychotics. Eur Arch Psychiatry Clin Neurosci 2011; 261(6):417–23.

104. Lam DD, Garfield AS, Marston OJ, et al. Brain serotonin system in the coordination of food intake and body weight. Pharmacol Biochem Behav 2010;97(1): 84–91.

105. Schreiber R, De Vry J. Role of 5-hT2C receptors in the hypophagic effect of m-CPP, ORG 37684 and CP-94,253 in the rat. Prog Neuropsychopharmacol Biol Psychiatry 2002;26(3):441–9.

106. Kitchener SJ, Dourish CT. An examination of the behavioural specificity of hypophagia induced by 5-HT1B, 5-HT1C and 5-HT2 receptor agonists using the post-prandial satiety sequence in rats. Psychopharmacology (Berl) 1994; 113(3–4):369–77.

107. Kirk SL, Glazebrook J, Grayson B, et al. Olanzapine-induced weight gain in the rat: role of 5-HT2C and histamine H1 receptors. Psychopharmacology (Berl) 2009;207(1):119–25.

108. Kim SH, Ivanova O, Abbasi FA, et al. Metabolic impact of switching antipsychotic therapy to aripiprazole after weight gain: a pilot study. J Clin Psychopharmacol 2007;27(4):365–8.

109. Davoodi N, Kalinichev M, Clifton PG. Comparative effects of olanzapine and ziprasidone on hypophagia induced by enhanced histamine neurotransmission in the rat. Behav Pharmacol 2008;19(2):121–8.

110. Deng C, Lian JM, Pai N, et al. Reducing olanzapine-induced weight gain side effect by using betahistine: a study in the rat model. J Psychopharmacol 2012;26(9):1271–9.

111. Poyurovsky M, Fuchs C, Pashinian A, et al. Reducing antipsychotic-induced weight gain in schizophrenia: a double-blind placebo-controlled study of reboxetine–betahistine combination. Psychopharmacology (Berl) 2013;226(3):615–22.

112. Poyurovsky M, Pashinian A, Levi A, et al. The effect of betahistine, a histamine H1 receptor agonist/H3 antagonist, on olanzapine-induced weight gain in first-episode schizophrenia patients. Int Clin Psychopharmacol 2005;20(2):101–3.

113. Silvestre JS, Prous J. Research on adverse drug events. I. Muscarinic M3 receptor binding affinity could predict the risk of antipsychotics to induce type 2 diabetes. Methods Find Exp Clin Pharmacol 2005;27(5):289–304.
114. Jindal R, Keshavan M. Critical role of M3 muscarinic receptor in insulin secretion: implications for psychopharmacology. J Clin Psychopharmacol 2006; 26(5):449–50 [editorial].
115. Starrenburg FC, Bogers JP. How can antipsychotics cause diabetes mellitus? Insights based on receptor-binding profiles, humoral factors and transporter proteins. Eur Psychiatry 2009;24(3):164–70.
116. Correll CU. From receptor pharmacology to improved outcomes: individualising the selection, dosing, and switching of antipsychotics. Eur Psychiatry 2010; 25(Suppl 2):S12–21.
117. Dockray GJ. The versatility of the vagus. Physiol Behav 2009;97(5):531–6.
118. Hahn M, Chintoh A, Giacca A, et al. Atypical antipsychotics and effects of muscarinic, serotonergic, dopaminergic and histaminergic receptor binding on insulin secretion in vivo: an animal model. Schizophr Res 2011;131(1–3): 90–5.
119. Renuka TR, Ani DV, Paulose CS. Alterations in the muscarinic M1 and M3 receptor gene expression in the brain stem during pancreatic regeneration and insulin secretion in weanling rats. Life Sci 2004;75(19):2269–80.
120. Li Y, Wu X, Zhu J, et al. Hypothalamic regulation of pancreatic secretion is mediated by central cholinergic pathways in the rat. J Physiol 2003;552(2):571–87.
121. Weston-Green K. Alterations in hypothalamic and brainstem neurotransmitter signalling associated with olanzapine-induced metabolic side-effects. Wollongong (Australia): University of Wollongong; 2012.
122. Martins PJF, Haas M, Obici S. Central nervous system delivery of the antipsychotic olanzapine induces hepatic insulin resistance. Diabetes 2010;59(10): 2418–25.
123. Lencz T, Robinson DG, Napolitano B, et al. DRD2 promoter region variation predicts antipsychotic-induced weight gain in first episode schizophrenia. Pharmacogenet Genomics 2010;20(9):569–72.
124. Volkow ND, Wang GJ, Baler RD. Reward, dopamine and the control of food intake: implications for obesity. Trends Cogn Sci 2011;15(1):37–46.
125. Huang X-F, Zavitsanou K, Huang X, et al. Dopamine transporter and D2 receptor binding densities in mice prone or resistant to chronic high fat diet-induced obesity. Behav Brain Res 2006;175(2):415–9.
126. Stahl S. Describing an atypical antipsychotic: receptor binding and its role in pathophysiology. Prim Care Companion J Clin Psychiatry 2003;5:9–13.
127. Elman I, Borsook D, Lukas SE. Food intake and reward mechanisms in patients with schizophrenia: implications for metabolic disturbances and treatment with second-generation antipsychotic agents. Neuropsychopharmacology 2006; 31(10):2091–120.
128. Grimm O, Vollstadt-Klein S, Krebs L, et al. Reduced striatal activation during reward anticipation due to appetite-provoking cues in chronic schizophrenia: a fMRI study. Schizophr Res 2012;134(2–3):151–7.
129. Rubi B, Ljubicic S, Pournourmohammadi S, et al. Dopamine D2-like receptors are expressed in pancreatic beta cells and mediate inhibition of insulin secretion. J Biol Chem 2005;280(44):36824–32.
130. Garcia-Tornadu I, Ornstein AM, Chamson-Reig A, et al. Disruption of the dopamine D2 receptor impairs insulin secretion and causes glucose intolerance. Endocrinology 2010;151(4):1441–50.

131. Haddad P. Weight change with atypical antipsychotics in the treatment of schizophrenia. J Psychopharmacol 2005;19(Suppl 6):16–27.

132. Lane H-Y, Liu Y-C, Huang C-L, et al. Risperidone-related weight gain: genetic and nongenetic predictors. J Clin Psychopharmacol 2006;26(2):128–34.

133. Gebhardt S, Haberhausen M, Heinzel-Gutenbrunner M, et al. Antipsychotic-induced body weight gain: predictors and a systematic categorization of the long-term weight course. J Psychiatr Res 2009;43(6):620–6.

134. Seeman MV. Secondary effects of antipsychotics: women at greater risk than men. Schizophr Bull 2009;35(5):937–48.

135. Treuer T, Pendlebury J, Lockman H, et al. Weight gain risk factor assessment checklist: overview and recommendation for use. Neuroendocrinol Lett 2011; 32(2):199–205.

136. Saddichha S, Ameen S, Akhtar S. Predictors of antipsychotic-induced weight gain in first-episode psychosis: conclusions from a randomized, double-blind, controlled prospective study of olanzapine, risperidone, and haloperidol. J Clin Psychopharmacol 2008;28(1):27–31.

The Impact of Traumatic Brain Injury on Pituitary Function

Nina K. Sundaram, MD[a], Eliza B. Geer, MD[a,*],
Brian D. Greenwald, MD[b,c]

KEYWORDS

- Traumatic brain injury • Hypopituitarism • Hormone replacement therapy
- Screening • Diagnosis • Pathophysiology • Neurocognitive impairment • Outcome

KEY POINTS

- The pituitary gland is vulnerable to both mechanical and ischemic injury, accounting for the estimated 27.5% prevalence of anterior hypopituitarism after traumatic brain injury (TBI).
- Although patients with severe TBI may be at increased risk of hypopituitarism, patients with mild TBI remain at significant risk, and overall there is a lack of reliable predictors.
- Somatotropin and gonadotropin deficiencies occur more commonly than thyrotropin and corticotrophin deficiencies.
- There is generally recovery of pituitary function over time, but the development of new pituitary deficiencies can occur.
- Posttraumatic hypopituitarism is associated with poor outcomes, and the impact of treatment on clinical outcomes is promising, although further investigation is needed.

BACKGROUND

The Centers for Disease Control and Prevention (CDC) estimate that each year 1.7 million Americans are seen in a hospital for a traumatic brain injury (TBI).[1] Of these patients, 52,000 die, 275,000 are hospitalized, and 1.365 million are treated and released from an emergency department. The number of people who sustain a TBI and do not seek medical care is unknown. Sports-related concussions are routinely underreported, and it has been estimated that there are 1.6 to 3.8 million cases each year.[1] It is estimated that 80,000 people in the United States are left with long-term

Disclosure statement: The authors have no disclosures or conflicts of interest to declare.
[a] Division of Endocrinology, Diabetes, and Bone Disease, Mount Sinai Medical Center, One Gustave L. Levy Place, Box 1055, New York, NY 10029, USA; [b] JFK Johnson Rehabilitation Center for Head Injuries, 65 James Street, Edison, NJ 08818, USA; [c] Department of Physical Medicine and Rehabilitation, UMDNJ-Robert Wood Johnson Medical School, JFK Johnson Rehabilitation Institute, 65 James Street, Edison, NJ 08818, USA
* Corresponding author.
E-mail address: eliza.geer@mssm.edu

disabilities from TBI annually.[2] The CDC estimates suggest that approximately 3.2 million to 5.3 million persons (1.1%–1.7% of the US population) live with long-term disabilities (the loss of 1 or more physical or mental functions) that result from an injury to the brain.[1]

TBI is traumatically induced physiologic disruption of brain function. The initial clinical presentation after brain injury is the determinant of the category of severity of brain injury. Mild brain injury (sometimes referred to as a concussion) often presents with a transient loss of consciousness (30 minutes or less), being dazed or confused, or posttraumatic amnesia.[3] Patients with moderate to severe TBI present with prolonged loss of consciousness and deeper levels of unconsciousness. At first, the depth of unconsciousness is measured by the Glasgow Coma Scale (GCS). Mild brain injury (GCS score of 13–15) represents 80% of all TBI, moderate brain injury (GCS score of 9–13) represents 10%, and severe brain injury (GCS score of 3–8) represents 10%.[4] As a broad generalization, the higher the GCS score is on admission to the emergency department, the more likely it is that a good outcome will result. Despite this, estimates are that 15% of those with mild brain injury have long-term sequelae.[5,6]

The pathophysiology of brain injury is classically broken up into primary and secondary injuries. Primary brain injury (including diffuse axonal injury, vascular tears, focal cortical contusions, and intracranial hemorrhage) results from the direct forces of impact and evolves in the early period after impact. Secondary brain injury includes complex pathways that are triggered shortly after the impact and continue to evolve and magnify the extent of damage. Examples include necrosis, apoptosis, ischemia, edema, and inflammation.

The spectrum of disability varies widely after moderate to severe TBI, ranging from cognitive impairment with no physical impairment to deep coma. Disabilities that commonly occur as a result of a TBI include problems with[1] cognition (memory, concentration, processing speed, and judgment),[2] motor skills (strength, coordination, and ambulation),[3] sensory impairment (special senses such as smell, vision, and hearing, as well as tactile sensation), and[4] emotional/mood issues (emotional instability, impulsivity, and irritability). The TBI population is not a cross section of society. Those with behavioral, psychiatric, and learning disabilities are disproportionately represented, and the premorbid personality may be magnified after a brain injury.[7]

After more than 25 years of prospective study of outcomes after TBI, there has been movement away from thinking of TBI as a one-time event and toward understanding it as the start of a lifelong process with ongoing medical care needs. In 2009, the Institute of Medicine (IOM) published a report regarding the long-term consequences of TBI.[8] The IOM reported that there is enough quality research to conclude that moderate to severe TBI is associated with neurocognitive deficits, dementia of Alzheimer type, Parkinson disease, and endocrine dysfunction. TBI is also associated with depression, aggressive behaviors, chronic traumatic encephalopathy, and unprovoked seizures.[8]

Persons with TBI are 1.5 to 17 times more likely to develop seizures than the general population.[9] TBI is a leading cause of epilepsy in the general population.[10] Sleep disturbance is significantly higher than in the general population, with long-term sleep complaints as high as 70% in persons after TBI.[11] In addition to the aggression, confusion, and agitation seen in the acute stages, TBI is associated with an increased risk of developing numerous psychiatric diseases, including obsessive-compulsive disorders, anxiety disorders, psychotic disorders, mood disorders, and major depression.[12] Persons who have severe TBI have 4 times the risk of Alzheimer-type dementia later in life.[13] Causes of this include changes to the blood-brain barrier, leakage of free oxygen radicals, loss of brain reserve capacity, and deposition of β-amyloid plaque or apoptosis.[14] Thus, traumatic brain injury is not a static, isolated process, but an ongoing process that has a significant impact on multiple organ systems.

PREVALENCE OF POSTTRAUMATIC HYPOPITUITARISM

Hypopituitarism following TBI was first reported in 1918.[15] Since this report almost a century ago, the phenomenon of both anterior and posterior pituitary deficiencies after TBI has been widely reported in case reports[16–20] and literature reviews.[21–23] However, this clinical entity remains largely underdiagnosed, with understanding of this condition improving only in recent years.

The prevalence of hypopituitarism following TBI has been reported to range from 15% to 68%.[24–35] Given that an estimated 1.7 million people are seen in hospitals for TBI each year, the incidence of posttraumatic hypopituitarism can therefore be estimated as affecting 255,000 to 1.1 million people, highlighting the magnitude of this problem. This broad range reported in the literature is likely caused by differences in trauma severity, time of evaluation after injury, and diagnostic criteria used to categorize hypopituitarism. The overall prevalence of anterior hypopituitarism after TBI is estimated to be 27.5%.[35] The deficiencies of each axis are estimated to be as follows[24–35]:

- Somatotrophin 12%
- Gonadotrophin 12%
- Corticotrophin 8%
- Thyrotrophin 5%

The role of trauma severity in predicting hypopituitarism has been frequently examined. Although many studies have shown no association between hypopituitarism and trauma severity,[24,26,28–32] others have reported it to be more frequent in cases of severe TBI.[25,27,34] The overall prevalence of hypopituitarism with severe TBI (35.3%) was higher than with moderate or mild TBI when analyzed in a large meta-analysis.[35] In the same way, markers of severe injury, such as diffuse axonal injury, basilar skull fracture, increased intracranial pressure, length of stay in the intensive care unit, and acute computed topography (CT) findings, specifically the presence of diffuse brain swelling, evacuated intracerebral hematoma, or multiple contusions, have been identified as predictors of hypopituitarism.[27,36,37]

Although patients with severe brain injury may be at increased risk for developing hypopituitarism, chronic hypopituitarism has been reported in 10% to 25% of patients with mild TBI.[24–35] Thus, the diagnosis cannot be overlooked in these patients. In fact, the repetitive mild injury that occurs in contact sports such as boxing may result in an even higher rate of hypopituitarism, particularly growth hormone deficiency.[38–40]

The presence of anterior pituitary deficiencies immediately following injury does not typically predict chronic hypopituitarism. In the acute phase, some hormonal changes, such as decreased luteinizing hormone (LH)/follicle-stimulating hormone (FSH), and thyroid stimulating hormone (TSH), may simply represent normal physiologic responses to critical illness. Furthermore, spontaneous recovery of pituitary function has been well-documented, with resolution of somatotropin and gonadotropin deficiency reported most frequently.[24,26,31,41,42] However, panhypopituitarism may serve as a predictor of chronic hypopituitarism.[24] Although the overall trend is toward recovery of pituitary deficits, the evolution of pituitary function over time remains unpredictable. As such, the development of new pituitary deficiencies and the progression from isolated to multiple deficiencies has been reported within the first 6 months and as far as 1 to 3 years following the initial injury.[24,26,31,42]

Posterior pituitary deficiency (ie, diabetes insipidus) has been reported to be as high as 26% in the acute phase, with the largest study reporting an incidence of 6.9% at long-term follow-up.[41,43] There is no known association between posttraumatic posterior pituitary deficiency and anterior hypopituitarism.[43] Age, gender, and body mass index (BMI) have also been examined but have not been uniformly identified as predictors.[25–29,31]

PATHOPHYSIOLOGY OF HYPOPITUITARISM AFTER TBI

The underlying mechanism of posttraumatic hypopituitarism remains unclear. It is likely that several factors are involved, most significantly the primary brain injury and the ischemic injury that can be caused by this primary event or by secondary events such as hypotension, increased intracranial pressure, hypoxia, or anemia.[44]

The pituitary gland is located within the bony sella turcica at the base of the skull and is covered by the dural diaphragma sellae, through which the stalk connects to the median eminence of the hypothalamus. Given these confinements, the pituitary gland, infundibulum and hypothalamus remain vulnerable to mechanical trauma, such as fractures through base of the skull and sella turcica.[45] The hemorrhage that often accompanies these traumatic injuries can also damage the pituitary gland, for example by directly impinging on the pituitary capsule.

The blood supply of the pituitary gland is primarily provided by the internal carotid artery (Fig. 1). The long hypophyseal portal vessels, which arise above the diaphragma from the superior hypophyseal arteries (a branch of the intracranial portion of the inferior carotid artery), travel down the infundibulum to provide the anterior pituitary with 70% to 90% of its blood supply. The short hypophyseal portal vessels arise from the inferior hypophyseal artery (a branch of the intracavernous internal carotid artery) and enter the sella from below the diaphragma sellae and supply the gland with less than 30% of its vascular supply, predominantly in the medial portion. Because the long portal vessels arise within the subarachnoid space and pass through the diaphragma sellae, they are particularly susceptible to mechanical trauma, low cerebral blood flow, and/or increased intracranial pressure. This increased risk of injury has been correlated by autopsy studies, including a study in which 35% of patients, all of whom survived at least 12 hours, had anterior lobe necrosis with an infarction pattern in the blood supply of the long hypophyseal portal veins, whereas tissue in the short portal veins survived.[16] Further supporting this vascular hypothesis is the pattern of hormonal loss seen in hypopituitarism following TBI.[44] The somatotrophs and gonadotrophs, located in territory perfused by the long portal vessels, are often the most predisposed to dysfunction following TBI.[24–35] In contrast, the corticotrophs and thyrotrophs are located more medially in the territory supplied by the less vulnerable short portal vessels, and thus deficiencies of these axes are less frequent after TBI.[24–35]

CLINICAL IMPACT OF POSTTRAUMATIC HYPOPITUITARISM

Untreated hypopituitarism is associated with increased morbidity and mortality, providing a compelling reason to improve awareness of this clinical entity. Arguably of greatest clinical significance is the identification of the relationship between posttraumatic hypopituitarism and the neurocognitive impairments that affect patients with TBI. As previously mentioned, patients with moderate to severe TBI experience a variety neuropsychiatric complaints including impairments of memory, concentration, judgment, and problem-solving, as well as fatigue, anxiety, depression, and social isolation.[7] These symptoms are also commonly reported by patients with

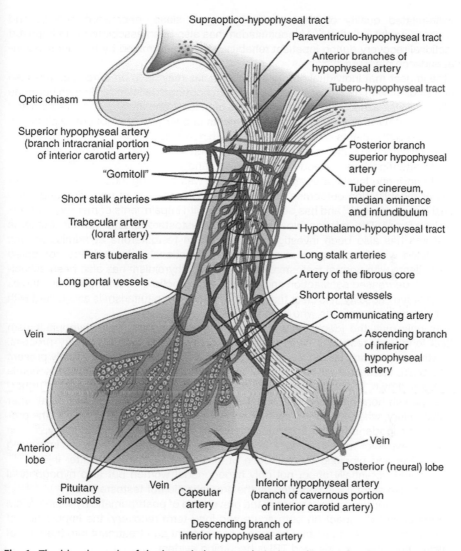

Supraoptico-hypophyseal tract

Paraventriculo-hypophyseal tract

Anterior branches of
hypophyseal artery

Tubero-hypophyseal tract

Optic chiasm

Superior hypophyseal artery
(branch intracranial portion
of interior carotid artery)

Posterior branch
superior hypophyseal
artery

"Gomitoll"

Tuber cinereum,
median eminence
and infundibulum

Short stalk arteries

Trabecular artery
(loral artery)

Hypothalamo-hypophyseal tract

Pars tuberalis

Long stalk arteries

Long portal vessels

Artery of the fibrous core

Short portal vessels

Communicating artery

Vein

Ascending branch
of inferior
hypophyseal
artery

Anterior
lobe

Vein

Pituitary
sinusoids

Vein

Capsular
artery

Posterior (neural) lobe

Inferior hypophyseal artery
(branch of cavernous portion
of interior carotid artery)

Descending branch of
inferior hypophyseal artery

Fig. 1. The blood supply of the hypothalamus and pituitary. (*From* Scheithauer BW. The hypothalamus and neurohypophysis. In: Kovacs K, Asa SL, eds. Functional Endocrine Pathology. Oxford, UK: Blackwell Scientific; 1991; with permission from John Wiley & Sons, Inc.)

hypopituitarism. Most notable is the overlap in symptoms between patients with growth hormone deficiency and those with moderate to severe TBI.[46] In addition, low levels of testosterone have been correlated with not only decreased quality of life but with impairments of verbal fluency, visual and verbal memory, and visuospatial processing.[47,48] Therefore, it is logical to suspect that untreated hypopituitarism may be a contributing factor in the neurocognitive impairments experienced by these patients, which negatively affect both quality of life and the ability to participate in rehabilitation.

As a result, the outcomes of patients with untreated posttraumatic hypopituitarism have been investigated. Hypopituitarism was an independent predictor of worsened health-related quality of life, specifically poorer sleep, decreased energy, and increased social isolation.[27] Hypopituitarism has also been associated with impaired functional recovery during inpatient rehabilitation as determined by the functional independence measure.[49–51]

The impact that individual hormonal deficiencies may have on outcomes has also been studied, with particular interest on growth hormone deficiency. Growth hormone deficiency was associated with higher rates of at least one marker of depression and reduced quality of life, specifically impairments in energy and emotional well-being, compared with patients with TBI without growth hormone deficiency.[37,52] Growth hormone deficiency in patients with TBI has also been associated with more severe deficits in attention level, executive functioning, and memory problems.[53] Low peak growth hormone levels after stimulation testing was a strong independent predictor of poor rehabilitation outcomes as determined by measures of cognition and functional independence[50] and has been associated with impairments of memory and verbal learning.[28] The relationship between low testosterone and various outcome measures has also been investigated. Low serum testosterone at admission was associated with long lengths of stay and low functional independence compared with patients with normal testosterone.[49,54,55] Hypothyroidism has also been associated with decreased satisfaction and performance function.[56] Although these studies do not prove causality, it is clear that posttraumatic hypopituitarism is associated with poor outcomes in patients who have had TBI.

Not only may the identification and treatment of posttraumatic hypopituitarism affect long-term recovery, it may also play a role in the acute recovery process. Growth hormone and insulin like growth factor 1 (IGF-1) receptors are widely present in the brain. Increased expression of growth hormone receptors after focal ischemia has been shown, suggesting its function in recovery after neuronal injury.[57] Furthermore, growth hormone may have direct effects on vascular function and repair after hypoxic injury, whereas IGF-1 may be involved in myelinating processes and the protection of oligodendrocytes from tumor necrosis factor-alpha induced injury.[58–64] In addition, estradiol may also have important neuroprotective effects by improving cell survival and blocking the secretion of inflammatory mediators after injury,[65,66] which could potentially affect not only hypogonadal women but also hypogonadal men because estradiol is provided by the aromatization of testosterone.

Thus, with improving awareness of the prevalence of posttraumatic hypopituitarism and the potential impact on both acute and long-term recovery, the importance of routinely incorporating pituitary hormonal assessment and treatment into the care of patients who have experienced TBI is becoming evident.

SCREENING FOR POSTTRAUMATIC HYPOPITUITARISM

As previously mentioned, the natural history of posttraumatic hypopituitarism varies such that deficiencies that are present immediately following the initial injury may resolve and new hormonal deficits may develop over time, necessitating periodic monitoring of pituitary function. Any patient with life-threatening signs or symptoms of hypopituitarism, such as adrenal insufficiency or diabetes insipidus, should be immediately tested for these deficiencies, the specifics of which are discussed later. Routine clinical evaluation for all hormonal deficiencies should be conducted 3 to 6 months following the initial trauma with a detailed history and physical examination. If any signs or symptoms of hypopituitarism are present (**Table 1**), pituitary testing should be carried out. Given the potential impact on recovery and the often indistinguishable clinical presentations of hypopituitarism and TBI, the threshold to proceed

Table 1
Clinical presentation of hypopituitarism

Hormone Deficiency	Symptoms	Clinical Findings
Somatotropin (GH)	Decreased energy, impaired quality of life, cognitive impairments, anxiety, depression, social isolation	Visceral adiposity, decreased lean muscle mass, dyslipidemia ($\uparrow$LDL and $\downarrow$HDL), osteoporosis
Gonadotropin (LH/FSH)	Mood symptoms, hot flashes, sexual dysfunction, reduced cognition, fatigue, menstrual disturbances	Infertility, osteoporosis, vaginal atrophy in women; reduced muscle mass, scant secondary hair, and anemia in men
Thyrotropin (TSH)	Cold intolerance, fatigue, constipation, depressed mood, weight gain, menstrual irregularities, myalgias	Dry skin, periorbital edema, bradycardia, hypertension, delayed relaxation phase of deep tendon reflexes, hyperlipidemia, anemia, increased creatine kinase, hyponatremia
Corticotropin (ACTH)	Fatigue, generalized weakness, postural dizziness, weight loss, anorexia, nausea, myalgias, arthralgias, decreased libido	Orthostatic hypotension, hypoglycemia, hyponatremia, eosinophilia, anemia
Posterior pituitary	Abrupt onset of polyuria, nocturia, polydipsia	High-normal sodium concentration, urine osmolality less than plasma osmolality

Abbreviations: ACTH, adrenocorticotropic hormone; GH, growth hormone; HDL, high-density lipoprotein; LDL, low-density lipoprotein.

with pituitary testing should be low, with the most recent consensus guidelines recommending routine hormonal testing at 3 and 12 months, irrespective of symptoms.[46]

If pituitary deficiencies are detected 3 to 6 months after the initial injury, pituitary testing should be repeated at 12 months to assess for recovery of any hormonal deficiencies, especially in the case of isolated somatotropin or gonadotropin deficiency, which are often transient in nature, as well as to evaluate for any new hormonal deficiencies that may have occurred. If no pituitary deficiency was initially identified at 3 to 6 months, a repeat clinical assessment should be performed at 12 months with the use of pituitary testing in those patients with signs and symptoms of hypopituitarism.

After 12 months from the initial injury, it is thought that any hormonal deficit still present is unlikely to be transient.[46] Therefore, in patients who have had a TBI for more than 1 year and have never undergone endocrine evaluation, pituitary testing at this time can serve as a one-time screening tool for chronic hypopituitarism. However, this recommendation is limited by the time of follow-up in current prospective studies. Thus far, the longest prospective study has followed patients for 3 years and has reported recovery of all anterior pituitary deficiencies, as well as new-onset corticotropin and somatotropin deficiencies, occurring between year 1 and year 3 after the injury.[42] Continuation of these studies will improve understanding as to how long after the initial injury pituitary deficiencies can develop or resolve. Therefore, a reasonable approach is to clinically assess these patients for signs and symptoms of hypopituitarism on a yearly basis and proceed to pituitary testing when indicated.

The subset of patients with TBI that should undergo routine screening must also be established, although this is difficult to determine because of a lack of reliable predictive factors. Although patients with severe TBI may be at increased risk of hypopituitarism, a substantial risk still exists for patients with mild TBI, at frequencies comparable with those with moderate TBI.[35] Thus, endocrine evaluation should ideally be pursued in every patient who has had TBI.[46] However, this approach may not be practical or cost-effective.[67–69] It has therefore been proposed that, among patients of all trauma severities, only those who are symptomatic of hypopituitarism, have been hospitalized, or display predictive radiologic findings as previously discussed, should undergo screening.[35,67] Others argue that screening should focus on those with moderate to severe injuries, because the most data are available for this cohort, and there is potential for more substantial benefit from hormone replacement because of the significant morbidity that they often experience.[68,69]

DIAGNOSTIC TESTING OF POSTTRAUMATIC HYPOPITUITARISM

The diagnostic tools used in posttraumatic hypopituitarism are the same as those used to diagnose hypopituitarism from any other cause. In the acute setting, adrenal insufficiency should be suspected in patients with hypotension, hyponatremia, and/or hypoglycemia. Dynamic testing is generally not performed in the acute phase of illness. A morning serum cortisol level less than 3.5 μg/dL strongly indicates adrenal insufficiency, whereas a level greater than 18 μg/dL makes the diagnosis less likely.[70] Given that the patient is in a state of acute stress, the morning cortisol levels should arguably be significantly higher than 3 μg/dL, with some advocating a morning cortisol level of less than 7.2 μg/dL consistent with adrenal insufficiency,[35,41,67] whereas others use a level less than 11 μg/dL to make the diagnosis.[69,71] Cortisol values between these cutoff values may still represent adrenal insufficiency, and the diagnosis should be considered in the right clinical setting. Because of the potential life-threatening consequences of corticotropin deficiency, the routine monitoring of morning cortisol levels in the first week after injury has also been proposed, regardless of clinical findings.[69]

Suspicion for posterior pituitary deficiency should be raised in patients with polyuria and hypernatremia, and this should also be immediately investigated. The diagnosis of diabetes insipidus in the acute phase can be made from the presence of high-normal serum sodium concentration (>145 mEq/L) and polyuria (typically >3.5 L/24 h) with dilute urine, defined by an osmolality less than plasma osmolality (usually <300 mOsm/kg).[43] Overt hypernatremia can also be present in the setting of an impaired thirst mechanism or lack of access to free water.

Recommended testing for hypopituitarism in the chronic phase is listed in **Table 2**. IGF-1 levels, matched for age and gender, are not considered a good screening test for growth hormone deficiency because of its low sensitivity. A significant percentage of patients with growth hormone deficiency have normal IGF-1 levels. However, a low IGF-1 level in the absence of catabolic states, liver disease, and oral estrogen therapy may predict growth hormone deficiency. An IGF-1 concentration that is less than the range of normal for the assay used can be used alone to make the diagnosis of growth hormone deficiency in patients with 3 other pituitary hormonal deficiencies.[74] In all other settings, a low IGF-1 level should warrant provocative testing for confirmation of the diagnosis. There are several methods of dynamic testing available for the diagnosis of growth hormone deficiency and the choice is often determined by clinician preference and safety profile that best suits the patient. For example, although the insulin tolerance test is considered the gold standard, its use is contraindicated in patients with ischemic heart disease or seizure disorder. Growth hormone–releasing hormone (GHRH)–arginine test, found to be most sensitive and specific when adjusted

Table 2
Diagnostic testing for hypopituitarism in the chronic phase after TBI

Hormonal Axis	Diagnostic Test	Criteria for Hormone Deficiency
Somatotropin (GH)	Insulin tolerance test	Peak GH at 120 min <5.1 µg/L[72]
	GHRH-arginine test	BMI-dependent peak GH levels at 30–60 min[58]:
		BMI<25: GH <11.5 µg/L
		BMI 25–30: GH <8 µg/L
		BMI>30: GH <4.2 µg/L
	Glucagon stimulation test	Peak GH at 180 min <3 µg/L[73]
	IGF-1 level[a]	Less than normal age-adjusted and gender-adjusted reference range
Gonadotropin (LH/FSH)	LH/FSH	Low or inappropriately normal[b]
	8 AM Testosterone (men)	Low[b]
	Estradiol (women)	Low[b]
Thyrotropin (TSH)	TSH	Low or inappropriately normal[b]
	Free thyroxine	Low[b]
Corticotropin (ACTH)	8 AM Cortisol	Cortisol <3.5 µg/dL[70]
	8 AM ACTH	Low or inappropriately normal[b]
	Cosyntropin stimulation test:	
	High dose (250 µg)	Cortisol at 60 min <18 µg/dL[74]
	Low dose (1 µg)	Cortisol at 30 min <18 µg/dL[75]
	Insulin tolerance test	Cortisol at 45 min <18 µg/dL[76]
Posterior pituitary	Random urine and plasma sample	High-normal serum sodium concentration (>145 mEq/L) with urine osmolality less than plasma osmolality (typically <300 mOsm/kg)[1J]
	Water restriction test	Urine osmolality <700 mOsm/kg or ratio of urine to plasma osmolality <2[43]

Abbreviation: GHRH, growth hormone–releasing hormone.

[a] IGF-1 levels may only be used to diagnose growth hormone deficiency when 3 additional pituitary hormone deficits are present.

[b] Specific values are not given because reference ranges depend on the laboratory and assay used.

for BMI, should be avoided in patients with suspected hypothalamic disease because this may result in a falsely normal growth hormone response.[77] The glucagon stimulation test is recommended as the diagnostic test of choice when the insulin tolerance test and GHRH-arginine test cannot be performed, because it is readily available, easy to perform, well-tolerated, and inexpensive.[74]

As previously discussed, morning serum cortisol levels may identify corticotroph dysfunction. In the chronic phase after injury, stimulation testing may also be used to make the diagnosis and can be particularly helpful when morning serum cortisol levels cannot definitively do so. The insulin tolerance test is again considered the gold standard for diagnosis, but its unpleasantness for patients and contraindication in patients with seizure disorder, which is of particular concern in this patient population, may preclude its use. The standard high-dose (250 µg) or low-dose (1 µg) cosyntropin stimulation test is therefore commonly used. Some studies have shown that the low-dose test may be a better diagnostic tool in cases of recent-onset adrenocorticotropic hormone (ACTH) deficiency and chronic partial ACTH deficiency in which the adrenal glands are still capable of responding to cosyntropin.[78–80] Provocative testing is not used to diagnose thyrotropin or gonadotropin deficiencies.

INITIATION OF TREATMENT OF POSTTRAUMATIC HYPOPITUITARISM

The decision to initiate hormone replacement in the first 3 to 6 months after injury depends on the specific deficiency present. Hormone replacement should be initiated for isolated deficiencies of posterior pituitary, thyrotroph, and corticotroph function at the time of diagnosis, because of the critical roles of these hormones. Isolated gonadotropin and somatotropin deficiencies that occur 3 to 6 months after the initial trauma are often transient; therefore, some suggest that pituitary testing be repeated at 12 months and hormone replacement be initiated at that time if the deficiency is still present. As further studies are conducted, it may be shown that growth hormone and/or gonadotropin replacement in this phase has a significant effect on recovery and rehabilitation, thus providing a compelling reason to treat even a transient deficiency.

Pituitary deficiencies that are identified 1 year after the initial injury are less likely to resolve and replacement should be initiated as appropriate. Again, this recommendation is based on the limited time of follow-up in current prospective studies. With the longest prospective study showing resolution of growth hormone deficiency in 20% of patients between year 1 and year 3 after injury, it might be reasonable to delay treatment if no signs or symptoms of severe growth hormone deficiency are present.[42,67] In the setting of panhypopituitarism, the diagnosis of growth hormone deficiency cannot be made until all other pituitary deficiencies have been adequately replaced. Therefore, treatment of growth hormone deficiency should only begin when the diagnosis has been confirmed 3 to 6 months after optimal replacement of other hormonal deficiencies.[74] An algorithm for screening and initiation of treatment of posttraumatic hypopituitarism is provided in **Fig. 2**.

CLINICAL BENEFITS OF TREATMENT OF HYPOPITUITARISM AND POTENTIAL IMPACT ON OUTCOMES

Appropriate hormone replacement for hypopituitarism in general has known clinical benefits as summarized in **Table 3**. In addition to resolution of symptoms that are caused by each hormonal deficiency, treatment has a significant impact on long-term outcomes, which is especially important given the young age of most patients with TBI.[81]

The effect that hormone replacement has on quality of life and neurocognitive impairments is of particular interest in this patient population. Treatment of each anterior pituitary deficiency has been shown to result in an improvement in fatigue and quality of life.[82–90] With respect to cognitive impairments, treatment with growth hormone has resulted in improvements in memory, attention, and processing speed.[91–96] In addition, testosterone and estradiol replacement have been shown to improve spatial abilities and verbal and visual memory.[48,97–104] Treatment of hypothyroidism can also improve cognitive deficits, with one study showing that specific memory retrieval deficits associated with hypothyroidism can resolve after 3 months of treatment.[105]

Treatment of hypopituitarism can also have significant effects on physical function, which may affect recovery. Treatment of growth hormone–deficient patients has been shown to affect body composition by increasing muscle mass, although not as robustly as it decreases fat mass.[106–109] Whether or not this increase in muscle mass has functional significance has been examined, with some studies showing increases in isometric strength and exercise capacity after growth hormone replacement.[110–112] Androgen replacement has been shown to have similar effects on body composition, including decreasing fat mass and increasing muscle mass and strength.[113–115] In addition, treatment with estradiol, testosterone, and growth hormone replacement have all been shown to improve bone density, an outcome that

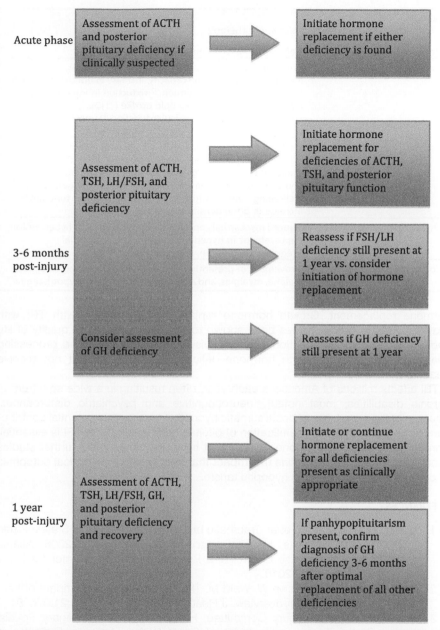

Fig. 2. Algorithm for screening and initiation of treatment of posttraumatic hypopituitarism.

may be particularly important in young patients who have not yet achieved peak bone mass.[116–129]

These improvements in quality of life, neurocognitive impairments, and physical function after treatment of hypopituitarism could improve the poorer outcomes that are observed in patients with posttraumatic hypopituitarism. However, there are limited studies examining this, all of which have focused on the effect of growth

Table 3
Clinical benefits of hormone replacement therapy

Hormonal Deficiency	Benefits of Hormone Replacement Therapy
Somatotropin (GH)	Decrease in visceral fat, increase in lean muscle mass, improvement in exercise capacity, increase in bone density, mild improvement of hypertension,[81] reduction in inflammatory markers,[82] more favorable lipid profile ($\uparrow$HDL, $\downarrow$LDL),[83] enhancement of left ventricular function,[84] improvement in energy
Gonadotropin (LH/FSH)	Testosterone: increased energy and libido, improvement in muscle strength and lean muscle mass, increase in bone density Estradiol: increased energy, amelioration of vasomotor symptoms and vaginal dryness, improvement in mood changes, sexual well-being, and cognition, enhanced endothelial function[85]; increase in bone density
Thyrotropin (TSH)	Enhanced myocardial contractility, better control of hypertension, improvement in hyperlipidemia, fatigue, menstrual irregularities, dry skin, and constipation[86]
Corticotropin (ACTH)	Improvement in presenting symptoms of generalized weakness, malaise, myalgias, and arthralgias; resolution of hypoglycemia[78]

hormone replacement. Growth hormone replacement in patients with TBI with growth hormone deficiency has been shown to improve measures of quality of life and cognition, such as attention, memory, visual-motor dexterity, and processing speed compared with growth hormone–deficient patients who did not receive treatment.[130–134]

TBI affects millions of Americans each year, often resulting in a wide spectrum of chronic disabilities, most notably neurocognitive and psychiatric disturbances. Because of the prevalence of posttraumatic hypopituitarism and its potential contribution to these impairments, identification of pituitary deficiencies after TBI is essential. Benefits of appropriate hormone replacement have been shown, but further studies should be conducted to examine the impact that treatment has on clinical outcomes of patients with posttraumatic hypopituitarism.

REFERENCES

1. Faul M, Xu L, Wald MM, et al. Traumatic brain injury in the United States: Emergency Department Visits, Hospitalizations, and Deaths 2002–2006. Atlanta (GA): Centers for Disease Control and Prevention, National Center for Injury Prevention and Control; 2010.
2. Langlois JA, Rutland-Brown W, Wald M. The epidemiology and impact of traumatic brain injury: a brief overview. J Head Trauma Rehabil 2006;21:375–8.
3. Mild Traumatic Brain Injury Committee, Head Injury Interdisciplinary Special Interest Group, American Congress of Rehabilitation Medicine. Definition of mild traumatic brain injury. J Head Trauma Rehabil 1993;8(3):86.
4. Bruns J, Hauser WA. The epidemiology of traumatic brain injury: a review. Epilepsia 2003;44(Suppl 10):2–10.
5. Kushner D. Mild traumatic brain injury. ARCH Intern Med 1998;158:1617–24.
6. Alexander MP. Mild traumatic brain injury: pathophysiology, natural history, and clinical management. Neurology 1995;45:1253–60.
7. Hibbard MR, Bogdany J, Uysal S, et al. Axis II psychopathology in individuals with traumatic brain injury. Brain Inj 2000;14:45–61.

8. Institute of Medicine. Gulf war and health, Vol. 7: longterm consequences of traumatic brain injury. Washington, DC: The National Academies Press; 2009.

9. Annegers JF, Hauser WA, Coan SP, et al. A population-based study of seizures after traumatic brain injury. N Engl J Med 1998;338:20–4.

10. Hauser WA, Annegers JF, Kurland LT. Prevalence of epilepsy in Rochester, Minnesota: 1940-1980. Epilepsia 1991;32:429–45.

11. Greenwald BD, Sabini RC. Sleep. In: Cristian A, editor. Medical management of adults with neurologic disabilities. New York: Demos Medical Publishing; 2009. p. 363–74.

12. McAllister TW. Emotional and behavioral sequelae of traumatic brain injury. In: Zasler ND, Katz DI, Zafonte RD, editors. Brain injury medicine: principles and practice. 2nd edition. New York: Demos Medical Publishing; 2013. p. 1039.

13. Plassman BL, Havlik RJ, Steffens DC, et al. Documented head injury in early adulthood and risk of Alzheimer's disease and other dementias. Neurology 2000;55:1158–66.

14. Lye TC, Shores EA. Traumatic brain injury as a risk factor for Alzheimer's disease: a review. Neuropsychol Rev 2000;10:115–29.

15. Cyran E. Hypohysenschadigung durch Schadelbasisfraktur. Dtsch Med Wochenschr 1918;44:1261.

16. Chou YC, Wang TY, Yang PY, et al. Permanent central diabetes insipidus after mild traumatic brain injury. Brain Inj 2009;23:1095–8.

17. Kornblum RN, Fisher RS. Pituitary lesions in craniocerebral injuries. Arch Pathol 1969;88:242–8.

18. Poomthavorn P, Zacharin M. Traumatic brain injury-mediated hypopituitarism. Report of four cases. Eur J Pediatr 2007;166:1163–8.

19. Klingbeil GE, Cline P. Anterior hypopituitarism: a consequence of head injury. Arch Phys Med Rehabil 1985;66:44–6.

20. Takala RS, Katila AJ, Sonninen P, et al. Panhypopituitarism after traumatic head injury. Neurocrit Care 2006;4:21–4.

21. Edwards OM, Clark JD. Post-traumatic hypopituitarism. Six cases and a review of the literature. Medicine (Baltimore) 1986;65:281–90.

22. Benvenga S, Campenní A, Ruggeri RM, et al. Clinical review 113: hypopituitarism secondary to head trauma. J Clin Endocrinol Metab 2000;85:1353–61.

23. Urban RJ, Harris P, Masel B. Anterior hypopituitarism following traumatic brain injury. Brain Inj 2005;19:349–58.

24. Aimaretti G, Ambrosio MR, Di Somma C, et al. Residual pituitary function after brain injury-induced hypopituitarism: a prospective 12-month study. J Clin Endocrinol Metab 2005;90:6085–92.

25. Bondanelli M, De Marinis L, Ambrosio MR, et al. Occurrence of pituitary dysfunction following traumatic brain injury. J Neurotrauma 2004;21:685–96.

26. Tanriverdi F, Senyurek H, Unluhizarci K, et al. High risk of hypopituitarism after traumatic brain injury: a prospective investigation of anterior pituitary function in the acute phase and 12 months after trauma. J Clin Endocrinol Metab 2006;91:2105–11.

27. Klose M, Juul A, Struck J, et al. Acute and long-term pituitary insufficiency in traumatic brain injury: a prospective single-centre study. Clin Endocrinol (Oxf) 2007;67:598–606.

28. Popovic V, Pekic S, Pavlovic D, et al. Hypopituitarism as a consequence of traumatic brain injury (TBI) and its possible relation with cognitive disabilities and mental distress. J Endocrinol Invest 2004;27:1048–54.

29. Agha A, Rogers B, Sherlock M, et al. Anterior pituitary dysfunction in survivors of traumatic brain injury. J Clin Endocrinol Metab 2004;89:4929–36.
30. Leal-Cerro A, Flores JM, Rincon M, et al. Prevalence of hypopituitarism and growth hormone deficiency in adults long-term after severe traumatic brain injury. Clin Endocrinol (Oxf) 2005;62:525–32.
31. Schneider HJ, Schneider M, Saller B, et al. Prevalence of anterior pituitary insufficiency 3 and 12 months after traumatic brain injury. Eur J Endocrinol 2006;154:259–65.
32. Herrmann BL, Rehder J, Kahlke S, et al. Hypopituitarism following severe traumatic brain injury. Exp Clin Endocrinol Diabetes 2006;114:316–21.
33. Lieberman SA, Oberoi AL, Gilkison CR, et al. Prevalence of neuroendocrine dysfunction in patients recovering from traumatic brain injury. J Clin Endocrinol Metab 2001;86:2752–6.
34. Kelly DF, Gonzalo IT, Cohan P, et al. Hypopituitarism following traumatic brain injury and aneurysmal subarachnoid hemorrhage: a preliminary report. J Neurosurg 2000;93:743–52.
35. Schneider HJ, Kreitschmann-Andermahr I, Ghigo E, et al. Hypothalamopituitary dysfunction following traumatic brain injury and aneurysmal subarachnoid hemorrhage: a systematic review. JAMA 2007;298:1429–38.
36. Schneider M, Schneider HJ, Yassouridis A, et al. Predictors of anterior pituitary insufficiency after traumatic brain injury. Clin Endocrinol (Oxf) 2008;68:206–12.
37. Bavisetty S, Bavisetty S, McArthur DL, et al. Chronic hypopituitarism after traumatic brain injury: risk assessment and relationship to outcome. Neurosurgery 2008;62:1080–93 [discussion: 1093–4].
38. Kelestimur F, Tanriverdi F, Atmaca H, et al. Boxing as a sport activity associated with isolated GH deficiency. J Endocrinol Invest 2004;27:28–32.
39. Ives JC, Alderman M, Stred SE. Hypopituitarism after multiple concussions: a retrospective case study in an adolescent male. J Athl Train 2007;42:431–9.
40. Tanriverdi F, Unluhizarci K, Coksevim B, et al. Kickboxing sport as a new cause of traumatic brain injury-mediated hypopituitarism. Clin Endocrinol (Oxf) 2007;66:360–6.
41. Agha A, Phillips J, O'Kelly P, et al. The natural history of post-traumatic hypopituitarism: implications for assessment and treatment. Am J Med 2005;118:1416.
42. Tanriverdi F, Ulutabanca H, Unluhizarci K, et al. Three years prospective investigation of anterior pituitary function after traumatic brain injury: a pilot study. Clin Endocrinol (Oxf) 2008;68:573–9.
43. Agha A, Thornton E, O'Kelly P, et al. Posterior pituitary dysfunction after traumatic brain injury. J Clin Endocrinol Metab 2004;89:5987–92.
44. Dusick J, Wang C, Cohan P, et al. Pathophysiology of hypopituitarism in the setting of brain injury. Pituitary 2012;15:2–9.
45. Bristritzer T, Theodor R, Inbar D, et al. Anterior hypopituitarism due to fracture of the sella turcica. Am J Dis Child 1981;135:966–8.
46. Ghigo E, Masel B, Aimaretti G, et al. Consensus guidelines on screening for hypopituitarism following traumatic brain injury. Brain Inj 2005;19:711–24.
47. Moffat SD, Zonderman AB, Metter EJ, et al. Longitudinal assessment of serum free testosterone concentration predicts memory performance and cognitive status in elderly men. J Clin Endocrinol Metab 2002;87:5001–7.
48. Janowsky JS, Chavez B, Orwoll E. Sex steroids modify working memory. J Cogn Neurosci 2000;12:407–14.

49. Rosario ER, Aqeel R, Brown MA, et al. Hypothalamic-pituitary dysfunction following traumatic brain injury affects functional improvement during acute inpatient rehabilitation. J Head Trauma Rehabil 2012;28(3):1–7.
50. Bondanelli M, Ambrosio MR, Cavazzini L, et al. Anterior pituitary function may predict functional and cognitive outcome in patients with traumatic brain injury undergoing rehabilitation. J Neurotrauma 2007;24:1687–97.
51. Park KD, Kim DY, Lee JK, et al. Anterior pituitary dysfunction in moderate-to-severe chronic traumatic brain injury patients and the influence on functional outcome. Brain Inj 2010;24:1330–5.
52. Kelly DF, McArthur DL, Levin H, et al. Neurobehavioral and quality of life changes associated with growth hormone insufficiency after complicated mild, moderate, or severe traumatic brain injury. J Neurotrauma 2006;23: 928–42.
53. León-Carrión J, Leal-Cerro A, Cabezas FM, et al. Cognitive deterioration due to GH deficiency in patients with traumatic brain injury: a preliminary report. Brain Inj 2007;21:871–5.
54. Young TP, Hoaglin HM, Burke DT. The role of serum testosterone and TBI in the in-patient rehabilitation setting. Brain Inj 2007;21:645–9.
55. Carlson NE, Brenner LA, Wierman ME, et al. Hypogonadism on admission to acute rehabilitation is correlated with lower functional status at admission and discharge. Brain Inj 2009;23:336–44.
56. Srinivasan L, Roberts B, Bushnik T, et al. The impact of hypopituitarism on function and performance in subjects with recent history of traumatic brain injury and aneurysmal subarachnoid haemorrhage. Brain Inj 2009;23:639–48.
57. Christophidis LJ, Gorba T, Gustavsson M, et al. Growth hormone receptor immunoreactivity is increased in the subventricular zone of juvenile rat brain after focal ischemia: a potential role for growth hormone in injury-induced neurogenesis. Growth Horm IGF Res 2009;19:497–506.
58. Silha JV, Krsek M, Hana V, et al. The effects of growth hormone status on circulating levels of vascular growth factors. Clin Endocrinol (Oxf) 2005;63:79–86.
59. Scheepens A, Williams CE, Breier BH, et al. A role for the somatotropic axis in neural development, injury and disease. J Pediatr Endocrinol Metab 2000; 13(Suppl 6):1483–91.
60. Napoli R, Guardasole V, Angelini V, et al. Acute effects of growth hormone on vascular function in human subjects. J Clin Endocrinol Metab 2003;88: 2817–20.
61. Hána V, Prázný M, Marek J, et al. Reduced microvascular perfusion and reactivity in adult GH deficient patients is restored by GH replacement. Eur J Endocrinol 2002;147:333–7.
62. Ye P, Li L, Richards RG, et al. Myelination is altered in insulin-like growth factor-I null mutant mice. J Neurosci 2002;22:6041–51.
63. Ye P, D'Ercole AJ. Insulin-like growth factor I protects oligodendrocytes from tumor necrosis factor-alpha-induced injury. Endocrinology 1999;140:3063–72.
64. Zhong J, Deng J, Phan J, et al. Insulin-like growth factor-I protects granule neurons from apoptosis and improves ataxia in weaver mice. J Neurosci Res 2005; 80:481–90.
65. Stein DG. Brain damage, sex hormones and recovery: a new role for progesterone and estrogen? Trends Neurosci 2001;24:386–91.
66. Vegeto E, Belcredito S, Etteri S, et al. Estrogen receptor-alpha mediates the brain antiinflammatory activity of estradiol. Proc Natl Acad Sci U S A 2003; 100:9614–9.

67. Tanriverdi F, Unluhizarci K, Kelestimur F. Pituitary function in subjects with mild traumatic brain injury: a review of literature and proposal of a screening strategy. Pituitary 2010;13:146–53.

68. Gasco V, Prodam F, Pagano L, et al. Hypopituitarism following brain injury: when does it occur and how best to test? Pituitary 2012;15:20–4.

69. Glynn N, Agha A. Which patient requires neuroendocrine assessment following traumatic brain injury, when and how? Clin Endocrinol (Oxf) 2013;78:17–20.

70. Schmidt IL, Lahner H, Mann K, et al. Diagnosis of adrenal insufficiency: evaluation of the corticotropin-releasing hormone test and basal serum cortisol in comparison to the insulin tolerance test in patients with hypothalamic-pituitary-adrenal disease. J Clin Endocrinol Metab 2003;88:4193–8.

71. Hannon MJ, Sherlock M, Thompson CJ. Pituitary dysfunction following traumatic brain injury or subarachnoid haemorrhage - in "Endocrine Management in the Intensive Care Unit". Best Pract Res Clin Endocrinol Metab 2011;25:783–98.

72. Biller BM, Samuels MH, Zagar A, et al. Sensitivity and specificity of six tests for the diagnosis of adult GH deficiency. J Clin Endocrinol Metab 2002;87:2067–79.

73. Conceição FL, Da Costa e Silva A, Leal Costa AJ, et al. Glucagon stimulation test for the diagnosis of GH deficiency in adults. J Endocrinol Invest 2003;26: 1065–70.

74. Molitch ME, Clemmons DR, Malozowski S, et al. Evaluation and treatment of adult growth hormone deficiency: an Endocrine Society clinical practice guideline. J Clin Endocrinol Metab 2011;96:1587–609.

75. Thaler LM, Blevins LS Jr. The low dose (1-microg) adrenocorticotropin stimulation test in the evaluation of patients with suspected central adrenal insufficiency. J Clin Endocrinol Metab 1998;83:2726–9.

76. Tuchelt H, Dekker K, Bähr V, et al. Dose-response relationship between plasma ACTH and serum cortisol in the insulin-hypoglycaemia test in 25 healthy subjects and 109 patients with pituitary disease. Clin Endocrinol 2000;53:301–7.

77. Corneli G, Di Somma C, Baldelli R, et al. The cut-off limits of the GH response to GH-releasing hormone-arginine test related to body mass index. Eur J Endocrinol 2005;153:257–64.

78. Streeten DH, Anderson GH Jr, Bonaventura MM. The potential for serious consequences from misinterpreting normal responses to the rapid adrenocorticotropin test. J Clin Endocrinol Metab 1996;81:285–90.

79. Dickstein G, Shechner C, Nicholson WE, et al. Adrenocorticotropin stimulation test: effects of basal cortisol level, time of day, and suggested new sensitive low dose test. J Clin Endocrinol Metab 1991;72:773–8.

80. Dökmetaş HS, Colak R, Keleştimur F, et al. A comparison between the 1-microg adrenocorticotropin (ACTH) test, the short ACTH (250 microg) test, and the insulin tolerance test in the assessment of hypothalamo-pituitary-adrenal axis immediately after pituitary surgery. J Clin Endocrinol Metab 2000;85:3713–9.

81. Maison P, Griffin S, Nicoue-Beglah M, et al. Impact of growth hormone (GH) treatment on cardiovascular risk factors in GH-deficient adults: a metaanalysis of blinded, randomized, placebo-controlled trials. J Clin Endocrinol Metab 2004;89:2192–9.

82. Bollerslev J, Ueland T, Jørgensen AP, et al. Positive effects of a physiological dose of GH on markers of atherogenesis: a placebo-controlled study in patients with adult-onset GH deficiency. Eur J Endocrinol 2006;154:537–43.

83. Abs R, Feldt-Rasmussen U, Mattsson AF, et al. Determinants of cardiovascular risk in 2589 hypopituitary GH-deficient adults - a KIMS database analysis. Eur J Endocrinol 2006;155:79–90.

84. Maison P, Chanson P. Cardiac effects of growth hormone in adults with growth hormone deficiency: a meta-analysis. Circulation 2003;108:2648–52.
85. Rosano GM, Vitale C, Fini M. Hormone replacement therapy and cardioprotection: what is good and what is bad for the cardiovascular system? Ann N Y Acad Sci 2006;1092:341–8.
86. Garber JR, Cobin RH, Gharib H, et al. Clinical practice guidelines for hypothyroidism in adults: cosponsored by the American Association of Clinical Endocrinologists and the American Thyroid Association. Thyroid 2012;22:1200–35.
87. Rutland-Brown W, Langlois JA, Thomas KE, et al. Incidence of traumatic brain injury in the United States, 2003. J Head Trauma Rehabil 2006;21:544–8.
88. Bleicken B, Hahner S, Loeffler M, et al. Influence of hydrocortisone dosage scheme on health-related quality of life in patients with adrenal insufficiency. Clin Endocrinol (Oxf) 2010;72:297–304.
89. Langenheim J, Ventz M, Hinz A, et al. Modified-release prednisone decreases complaints and fatigue compared to standard prednisolone in patients with adrenal insufficiency. Horm Metab Res 2013;45:96–101.
90. Samuels MH, Schuff KG, Carlson NE, et al. Health status, psychological symptoms, mood, and cognition in L-thyroxine-treated hypothyroid subjects. Thyroid 2007;17:249–58.
91. Dugbartey AT. Neurocognitive aspects of hypothyroidism. Arch Intern Med 1998;158:1413–8.
92. Soares CN, Almeida OP, Joffe H, et al. Efficacy of estradiol for the treatment of depressive disorders in perimenopausal women: a double-blind, randomized, placebo-controlled trial. Arch Gen Psychiatry 2001;58:529–34.
93. Zweifel JE, O'Brien WH. A meta-analysis of the effect of hormone replacement therapy upon depressed mood. Psychoneuroendocrinology 1997;22:189–212.
94. Rosilio M, Blum WF, Edwards DJ, et al. Long-term improvement of quality of life during growth hormone (GH) replacement therapy in adults with GH deficiency, as measured by questions on life satisfaction-hypopituitarism (QLS-H). J Clin Endocrinol Metab 2004;89:1684–93.
95. Wirén L, Bengtsson BÅ, Johannsson G. Beneficial effects of long-term GH replacement therapy on quality of life in adults with GH deficiency. Clin Endocrinol 1998;48:613–20.
96. Murray RD, Skillicorn CJ, Howell SJ, et al. Influences on quality of life in GH deficient adults and their effect on response to treatment. Clin Endocrinol 1999;51:565–73.
97. Maruff P, Falleti M. Cognitive function in growth hormone deficiency and growth hormone replacement. Horm Res 2005;64(Suppl 3):100–8.
98. Falleti MG, Maruff P, Burman P, et al. The effects of growth hormone (GH) deficiency and GH replacement on cognitive performance in adults: a meta-analysis of the current literature. Psychoneuroendocrinology 2006;31:681–91.
99. Deijen JB, De Boer H, Van der Veen EA. Cognitive changes during growth hormone replacement in adult men. Psychoneuroendocrinology 1998;23:45–55.
100. Arwert LI, Veltman DJ, Deijen JB, et al. Effects of growth hormone substitution therapy on cognitive functioning in growth hormone deficient patients: a functional MRI study. Neuroendocrinology 2006;83:12–9.
101. Sathiavageeswaran M, Burman P, Lawrence D, et al. Effects of GH on cognitive function in elderly patients with adult-onset GH deficiency: a placebo-controlled 12-month study. Eur J Endocrinol 2007;156:439–47.

102. Oertel H, Schneider HJ, Stalla GK, et al. The effect of growth hormone substitution on cognitive performance in adult patients with hypopituitarism. Psychoneuroendocrinology 2004;29:839–50.
103. Janowsky JS, Oviatt SK, Orwoll ES. Testosterone influences spatial cognition in older men. Behav Neurosci 1994;108:325–32.
104. Cherrier MM, Craft S, Matsumoto AH. Cognitive changes associated with supplementation of testosterone or dihydrotestosterone in mildly hypogonadal men: a preliminary report. J Androl 2003;24:568–76.
105. Alexander GM, Swerdloff RS, Wang C, et al. Androgen-behavior correlations in hypogonadal men and eugonadal men. II. Cognitive abilities. Horm Behav 1998; 33:85–94.
106. Ross JL, Roeltgen D, Feuillan P, et al. Effects of estrogen on nonverbal processing speed and motor function in girls with Turner's syndrome. J Clin Endocrinol Metab 1998;83:3198–204.
107. Ross JL, Roeltgen D, Feuillan P, et al. Use of estrogen in young girls with Turner syndrome: effects on memory. Neurology 2000;54:164–70.
108. Sherwin BB. Estrogenic effects on memory in women. Ann N Y Acad Sci 1994; 743:213–30.
109. Schmidt R, Fazekas F, Reinhart B, et al. Estrogen replacement therapy in older women: a neuropsychological and brain MRI study. J Am Geriatr Soc 1996;44: 1307–13.
110. Jacobs DM, Tang MX, Stern Y, et al. Cognitive function in nondemented older women who took estrogen after menopause. Neurology 1998;50:368–73.
111. Miller KJ, Parsons TD, Whybrow PC, et al. Memory improvement with treatment of hypothyroidism. Int J Neurosci 2006;116:895–906.
112. Attanasio AF, Howell S, Bates PC, et al. Body composition, IGF-I and IGFBP-3 concentrations as outcome measures in severely GH-deficient (GHD) patients after childhood GH treatment: a comparison with adult onset GHD patients. J Clin Endocrinol Metab 2002;87:3368–72.
113. Attanasio AF, Bates PC, Ho KK, et al. Human growth hormone replacement in adult hypopituitary patients: long-term effects on body composition and lipid status–3-year results from the HypoCCS Database. J Clin Endocrinol Metab 2002;87:1600–6.
114. Hoffman AR, Kuntze JE, Baptista J, et al. Growth hormone (GH) replacement therapy in adult-onset GH deficiency: effects on body composition in men and women in a double-blind, randomized, placebo-controlled trial. J Clin Endocrinol Metab 2004;89:2048–56.
115. Gibney J, Wallace JD, Spinks T, et al. The effects of 10 years of recombinant human growth hormone (GH) in adult GH-deficient patients. J Clin Endocrinol Metab 1999;84:2596–602.
116. Widdowson WM, Gibney J. The effect of growth hormone replacement on exercise capacity in patients with GH deficiency: a metaanalysis. J Clin Endocrinol Metab 2008;93:4413–7.
117. Woodhouse LJ, Asa SL, Thomas SG, et al. Measures of submaximal aerobic performance evaluate and predict functional response to growth hormone (GH) treatment in GH-deficient adults. J Clin Endocrinol Metab 1998;84: 4570–7.
118. Götherström G, Elbornsson M, Stibrant-Sunnerhagen K, et al. Ten years of growth hormone (GH) replacement normalizes muscle strength in GH-deficient adults. J Clin Endocrinol Metab 2009;94:809–16.

119. Page ST, Amory JK, Bowman FD, et al. Exogenous testosterone (T) alone or with finasteride increases physical performance, grip strength, and lean body mass in older men with low serum T. J Clin Endocrinol Metab 2005;90:1502–10.

120. Snyder PJ, Peachey H, Hannoush P, et al. Effect of testosterone treatment on body composition and muscle strength in men over 65 years of age. J Clin Endocrinol Metab 1999;84:2647–53.

121. Sih R, Morley JE, Kaiser FE, et al. Testosterone replacement in older hypogonadal men: a 12-month randomized controlled trial. J Clin Endocrinol Metab 1997; 82:1661–7.

122. Cleemann L, Hjerrild BE, Lauridsen AL, et al. Long-term hormone replacement therapy preserves bone mineral density in Turner syndrome. Eur J Endocrinol 2009;161:251–7.

123. Khastgir G, Studd JW, Fox SW, et al. A longitudinal study of the effect of subcutaneous estrogen replacement on bone in young women with Turner's syndrome. J Bone Miner Res 2003;18:925–32.

124. Behre HH, Kliesch S, Leifke E, et al. Long term effect of testosterone therapy on bone mineral density in hypogonadal men. J Clin Endocrinol Metab 1997;82: 2386–90.

125. Amory JK, Watts NB, Easley KA, et al. Exogenous testosterone or testosterone with finasteride increases bone mineral density in older men with low serum testosterone. J Clin Endocrinol Metab 2004;89:503–10.

126. Tracz M, Sideras K, Bolon ER. Clinical review: testosterone use in men and its effects on bone health. A systematic review and meta-analysis of randomized placebo-controlled trials. J Clin Endocrinol Metab 2006;91:2011–6.

127. Biller BM, Sesmilo G, Baum HB, et al. Withdrawal of long-term physiological growth hormone (GH) administration: differential effects on bone density and body composition in men with adult-onset GH deficiency. J Clin Endocrinol Metab 2000;85:970–6.

128. Shalet SM, Shavrikova E, Cromer M, et al. Effect of growth hormone (GH) treatment on bone in postpubertal GH-deficient patients: a 2-year randomized, controlled, dose-ranging study. J Clin Endocrinol Metab 2003;88:4124–9.

129. Götherström G, Bengtsson BA, Bosaeus I, et al. Ten-year GH replacement increases bone mineral density in hypopituitary patients with adult onset GH deficiency. Eur J Endocrinol 2007;156:55–64.

130. Reimunde P, Quintana A, Castañón B, et al. Effects of growth hormone (GH) replacement and cognitive rehabilitation in patients with cognitive disorders after traumatic brain injury. Brain Inj 2011;25:65–73.

131. Kozlowski O, Cortet-Rudelli C, Yollin E, et al. Growth hormone replacement therapy in patients with traumatic brain injury. J Neurotrauma 2013;30(11): 998–1006.

132. Kreitschmann-Andermahr I, Poll EM, Reineke A, et al. Growth hormone deficient patients after traumatic brain injury–baseline characteristics and benefits after growth hormone replacement–an analysis of the German KIMS database. Growth Horm IGF Res 2008;18:472–8.

133. High WM Jr, Briones-Galang M, Clark JA, et al. Effect of growth hormone replacement therapy on cognition after traumatic brain injury. J Neurotrauma 2010;27:1565–75.

134. Tanriverdi F, Unluhizarci K, Karaca Z, et al. Hypopituitarism due to sports related head trauma and the effects of growth hormone replacement in retired amateur boxers. Pituitary 2010;13:111–4.

Drug Addiction and Sexual Dysfunction

Adham Zaazaa, MD, PhD, FECSM[a], Anthony J. Bella, MD, FRCSC[b],
Rany Shamloul, MD, PhD[a,c,*]

KEYWORDS

- Drug addiction • Sexual dysfunction • Heroin • Cocaine

KEY POINTS

- Even though alcohol is prevalent in many societies with many myths surrounding its sexual-enhancing effects, current scientific research cannot provide a solid conclusion on its effect on sexual function. The same concept applies to tobacco smoking; however, most of the current knowledge tends to support the notion that it, indeed, can negatively affect sexual function.
- Cannabinoid receptors in the human cavernous report the nonrelaxing effects of marijuana.
- Heroin exerts a depletion effect on plasma levels of free testosterone and raises testosterone-binding globulin levels, irrespective of age, amount of heroin intake per day, and period of contact with the drug with no effect on the pituitary gonadotropins.
- Initially, the use of cocaine may enhance the sexual functioning of men, but prolonged use may diminish sexual desire and performance and may contribute to difficulty in achieving orgasm.

INTRODUCTION

Throughout history the search for sex-enhancing drugs or aphrodisiacs has been a human obsession. In a review by Shah, different civilizations' thoughts and reactions concerning this goal is eloquently discussed.[1] For example, poems from the Hindu civilization dating back 3000 to 4000 years are the earliest recordings of the human eternal search for substances that can enhance sexual experiences lead to the much unknown, "supersex," and/or treat erectile dysfunction (ED).[2] The ancient Egyptians had their share of aphrodisiacs with several papyri describing many medications

[a] Department of Andrology, Cairo University, Cairo, Egypt; [b] Greta and John Hansen Chair in Men's Health Research, Department of Surgery and Neuroscience, University of Ottawa, Ottawa, Ontario, Canada; [c] Department of Surgery, Division of Urology, University of Ottawa, Ottawa, Ontario, Canada
* Corresponding author. Ottawa Hospital Research Institute, 725 Parkdale Avenue, Ottawa, ON K1Y 4E9, Canada.
E-mail address: ranyshamloul@gmail.com

Endocrinol Metab Clin N Am 42 (2013) 585–592
http://dx.doi.org/10.1016/j.ecl.2013.06.003
0889-8529/13/$ – see front matter © 2013 Elsevier Inc. All rights reserved.

for ED, including local penile application of oiled baby crocodile hearts, and ingestion of pine, salt, and watermelon.[3,4] Nevertheless, a recent review evaluating the use of natural aphrodisiacs concluded that there seems to be no strong evidence to support their use in the treatment of male or female sexual dysfunction (SD).[5]

Pharmaceutical agents, on the other hand, used to treat various medical diseases have had their own positive and negative effects on sexual function. Furthermore, there has been continued interest in studying the effect of drug addiction on human sexual function.[6] This article examines the effects of drugs of abuse on male and female sexual function. Because of the very wide range of drugs of abuse, the most common of them, namely, alcohol, cannabis, cocaine, tobacco, amphetamines, opioids, and antidepressant drugs, are focused on.

ALCOHOL

Alcohol, the most commonly used recreational drug, has been associated with sexuality for a long time. In Shakespeare's *Macbeth,* Act 2, Scene 3, it is stated, "What three things does drink especially provoke... lechery, sir, it provokes, and unprovokes; it provokes the desire, but it takes away the performance." Indeed, scientific evidence does support some of the historical claims. Alcohol is a central nervous system depressant that acts by increasing the levels of the inhibitory neurotransmitter, gamma amino butyric acid.[7] Alcohol is also known to cause disinhibition and thus can potentiate sexual desire. Indeed, several studies did confirm the potential harmful effects chronic alcohol drinking has on male and female sexual functions, which can be attributed to its effects on the cardiovascular and the neurologic systems.[8–10] In their excellent meta-analysis Chew and colleagues[11] demonstrated that chronic alcohol significantly increased the odds of ED among alcohol drinkers in 7 of the 11 cross-sectional studies cited. Although drinking less than 8 drinks per week had the lowest, but nonsignificant, risk for ED, drinking more than 8 standard drinks a week was associated with a statistically significant, but with higher ED, risk. Similar results were reported from other studies. Unfortunately, studies examining the effect of alcohol on female sexual function are very limited with inconclusive results.[12] Taken collectively, the current body of evidence from various epidemiologies is not sufficient to make a solid conclusion regarding the role of alcohol consumption on sexual function.

TOBACCO

Research concerning the relationship between tobacco smoking and sexual function has been abundant in the past few years, particularly in male sexuality.[13–17] The impact of smoking on erectile function, although more evident in older men, can be found in men under the age of 45 years.[14–16] There are several reasons smoking affects sexual function.[6,13] First, nicotine is considered a strong vasoconstrictor and therefore can significantly reduce blood flow to the male and female genitals during sexual activity.[6,13] In an excellent review, it was reported that nicotine, in fact, that can significantly reduce vasoactive substances, such as endothelium-derived relaxing factor, nitric oxide, prostaglandin, prostacycline, and thromboxane, in the vascular endothelium of the male and female genital tract.[18] In addition, it was shown that nicotine can negatively affect the levels of sex hormones, testosterone and estrogen, in male and female smokers.[15,19] However, other studies did not report similar findings.[20,21] Clinical studies examining the effects of smoking on male erectile function reported its negative impact on the ability of a man to initiate or maintain an erection.[22,23] Unfortunately, similar effects of nicotine on female sexual function have not been adequately studied. Although smoking does indeed negatively affect sexual function, stopping smoking, even for short periods of time, can improve sexual function. Furthermore, there is evidence that quitting smoking can have a sustained benefit on sexual function.[24,25]

CANNABIS

Cannabis (marijuana) is the most widely used illicit drug globally.[26] In 2004, the United Nations Office on Drugs and Crime estimated that approximately 4% of the world's adult population (162 million people) use cannabis annually, with 0.6% (22.5 million) reporting daily use.[27] Tetrahydrocannabinol, the active metabolite of cannabis, may serve as a central nervous system stimulant, depressant, and/or a hallucinogen. There are significant data from animal and in vitro studies to support the inhibitory role of the endocannabinoid system on male sexual function.[28–30] It is also well established that a group of oxytocinergic neurons containing cannabinoid (CB1) receptors in the paraventricular nucleus of the hypothalamus (PVN) regulate erectile function and copulatory behavior of men.[31] Furthermore, another study demonstrated that erections could be induced in male rats by injecting the CB1 receptor antagonist SR 141716A into the PVN.[32] Other studies reported that intracerebral microdialysis revealed that the proerectile effect of SR 141716A in the PVN occurred concomitantly with an increase in the concentration of glutamic acid, NO_2^-, and NO_3^-, in the paraventricular dialysate.[29] There is also emerging evidence for peripheral effects of CBs on penile erection. Relaxation of cavernous smooth muscle in the corpus cavernosum (CC) is critical for inducing and maintaining penile erections. CB1 receptors have been shown to be expressed in the CC of the rat[29] and CB1 and CB2 receptors have been shown to be expressed in the CC of rhesus monkeys and humans.[28] Several years after the discovery of the CB1 receptor, a second cannabinoid receptor, CB2, was identified.[33] In contrast to CB1, CB2 receptor has a more limited central distribution and is more abundant in the peripheral tissue, such as thymus, spleen, and immune cells.[33] A breakthrough study by Gratzke and colleagues[28] was published on the role of CBs for peripheral neurotransmission, including controlling of penile erection. CB1 and CB2 receptors were colocalized with nitric oxide synthase and with the vanilloid transient receptor potential 1; expression was primarily in the sensory nerves of human and monkey CC, in association with nitrergic nerves. In addition, functional studies showed that the endogenous CB1 and CB2 agonist, anandamide, depresses the nonadrenergic noncholinergic relaxations of the primate CC.[28] These exciting data may result in further research, as the role of CBs in regulating sexual function is incompletely elucidated.

OPIOIDS

The effects of opioids' abuse on sexual function may be of dual mode. At the beginning, many patients experience an improvement in their sexual function, with delayed ejaculation in men and improvement of vaginismus in women.[6] However, later on, both men and women report decreased libido and orgasmic functions. A recent study of 101 heroin addicts compared with a control group of matched healthy subjects found a significant decrease in weekly sexual intercourse and masturbatory activity in men, but not in women. Seventy-five percent of men and 68% of women thought that heroin decreased their interest in sex.[34] In addition, 71% of men and 60% of women thought that drug use worsened their sexual arousal. Also, about 60% of the addicts of both sexes thought that drug use decreased their ability to experience orgasm. When questioned about the first 6 months of heroin use, 21% of men and 28% of women thought their sexual satisfaction had increased.[34]

The mechanisms underlying the negative effects of opioids on sexual function remain unclear. However, specific biologic actions of heroin may help shed some light on opioids-induced SDs. Heroin exerts a depletion effect on plasma levels of free testosterone and raises testosterone-binding globulin levels, irrespective of age, amount of heroin intake per day, and period of contact with the drug with no effect on the pituitary gonadotropins,[6] suggesting that chronic heroin abuse depresses testicular function via the hypothalamus or higher centers. These hormonal changes returned promptly to normal after withdrawal.[35] Another theory explaining heroin effects on sexual function is through the action of opioids on the mesolimbic dopamine reward pathway. This system promotes behavior and actions deemed useful to the individual or the species. Certain drugs exert fast and significant control over behavior (eg, heroin) with deterioration in the ability of normal rewards (including sex) to control behavior.[6]

COCAINE

Cocaine has been correlated with both increased and inhibited desire.[36] Many cocaine-using men have a powerful association between sexual arousal and cocaine use, but frequently by the time they enter treatment, they have difficulty functioning sexually when under the influence of cocaine.[36] Indeed, although, initially, the use of cocaine may enhance the sexual functioning of men,[37] prolonged use may diminish sexual desire and performance and may contribute to difficulty in achieving orgasm.[38]

In one study of regular cocaine users, 66% of men who had been using the drug for 1 year or longer reported that they had difficulty getting erections.[39] It is common for regular cocaine users to also be heavy drinkers of alcohol. In a study of men who were dually addicted to alcohol and cocaine, 62% reported low sexual desire; 52% reported erectile dysfunction, and 30% experienced delayed ejaculation.[40]

The link between cocaine and sex is far less typical of female cocaine users, but contrary to the notion that crack cocaine may act as an aphrodisiac for women, a study of female crack cocaine users found that the drug diminished sexual desire and increased the likelihood of SD.[40] There are also reports of cases of priapism associated with intracavernosal injection of cocaine.[41]

AMPHETAMINES

Amphetamine is a highly addictive drug and it is well known that its long-term use is associated with increased risk for serious cardiovascular and lung disease, depression, psychosis, and cognitive impairment.[42] Concerning sexual function, amphetamines have a popular characteristic of being a potent aphrodisiac.[43] However, human observational studies revealed a variety of amphetamine-related SDs.[44] These variations may depend on several factors: dosage, route of administration, habits of the drug user, and social setting. It is postulated that low doses can increase enjoyment and lower inhibitions, whereas delayed orgasm may be useful to men with already established rapid ejaculation. On the other hand, high doses of amphetamines are associated with anorgasmia and low sex drive.[45] A potent well-known amphetamine, methamphetamine, has been strongly linked to heightened sexual behavior.[46,47] This appears to be due to the combination of increased social confidence, sexual disinhibition, and heightened sense of physical energy, perceived as sexual enhancement effects by its users.[48,49] There is no scientific evidence linking methamphetamine to direct action on specific receptors that can enhance sexuality;

it is thought to enhance sexual experience by enhancing one's general sense of well-being.[47] Prolonged use of amphetamine-based drugs has been associated with ED and delayed ejaculation in men as well as delayed orgasm in women.[48,49] A unique phenomenon related to the prolonged use of methamphetamine is its ability to induce a prolonged state of strong sex drive in men but with inadequate erections, which is popularly called "crystal dick."[50] In addition, several studies pointed out that methamphetamine can increase the likelihood for gay, bisexual, and heterosexual methamphetamine users to engage in very high HIV/sexually transmitted infection sexual risk behaviors.[51,52] A valid explanation for this peculiar phenomenon is that the combination of lowered sexual inhibitions, high libido and energy, and the highly charged sexual context in which methamphetamine use often takes place may predispose the abuse to such risky behaviors.[53]

PSYCHOTROPIC DRUGS

Psychotropic drugs are often associated with the development of SD. Of the commonly abused psychotropic drugs are tricyclic antidepressants, monoamine oxidase inhibitors, and selective serotonin reuptake inhibitors.

Antidepressant treatment is associated with significant rates of SD in men and women,[54] and there are also significant variations among the effects produced by different drugs in this class,[55] reflecting specific differences in the pharmacologic profiles of these different antidepressant drugs. A recent meta-analysis that analyzed data from selected studies investigating treatment-emergent SD by means of structured interviews and standardized SD questionnaires, drugs with a predominant serotonergic action, including selective serotonin reuptake inhibitors and venlafaxine, had the highest likelihood of inducing treatment-related SD (ranging from 26% for fluvoxamine to 80% for sertraline and venlafaxine).[54] On the other hand, several points need to be addressed here. First, it is unclear if the lower rates of SD associated with fluvoxamine and escitalopram are attributed to the specific characteristics of these drugs or whether they could simply reflect differences in the methods of inquiry. Also, it is again unclear how antidepressants that have an overall association with SD affect all 3 phases of the sexual cycle. Moreover, duloxetine, imipramine, and phenelzine, compared with placebo, could be significantly related to SD rates, whereas no significant difference was observed between the effects of placebo and those of moclobemide, agomelatine, amineptine, nefazodone, bupropion, or mirtazapine.[54]

Mechanisms behind these well-documented drug-mediated SD are largely unknown. A widely appreciated hypothesis is that selective serotonin reuptake inhibitors and venlafaxine do reduce dopaminergic transmission via serotonin receptors in the mesolimbic area, which is primarily associated with sexual desire and orgasm, and thus SD associated with these drugs is expected.[56] This hypothesis is further supported by the suggestion that serotonergic agents, such as mirtazapine and nefazodone, with antagonist rather than agonist action on 5HTR2, do not induce SD.[57] Other mechanisms proposed include reduction of the nitric oxidase synthase and the anticholinergic effects related to paroxetine could also be involved in antidepressant-related SD.[56]

SUMMARY

Despite the advancement in the understanding of the male and female sexual function,[58] research involving the effects of substance abuse on sexual function, especially the female component, still suffers major knowledge gaps. Unfortunately, not only is there limited research in this area but much of what is already known seems to be unclear or theoretical at best.[12]

This article attempted to review the most current and the well-established facts in this area. Surprisingly, even though alcohol is prevalent in many societies with many myths surrounding its sexual-enhancing effects, current scientific research cannot provide a solid conclusion on its effect on sexual function. Unfortunately, the same concept applies to tobacco smoking; however, most of current knowledge tends to support the notion that it, indeed, can negatively affect sexual function. Similar ambiguities also prevail with substance of abuse.

Scientific research concerning substance abuse–induced SD is not entirely ambiguous; there are recent encouraging signs. For example, research examining the sexual effects of marijuana has recently gained momentum. The discovery of cannabinoid receptors in the human cavernous tissue with its related in vitro data reporting the non-relaxing effects of marijuana on human cavernous tissue is very promising and encouraging. Rigorous basic and clinical research is key for the understanding of the mechanisms underlying the sexual effects of the drugs of abuse.

REFERENCES

1. Shah J. Erectile dysfunction through the ages. BJU Int 2002;90:433–41.
2. Bhishagratna KK. The Sushruta Samhita. An English translation based on original Sanskrit text. 2nd edition. Varanasi (India): Chowkhamba Sanskrit Series Office; 1963.
3. Smith GE. Papyrus Ebers. English translation. Chicago: Ares Publishers; 1974.
4. Nunn JF. Ancient Egyptian medicine. London: British Museum; 1996.
5. Shamloul R. Natural aphrodisiacs. J Sex Med 2010;7(1 Pt 1):39–49.
6. Palha AP, Esteves M. Drugs of abuse and sexual functioning. Adv Psychosom Med 2008;29:131–49.
7. Sadock BJ, Sadock VA. Abnormal Sexuality and Sexual Dysfunctions. In: Synopsis of Psychiatry. Philadelphia: Lippincott Williams & Wilkins; 2007. p. 689–705.
8. Schiavi RC. Chronic alcoholism and male sexual dysfunction. J Sex Marital Ther 1990;16:23–33.
9. Smith DE. Alcoholism, recovery, and sexual dysfunction. Psychiatr Med 1985;3: 163–72.
10. Okulate G, Olayinka O, Dogunro AS. Erectile dysfunction: prevalence and relationship to depression, alcohol abuse and panic disorder. Gen Hosp Psychiatry 2003;25:209–13.
11. Chew KK, Bremner A, Stuckey B, et al. Alcohol consumption and male erectile dysfunction: an unfounded reputation for risk? J Sex Med 2009;6: 1386–94.
12. Peugh J, Belenko S. Alcohol, drugs and sexual function: a review. J Psychoactive Drugs 2001;33(3):223–32.
13. Cao S, Yin X, Wang Y, et al. Smoking and risk of erectile dysfunction: systematic review of observational studies with meta-analysis. PLoS One 2013;8(4): e60443.
14. Hart TA, Moskowitz D, Cox C, et al. The cumulative effects of medication use, drug use, and smoking on erectile dysfunction among men who have sex with men. J Sex Med 2012;9(4):1106–13.
15. Park MG, Ko KW, Oh MM, et al. Effects of smoking on plasma testosterone level and erectile function in rats. J Sex Med 2012;9:472–81.

16. Harte CB, Meston CM. Association between smoking cessation and sexual health in men. BJU Int 2012;109:888–96.
17. Wu C, Zhang H, Gao Y, et al. The association of smoking and erectile dysfunction: results from the Fangchenggang Area Male Health and Examination Survey (FAMHES). J Androl 2012;33:59–65.
18. Wolf R, Schulman A. Erectile dysfunction and fertility related to cigarette smoking. J Eur Acad Dermatol Venereol 1996;6:209–16.
19. Society of Obstetricians and Gynaecologists of Canada. SOGC clinical practice guidelines. The detection and management of vaginal atrophy. Int J Gynaecol Obstet 2005;88:222–8.
20. Halmenschlager G, Rossetto S, Lara GM, et al. Evaluation of the effects of cigarette smoking on testosterone levels in adult men. J Sex Med 2009;6:1763–72.
21. Trummer H, Habermann H, Haas J, et al. The impact of cigarette smoking on human semen parameters and hormones. Hum Reprod 2002;17:1554–9.
22. Gades NM, Nehra A, Jacobson DJ, et al. Association between smoking and erectile dysfunction: a population-based study. Am J Epidemiol 2005;161(4):346–51.
23. He J, Reynolds K, Chen J, et al. Cigarette smoking and erectile dysfunction among Chinese men without clinical vascular disease. Am J Epidemiol 2007;166:803–9.
24. Glina S, Sharlip ID, Hellstrom WJ. Modifying risk factors to prevent and treat erectile dysfunction. J Sex Med 2013;10:115–9.
25. Chan SS, Leung DY, Abdullah AS, et al. Smoking-cessation and adherence intervention among Chinese patients with erectile dysfunction. Am J Prev Med 2010;39:251–8.
26. UNODC. World drug report. Vienna, Austria: United Nations Publication; 2010. p. 198.
27. United Nations Office on Drugs and Crime. Cannabis: why we should care. vol 1; Analysis. United Nations; 2006. p. 155–206.
28. Gratzke C, Christ GJ, Stief CG, et al. Localization and function of cannabinoid receptors in the corpus cavernosum: basis for modulation of nitric oxide synthase nerve activity. Eur Urol 2010;57:342–8.
29. Melis MR, Succu S, Mascia MS, et al. The cannabinoid receptor antagonist SR-141716A induces penile erection in male rats: involvement of paraventricular glutamic acid and nitric oxide. Neuropharmacology 2006;50:219–28.
30. Ghasemi M, Sadeghipour H, Mani AR, et al. Effect of anandamide on nonadrenergic noncholinergic mediated relaxation of rat corpus cavernosum. Eur J Pharmacol 2006;544:138–45.
31. Argiolas A, Melis MR. Central control of penile erection: role of the paraventricular nucleus of the hypothalamus. Prog Neurobiol 2005;76:1–21.
32. Melis MR, Succu S, Mascia MS, et al. Antagonism of cannabinoid CB1 receptors in the paraventricular nucleus of male rats induces penile erection. Neurosci Lett 2004;359:17–20.
33. Munro S, Thomas KL, Abu-Shaar M. Molecular characterization of a peripheral receptor for cannabinoids. Nature 1993;365:61–5.
34. Palha AP, Esteves M. A study of the sexuality of opiate addicts. J Sex Marital Ther 2002;28(5):427–37.
35. Roberts LJ, Finch PM, Pullan PT, et al. Sex hormone suppression by intrathecal opioids: a prospective study. Clin J Pain 2002;18:144–8.
36. Warner EA. Cocaine abuse. Ann Intern Med 1993;119(3):226–35.

37. Weatherby NL, Shultz JM, Chitwood DD, et al. Crack cocaine use and sexual activity in Miami, Florida. J Psychoactive Drugs 1992;24:373–80.
38. Rawson RA, Washton A, Domier CP, et al. Drugs and sexual effects: role of drug type and gender. J Subst Abuse Treat 2002;22:103–8.
39. Cocores JA, Miller NS, Pottash AC, et al. Sexual dysfunction in abusers of cocaine and alcohol. Am J Drug Alcohol Abuse 1988;14:169–73.
40. Henderson DJ, Boyd CJ, Whitmarsh J. Women and illicit drugs: sexuality and crack cocaine. Health Care Women Int 1995;16:113–24.
41. Mireku-Boateng AO, Tasie B. Priapism associated with intracavernosal injection of cocaine. Urol Int 2001;67:109–10.
42. Maxwell JC. Emerging research on methamphetamine. Curr Opin Psychiatry 2005;18:235–42.
43. Jansen KL, Theron L. Ecstasy (MDMA), methamphetamine, and date rape (drug-facilitated sexual assault): a consideration of the issues. J Psychoactive Drugs 2006;38:1–12.
44. Bang-Ping J. Sexual dysfunction in men who abuse illicit drugs: a preliminary report. J Sex Med 2009;6:1072–80.
45. Käll KI. Effects of amphetamine on sexual behavior of male i.v. drug users in Stockholm–a pilot study. AIDS Educ Prev 1992;4:6–17.
46. Gonzales R, Mooney L, Rawson RA. The methamphetamine problem in the United States. Annu Rev Public Health 2010;31:385–98.
47. Fisher DG, Reynolds GL, Napper LE. Use of crystal methamphetamine, Viagra, and sexual behavior. Curr Opin Infect Dis 2010;23:53–6.
48. Russell K, Dryden DM, Liang Y, et al. Risk factors for methamphetamine use in youth: a systematic review. BMC Pediatr 2008;8:48.
49. Winslow BT, Voorhees KI, Pehl KA. Methamphetamine abuse. Am Fam Physician 2007;76:1169–74.
50. Hirshfield S, Remien RH, Walavalkar I, et al. Crystal methamphetamine use predicts incident STD infection among men who have sex with men recruited online: a nested case-control study. J Med Internet Res 2004;6:e41.
51. Forrest DW, Metsch LR, LaLota M, et al. Crystal methamphetamine use and sexual risk behaviors among HIV-positive and HIV-negative men who have sex with men in South Florida. J Urban Health 2010;87:480–5.
52. Semple SJ, Zians J, Grant I, et al. Sexual risk behavior of HIV-positive methamphetamine-using men who have sex with men: the role of partner serostatus and partner type. Arch Sex Behav 2006;35:461–71.
53. Mckay A. Sexuality and substance use: the impact of tobacco, alcohol, and selected recreational drugs on sexual function. Can J Hum Sex 2005;14:47–56.
54. Angst J. Sexual problems in healthy and depressed persons. Int Clin Psychopharmacol 1998;13(Suppl 6):S1–4.
55. Cyranowski JM, Bromberger J, Youk A, et al. Lifetime depression history and sexual function in women at midlife. Arch Sex Behav 2004;33:539–48.
56. Kennedy S, Fulton K, Bagby R, et al. Sexual function during bupropion or paroxetine treatment. Can J Psychiatry 2006;51:45–52.
57. Baldwin D. Depression and sexual dysfunction. Br Med Bull 2001;57:81–99.
58. Shamloul R, Ghanem H. Erectile dysfunction. Lancet 2013;381:153–65.

Effects of Alcohol on the Endocrine System

Nadia Rachdaoui, PhD, Dipak K. Sarkar, PhD, DPhil*

KEYWORDS

- Alcoholism • Endocrine disorders
- Circadian dysfunction • Immune abnormalities

KEY POINTS

- Chronic consumption of a large amount of alcohol disrupts the communication between nervous, endocrine, and immune system and causes hormonal disturbances that lead to profound and serious consequences at physiologic and behavioral levels.
- These alcohol-induced hormonal dysregulations affect the entire body and can result in various disorders such as stress abnormalities, reproductive deficits, body growth defect, thyroid problems, immune dysfunction, cancers, bone disease, and psychological and behavioral disorders.

INTRODUCTION

Alcohol consumption is one of the most serious substance abuse disorders worldwide. Alcohol-related deaths, diseases, and disabilities are higher in men than women and are highest in developed countries, where they range from 8% to 18% for men and 2% to 4% for women. According to the National Institute of Alcohol Abuse and Alcoholism, each year, approximately 80,000 people die from alcohol-related causes, making it the third leading cause of death in the United States. Approximately 14 million of Americans (7.4%) have an alcohol use disorder that is classified as either alcoholism (alcohol dependency) or alcohol abuse.[1] There is considerable evidence, from human genome-wide association studies of individuals with family history of alcoholism and twin studies that several susceptibility genes are linked to the vulnerability and risk of developing alcohol-related disorders. Heritability of alcohol abuse, from twin studies, was estimated to range from 50% to 60%.[2,3] However, alcoholism

Funding: Supported by NIAAA grants 5R37 AA08757, AA11591, U24 AA014811.

Conflict of Interest: We have nothing to disclose.

Rutgers Endocrine Research Program, Department of Animal Sciences, Rutgers University, 67 Poultry Farm Lane, New Brunswick, NJ 08901, USA

* Corresponding author.

E-mail address: sarkar@aesop.rutgers.edu

Endocrinol Metab Clin N Am 42 (2013) 593–615

is a multifactorial and polygenic disorder, in which complex gene-to-gene and gene-to-environment interactions occur, resulting in a variety of addiction phenotypes. Environmental factors play an equally important role in the development of alcohol-related disorders (ie, stressful life events have been shown to influence alcohol-drinking and relapse behaviors) (**Table 1**).[4]

Excessive alcohol drinking has been recognized as having several adverse health consequences. Heavy alcohol drinking increases the risk of cardiovascular and liver disease, metabolic disturbances, nutritional deficiencies, cancers (ie, mouth, stomach, colon, liver, and breast cancer), neurobiological disorders, and fetal abnormalities.[5] In contrast to heavy alcohol use, light to moderate drinking, especially of alcoholic beverages rich in polyphenols such as red wine, was reported to lower the risk of coronary heart disease,[6] stroke,[7] and osteoporosis.[8] In this article, some of the literature is discussed surrounding studies in humans and animal models regarding the effects of both acute and chronic alcohol consumption on one of the body's most important systems, the endocrine system.

THE ENDOCRINE SYSTEM

Along with the nervous system, the endocrine system ensures a proper communication between various organs of the body to maintain a constant internal environment, also called homeostasis. The nervous system allows rapid transmission of information between different body regions, whereas the endocrine system, which is a complex system of glands that produce and secrete hormones directly into the blood circulation, have longer-lasting actions. Almost every organ and cell in the body is affected by the endocrine system. The endocrine system controls metabolism and energy levels, electrolyte balance, growth and development, and reproduction. The endocrine

Table 1
Summary of hormonal changes induced by acute and chronic alcohol exposure

Endocrine Gland	Hormone	Acute Alcohol		Chronic Alcohol	
		Male	Female	Male	Female
Hypothalamus	CRH	↑	↑	↔	↔
	LHRH	↑	↑	↔	↔
	TRH	↔	↔	↓	↓
	GHRH	↓	↓	↓	↓
	Somatostatin	↔	↔	↔	↔
Anterior pituitary gland	ACTH	↑	↑	↓	↓
	LH	↑	↑	↔	↓ ↔
	FSH	↑	↑	↓	↑
	TSH	↔	↔	↔ ↓	↔ ↑
	GH	↓	↓	↓	↓
	Prolactin			↑	↑
Adrenal cortex	Cortisol	↑	↑	↑	↑
Testes	Testosterone	↓	↔	↓	↑
Ovaries	Estrogen	↑	↑	↑	↑
	Progesterone		↓		↓
Thyroid gland	T4	↔	↔	↓	↓
	T3	↔	↔	↓	↓
Pancreas	Insulin	↓ ↔	↓ ↔	↓	↓

↑ increased hormone release; ↓ decreased hormone release; ↔ unchanged hormone release.

system also plays an essential role in enabling the body to respond and appropriately cope with changes in the internal or external environments, such as changes in the body's temperature or in the electrolyte composition of the body's fluids as well as responding to stress and injury. Substance abuse, such as chronic alcohol consumption, was shown to have serious adverse effects on the different components of the endocrine system.[9] The effects of alcohol induce hormonal disturbances that lead to profound and serious consequences at physiologic and behavioral levels. These alcohol-induced hormonal dysregulations affect the entire body and can result in various disorders such as cardiovascular diseases, reproductive deficits, immune dysfunction, certain cancers, bone disease, and psychological and behavioral disorders.

The goal in this review is to discuss the effects of both acute and chronic alcohol exposures on the different components of the endocrine system. The findings from human and animal studies are summarized, which provide consistent evidence on the various effects of alcohol abuse on the endocrine system and on how the latter might have a role in the initiation, the development, and the maintenance of alcohol-drinking disorders and relapse. The impact of alcohol on the primary hormonal center of the endocrine system, the hypothalamic-pituitary axis, is first discussed, and how its different components, the adrenal axis (hypothalamic-pituitary-adrenal [HPA] axis), the gonadal axis (hypothalamic-pituitary-gonadal [HPG] axis) and the thyroid axis (hypothalamic-pituitary-thyroid [HPT] axis) are affected by alcohol consumption is reviewed. The role that the HPA axis plays in alcohol-seeking behavior and dependence is also reviewed, and the effects of alcohol consumption on the activity of the HPA axis are discussed. Second, the recent literature on the effects of alcohol on body growth, circadian mechanism and the pancreas is reviewed. Because it is well documented that there is an overlap between the endocrine and the immune systems, how dysregulation in the hypothalamic-pituitary axis can negatively affect the body's immune response is discussed.

Alcohol and the HPA Axis

The HPA axis, also called the stress axis, is a major component of the neuroendocrine system, which controls the body's response to environmental stressors (psychological, physical, or infectious) and regulates many of the body's physiologic processes such as metabolism, reproduction, growth, mood and emotions, and the immune function. In response to any type of stress, release of corticotropin-releasing hormone (CRH) and increased peripheral glucocorticoid levels initiate a cascade of biological responses that help counteract the altered homeostatic state. Parvocellular neurons in the paraventricular nucleus (PVN) of the hypothalamus synthesize and secrete CRH into the hypothalamic-pituitary portal network that connects the hypothalamus and the anterior pituitary. At the anterior pituitary, CRH stimulates the synthesis and secretion of a pro-opiomelanocortin (POMC)-derived peptide called adrenocorticotropic hormone (ACTH) from corticotropic cells. ACTH is then transported through the blood circulation to the adrenal glands, where it acts on the zona fasciculata cells in the adrenal cortex to stimulate the production of glucocorticoids, mainly cortisol in humans and corticosterone in rodents. Glucocorticoids then, through a negative feedback loop, act on the hypothalamus, hippocampus, and the pituitary to decrease CRH and ACTH production. This decrease is regulated by a feedback system via glucocorticoid receptors (GR) in the PVN, and mineralocorticoid receptors (MR) and GR in the hippocampus. GR inhibit HPA activity, because at basal levels of cortisol, the MR are occupied, whereas GR are mostly unoccupied. However, when there are increased levels of plasma cortisol, like during a period of stress, there is an increased occupation of GR. It is the increased occupation of GR that triggers the negative feedback. The glucocorticoids released by the adrenal cortex interact with the GR in the pituitary, hypothalamus, and hippocampus; so any overactivity results in feedback, causing a reduction in circulating CRH, thereby switching off the stress response. In addition to their main function in restoring homeostasis after exposure to stress, glucocorticoids influence carbohydrate, lipid and nucleic acid metabolism, bone and calcium metabolism, growth and development and also have immunosuppressive and antiinflammatory effects.[10] Perturbations of the HPA axis may, therefore, have serious long-term health consequences.

The other main physiologic aspect of the stress response is the autonomic nervous system (ANS). The ANS has the capacity to trigger 2 opposing responses: the fight or flight of the sympathetic nervous system or the tend and mend of the parasympathetic nervous system. The release of ACTH from the pituitary signals induces not only the synthesis of glucocorticoids but also the release of catecholamines from the adrenal glands. Catecholamines such as epinephrine and norepinephrine trigger the activation of the sympathetic nervous system (SNS), which results in the familiar feeling of decreased saliva, increased perspiration, and heart rate. The SNS is the first line of defense against the stressor, traditionally allowing escape from the immediate threat. However, such a response cannot be physiologically maintained for long periods.

As part of the SNS response to stress, the opioid peptide β-endorphin (BEP) is synthesized by POMC and is implicated in the behavioral as well as the biological response associated with stress stimuli. The most well-studied effect of BEP is its ability to modulate pain, but the peptide has also been implicated in the central regulation of ACTH and hypothalamic CRH. BEP has been shown to play a critical role in bringing the stress response to a state of homoeostasis. In response to stress, the secretion of CRH and catecholamines stimulates the synthesis of BEP and other POMC-derived peptides from the hypothalamus, which in turn inhibit the activity of the HPA axis. Central BEP binds to δ and μ opioid receptors and modulates the ANS via neurons within the PVN. BEP produced from pituitary POMC that circulates in the periphery is primarily regulated by CRH and arginine vasopressin and has less impact on ANS function.[11]

Considerable evidence, from human and animal studies, has shown that alcohol administration affects the HPA axis activity. An acute exposure to alcohol activates the HPA stress axis, leading to a dose-related increase in circulating ACTH and glucocorticoid levels. In rats, an acute administration of ethanol increases plasma ACTH and corticosterone levels, with females showing a higher response then males.[12] These ethanol effects are primarily mediated through an enhanced release of CRH from the hypothalamus. Neutralization of circulating CRH with antibodies interrupts the stimulatory effects of ethanol on ACTH and corticosterone secretion.[13] Lesions of the PVN attenuate, but do not abolish, the stimulatory effects of ethanol on ACTH release, suggesting that extra PVN regions, or other ACTH secretagogues, such as vasopressin, mediate the ethanol stimulation of ACTH release. Neutralization of endogenous vasopressin, using antibodies, decreased the ethanol-induced ACTH secretion in both sham-operated and PVN-sectioned rats, indicating that vasopressin from outside the PVN partially mediates the pituitary-adrenocortical response to ethanol.[14]

In humans, several studies have also reported the stimulatory effect of alcohol on the HPA axis. In an early study, Jenkins and Connolly[15] showed that plasma cortisol levels significantly increased in healthy individuals at alcohol doses exceeding 100 mg/100 mL. In a recent study by Thayer and colleagues,[16] it was shown that healthy men who self-reported alcohol consumption had higher levels of excreted cortisol in urine. These investigators also reported that in heavy drinkers, the inhibitory control of the HPA axis was impaired. Richardson and colleagues,[17] using an operant self-administration animal model of alcohol dependence, showed that the HPA responses to several weeks of daily 30-minute self-administration of alcohol were higher in low-responding nondependent animals (<0.2 mg/kg/session), intermediate in nondependent animals (~0.4 mg/kg/session), and most blunted in dependent animals (~1.0 mg/kg/session). This and several other studies have all shown that basal ACTH and corticosterone levels are attenuated in response to chronic exposure to alcohol.

A decrease in CRH messenger RNA (mRNA) expression in the PVN[18] and a reduced responsiveness of the pituitary to CRH[19] were also observed. Low CRH levels were associated with more intense craving and increased probability of relapse after acute abstinence, suggesting that the CRH system plays an important role in the control of long-term alcohol drinking and dependence. In CRH knockout mice, ethanol intake was doubled, and the behavioral response to ethanol was diminished.[20] In rhesus macaques, which had a single nucleotide polymorphism in the promoter region of CRH (-248C $\rightarrow$ T), which confers increased stress reactivity, it was shown that release of ACTH and cortisol and suppression of environmental exploration (a behavioral response to social separation stress) were higher in those with the T allele.[21] These animals consumed more alcohol in a limited-access paradigm, suggesting that the CRH promoter variation that conferred increased stress responsivity also increased the risk for alcohol dependence. It has also been shown that in mice lacking a functional CRH1 receptor, repeated stress leads to enhanced and progressively increasing ethanol consumption, which seems to persist throughout their life.[22] This effect was associated with enhanced protein levels of NR2B subunit of the N-methyl-D-aspartate receptor of the glutamatergic system also known to be involved in addiction behavior.[23] As reported by Koob and colleagues,[24] disruptions in the CRH system develop over time and are worsened by prolonged exposure to excessive alcohol drinking. This phenomenon is seen only in rat strains that are prone to self-administer alcohol; in nondependent rats, the CRH system does not significantly modulate ethanol consumption.[25,26]

A role for ACTH and corticosteroids has also been documented in alcohol consumption behavior. Injections of ACTH analogues to rats exposed to free-choice ethanol consumption (10% ethanol) led to a reduction in ethanol consumption.[27] In another study by Fahlke and Eriksson,[28] male rats of alcohol-preferring (AA) and alcohol-avoiding (ANA) strains were adrenalectomized, then given access to 10% (v/v) ethanol or water for 2 weeks. This study showed that adrenalectomy results in decreased ethanol consumption in AA rats compared with sham-operated AA controls and injection with corticosterone restores the ethanol consumption. In contrast, no alterations in ethanol intake after adrenalectomy and after corticosterone injection were observed in the ANA rats. These data suggest that corticosterone stimulates ethanol consumption in animals with a high preference for alcohol.[28] In a subsequent study,[29] the same investigators found that intracerebroventricular infusions of corticosterone restore ethanol intake in adrenalectomized animals to levels similar to sham-operated controls. These data suggest that differences in the activity of the HPA axis may help determine whether certain individuals are at high risk for developing alcohol-related disorders and alcoholism.

A relationship between the endogenous opioid system, the HPA axis and reward has been proposed.[30] BEP neurons in the arcuate nucleus of the hypothalamus both inhibit CRH release in the PVN of the hypothalamus[31] and simultaneously stimulate dopamine release in the nucleus accumbens.[32] Because the opioids are involved in regulating both of these systems, it is proposed that a deficit in opioid neurotransmission may cause a simultaneous derangement of both physiologic processes. In recent years, a body of research has accumulated that provides evidence of deranged HPA axis function in drinking alcoholics[33] in acute withdrawal and more prolonged abstinence,[17] as well as in nondependent individuals with a family history of alcoholism.[34] Also, glucocorticoids, which are released during stress and after ethanol-induced activation of the HPA axis, modulate the activities of the opioidergic, CRH, and mesolimbic dopaminergic systems[35] and have been shown to interact with the rewarding properties of alcohol abuse.[36] It is believed that diminished opioid activity, which is either the result of alcoholism or genetically linked to the risk of alcoholism, could induce hypercortisolemia, alter mesolimbic dopamine production, and lead to abnormal ethanol reinforcement.[32,33]

Alcohol and the HPG Axis

Alcohol abuse and alcoholism are associated with disorders of reproductive function in both men and women. The HPG axis and its hormones are essential for proper functioning of the reproductive system. In alcohol abusers, the HPG dysfunction was shown to be associated with a decrease in libido, infertility, and gonadal atrophy. Several studies have clearly documented that alcohol has deleterious effects on all 3 components of the HPG axis (the hypothalamus, pituitary, and gonads). Some of these studies on the acute and chronic effects of alcohol on male and female reproductive systems are reviewed.

Overview of male and female HPG axis

The hypothalamus in a pulsatile way produces and secretes the hormone called luteinizing hormone-releasing hormone (LHRH), also called gonadotropin-releasing hormone, into the hypothalamic-pituitary portal network.[37] At the anterior pituitary, LHRH binds to specific receptors on gonadotropic cells and stimulates a cascade of events that lead to production and secretion of 2 important gonadotropin hormones (follicle-stimulating hormone [FSH] and luteinizing hormone [LH]) into the general circulation. In the ovary, during the follicular phase of each reproductive cycle (28 days in the human cycle), FSH stimulates the development of a dominant follicle, which, as it matures, produces and secretes increasing amounts of the estrogen called estradiol. Both FSH and LH stimulate estradiol secretion, and this increase in estradiol is responsible for the LH and FSH surge seen in midcycle. LH then stimulates ovulation and the development of the corpus luteum during the luteal phase, which then produces and secretes progesterone, an important hormone in the preparation of the uterine wall for the fertilized egg and for the maintenance of the pregnancy. In the testis, LH stimulates testosterone secretion, whereas FSH controls the initiation and maintenance of spermatogenesis. In addition, testosterone, estrogen, and progesterone control their own production through a feedback loop mechanism and can act on the hypothalamus and the pituitary to either inhibit or stimulate the release of LHRH, LH, and FSH.[38]

Although sex hormones are essential to reproductive processes, they can also act on other organs in the body and trigger numerous physiologic processes. For example, estrogen, progesterone, and testosterone were shown to play an important role in maintaining normal bone mass.[39,40] Estrogen is a vasodilator agent that can induce vascular relaxation[41] and was shown to reduce the risk of atherosclerosis and therefore cardiovascular disease in menopausal women by decreasing circulating low-density lipoproteins and inflammatory processes in the vasculature.[42] Testosterone was also shown to affect muscle mass and adiposity in adult men[43] and to affect emotional and cognitive behavior.[44] Dysregulation of the HPG axis, therefore, can lead not only to reproductive dysfunction but also to other serious health problems such as mood and memory disorders, osteoporosis, and muscle atrophy.

Alcohol and HPG axis in puberty

Normal initiation and progression of puberty is under the control and is mediated by central inputs that stimulate the pulsatile diurnal secretion of LHRH into the hypothalamic-pituitary portal system. LHRH then stimulates the pituitary gonadotropin secretion and subsequent ovarian maturation.[45] This LHRH surge, which is normally inhibited during childhood through hypothalamic inhibitory inputs such as γ aminobutyric acid and opioid peptides is triggered at puberty by stimulatory agents such as insulin like growth factor 1 (IGF1), norepinephrine, leptin, transforming growth factor α, and the kisspeptins.[46–48]

Little research has been carried out on the impact of alcohol consumption during puberty in humans. However, numerous studies documented decrease in estrogen levels in adolescent girls and that this decrease was sustained for prolonged periods after consumption of a moderate amount of alcohol.[49] Alcohol abuse was also shown to induce alterations in puberty-related hormones in adolescent boys, shown by significant reductions in testosterone, LH, and FSH levels.[50] However, in the last decade or so, the use of animal models such as rodents and monkeys has helped in understanding and identifying some of the mechanisms by which alcohol abuse affects puberty-related processes. In early studies on female rats, Bo and colleagues[51] reported that puberty, measured by vaginal opening, was markedly delayed in prepubertal female rats administered alcohol. Naltrexone, which is a blocker of the opioid receptors, completely prevented the alcohol-induced delay in vaginal opening,[52] which suggests that alcohol-induced pubertal delay might in part be caused by an increased opioid restraint on the normal progression of pubertal processes. It was also documented that alcohol decreased hypothalamic secretion of LHRH levels.[53] Moreover, these same investigators reported that alcohol increased hypothalamic growth hormone-releasing hormone (GHRH) content, which was associated with a decrease in circulating growth hormone (GH),[54] suggesting that alcohol decreased GH secretion as a result of decreased GHRH release from the hypothalamus. This alcohol-induced decrease in GH was also associated with a decrease in circulating IGF1, which could explain the growth impairments observed in animals administered alcohol.[55]

In another study on immature female rhesus macaques, it was shown that alcohol consumption (2 g/kg) for 12 months resulted in the suppression of the night-related increase in circulating GH that is expected to occur during late juvenile development. This effect of alcohol was associated with a significant decline in circulating IGF1, LH, and estrogen levels, which were most pronounced at 32 months of age. However, FSH and leptin levels were not altered by alcohol consumption. The investigators[56] also found that alcohol affected the monthly pattern of menstruation, which was reflected by lengthening of the intervals between menses. In a more recent study,[57] the same group of researchers suggested that the alcohol-damaging action on ovaries is partly mediated through an increased ovarian nitric oxide (NO) synthase and suppressed steroidogenic acute regulatory protein 2, important intermediates in steroid hormone production. These studies show that alcohol abuse induces hormonal alterations of HPG axis and GH-IGF1 axis during puberty. HPG activity and GH-IGF1 secretion during this stage of development are closely interconnected. Estrogen can stimulate GH secretion[58] and IGF1 can stimulate LHRH secretion,[59] suggesting that HPG axis activation leads to both sexual maturation and a growth spurt mediated through estrogen-induced stimulation of the GH-IGF axis. Therefore, alcohol-induced disturbances in HPG axis activity, during this critical stage of development, could have far-reaching consequences on reproductive function as well as growth, which might persist through adult life.

Alcohol and the female HPG axis

Alcohol use in premenopausal women, even in moderate amounts, was linked to a multitude of reproductive disorders such as irregular menstrual cycles, anovulation, increased risk of spontaneous abortions, and early menopause. Jensen and colleagues[60] in a study on 430 healthy women aged 20 to 35 years who were trying to conceive for the first time found that alcohol intake, even as few as 5 or fewer drinks per week, was associated with decreased fecundability. In another study on 26 healthy nonalcoholic women who were classified as heavy ($\sim$7.81 drinks/d), social ($\sim$3.84 drinks/d), and occasional ($\sim$1.22 drinks/d) alcohol users, Mendelson and Mello and colleagues[61,62] found that 50% of social drinkers and 60% of heavy drinkers had significant disturbances of reproductive hormones and of menstrual cycle compared with occasional drinkers and the social drinkers who consumed fewer than 3 drinks/d. Social drinkers had anovulatory cycles and heavy drinkers had hyperprolactinemia. It was reported that alcohol intake increases estradiol levels in humans[63] and in rodents.[64] The increased estradiol level may in part explain the negative effect of alcohol on menstrual cycle and on its irregularity. Long-term moderate alcohol consumption was also shown to decrease ovarian reserve, which was associated with increased FSH levels.[65] Faut and colleagues[66] have suggested that an in situ metabolism of ethanol to acetaldehyde increases the susceptibility of rat ovarian tissue to oxidative stress and leads to cell damage and ovarian dysfunction.

In postmenopausal women receiving hormone therapy, acute exposure to alcohol induces a temporary increase in estradiol levels, which might be caused by impaired estradiol metabolism, with decreased conversion of estradiol to estrone. In contrast, alcohol exposure had no effect on estradiol levels in women who were not receiving hormone therapy.[67]

Alcohol and the male HPG axis

There are numerous studies in animals and humans that amply document the deleterious effects of alcohol on male reproductive function. Associations between both acute and chronic alcohol consumption and lower testosterone levels have been clearly shown. Muthusami and Chinnaswamy,[68] in a study on 66 alcoholic and 30 nonalcoholic men, found that chronic alcohol consumption significantly increased FSH, LH, and estrogen levels, whereas testosterone and progesterone were significantly decreased and prolactin (PRL) unchanged. Semen volume, sperm count, motility, and number of morphologically normal sperm were also significantly lower in the alcoholic group. Alcohol abuse results in hypogonadism even in the absence of liver disease. Alcoholic men with cirrhosis have increased circulating estradiol and estrone levels.[69] Ethanol increases aromatase activity, an enzyme that converts androgens to estrogens, especially in the liver.[70] A decrease in IGF1 bioavailability as a result of liver disease, contributes at least in part to the development of hypogonadism associated with cirrhosis[71] because IGF1 is known to stimulate testosterone synthesis and spermatogenesis.[72]

Both acute and chronic exposure of pubertal young male rats to alcohol induced a profound decrease in testosterone concentration, which was associated with lower or normal LH and FSH levels, which is abnormal given that low testosterone in normal conditions signals to the hypothalamus to produce LHRH, which in turn stimulates LH and FSH secretion and therefore stimulation of the testis to produce testosterone.[73] However, in an another study,[74] these investigators found that chronic ethanol feeding in pubertal male rats significantly decreased testosterone but did not produce any changes in circulating FSH and LH levels. These investigators also found that chronic ethanol exposure induced an increase in free radical damage at the pituitary level, resulting in inappropriate serum levels of FSH and LH in response to lower testosterone.[74]

Alcohol metabolism, by generating highly toxic reactive oxygen species (ROS), such as anion superoxide, hydrogen peroxide, and hydroxyl radicals, can induce cell damage in the testes. It was shown that acetaldehyde, a metabolite of alcohol, was more toxic than alcohol and altered testosterone production by inhibiting protein kinase C, a key enzyme in testosterone synthesis.[75,76] NO, also synthesized in the testes, has been suggested as another player in the alcoholic's reduced production of testosterone. Inhibition of nitric oxide synthase, the enzyme responsible for NO synthesis, prevents the decrease in testosterone associated with alcohol drinking.[77]

Alcohol and pituitary PRL

The action of PRL action on the mammary gland and in the maintenance of lactation has long been known and is the source of the name for this hormone. It is one of the most abundant hormones in the pituitary gland and is produced and secreted by lactrope cells. Common manifestations of increase of plasma PRL (hyperprolactinemia) in women include amenorrhea (lack of menstrual cycles) and galactorrhea (excessive secretion of milk). Men with hyperprolactinemia typically show hypogonadism, with decreased sex drive, low sperm production, and impotence. Such men often show breast enlargement (gynecomastia), but rarely produce milk. A pituitary microadenoma or hyperplasia is the cause of hyperprolactinemia in most patients.[78]

There are several reports showing evidence for the existence of hyperprolactinemia in chronic alcoholic men and women. In a study conducted by European scientists,[79] persistent hyperprolactinemia was observed in 16 alcoholic women during a 6-week treatment trial. These patients reported daily alcohol intake of 170 g for a 2-year to 16-year period but had no clinical evidence of alcoholic liver cirrhosis. In a study reported by Japanese scientists, 22 of 23 women admitted for alcoholism treatment had PRL levels higher than normal, ranging between 27 and 184 ng/mL. These women reported drinking an average of 84 g of alcohol each day for at least 7 years. None of these patients showed liver cirrhosis, but 10 had hepatitis and the rest had fatty liver.[80] Studies conducted in a Massachusetts hospital[81] reported hyperprolactinemia (22–87 ng/mL) in 6 of 12 alcohol-dependent women who had a history of drinking 75 to 247 g of alcohol per day for a minimum period of 7 years. Alcohol-induced hyperprolactinemia was also reported in healthy, well-nourished women during residence on a clinical research ward for 35 days.[62] Sixty percent of women in the heavy drinker category (blood alcohol content [BAC]: 109–199 mg/dL) and 50% of moderate drinkers (BAC: 48–87 mg/dL) showed increased PRL levels, and many of these drinkers had increased PRL several days after cessation of drinking. Alcohol-induced hyperprolactinemia was also evident in 66 postmenopausal women.[82] Alcoholic men also showed increased plasma levels of PRL.[83,84] Thus, it seems that chronic alcohol intake in humans promotes hyperprolactinemia.

Alcohol-induced hyperprolactinemia has also been shown in nonhuman primates and laboratory animals. Studies conducted in macaque female monkeys showed that the PRL levels were increased after chronic self-administration of alcohol (3.4 g/kg/d).[85,86] Histologic examination of the pituitary gland of 1 monkey showed apparent pituitary hyperplasia.[86] Using the laboratory rats, it has been shown that ethanol increases plasma PRL levels and pituitary weight in cyclic female rats and ovariectomized rats,[87] and promotes estradiol-induced development of prolactinomas.[88] Therefore, the clinical data as well as animal data suggest that ethanol consumption is a positive risk factor for prolactinomas and hyperprolactinemia.

Alcohol and the HPT Axis

The HPT axis is responsible for the regulation of metabolism in every cell in the body. When circulating levels of thyroid hormones, thyroxin (T4) and triiodothyronine (T3) are low, the hypothalamus responds by releasing thyrotropin-releasing hormone (TRH), which then stimulates thyrotrope cells in the anterior pituitary to produce and secrete thyroid-stimulating hormone (TSH). TSH then stimulates the synthesis and secretion of T4 and T3 from the thyroid gland. T3 is the active form of thyroid hormones, and although T4 and T3 are both secreted after TSH stimulation, 80% of circulating T3 comes from liver conversion of T4 by enzymes called deiodinases. T4, but primarily T3 by negative feedback at the hypothalamus and the pituitary, can control their own release by inhibiting release of TRH and TSH.[89]

Alcoholic individuals often show dysregulations of the HPT axis. A significant reduction in T4 and T3 concentrations was observed in the alcoholic groups during withdrawal and early abstinence, compared with nonalcoholic healthy groups.[90] In addition, a blunted response of TSH to TRH has been consistently reported in alcoholics and during early withdrawal and was positively correlated with severity of withdrawal symptoms.[91] It was also documented that, after longer periods of abstinence, thyroid dysfunction recovers and thyroid hormones and TSH response to TRH return to normal levels.[91] However, in individuals who relapsed and returned to their alcohol-drinking behavior, lower T4 and T3 levels and a blunted TSH response to TRH were again observed.[92]

Similar results were found in studies performed on animal models. For example, chronic alcohol administration to adult male rats in a liquid diet containing 10% (w/v) ethanol for 40 days induced a significant decrease in total T4 and T3 and free T4 and T3 as well as basal TSH levels when compared with control animals fed an isocaloric diet.[93] In addition, chronic ethanol treatment was shown to induce an increase in TRH mRNA content in neurons of the PVN; however, the peripheral stimulation of thyroid hormones by cold exposure was absent in rats,[94] suggesting that chronic exposure to ethanol induces thyroid gland dysfunction, which is no longer able to properly respond to TRH stimulation. Furthermore, downregulation of TRH receptors in the pituitary has been proposed as a mechanism by which chronic alcohol induces the blunted TSH response to TRH.

Other mechanisms for ethanol action on HPT axis have been proposed, which focused on thyroid hormone metabolism and on the activity of enzymes that catalyze the conversion of T4 to T3 (5'-II-deiodinase) and inactivate T3 to 3,3''-T2 (5'II deiodinase). Baumgartner and colleagues[95] in a study in behaviorally dependent and ethanol-exposed but not ethanol-dependent rats, found that the activity of the 5'II deiodinase isoenzyme was increased in the frontal cortex in both groups of rats. However, the activity of the 5'II deiodinase isoenzyme was selectively inhibited in the amygdala of the rats that were behaviorally dependent on ethanol, but was normal in the nondependent rats. These investigators suggested that increases in intracellular concentrations of T3 in the amygdala may be involved in the development of dependence behaviors to alcohol.

Alcohol and GH-IGF1 Axis

In the hypothalamic-pituitary-GH-IGF1 axis, GHRH is secreted from cells in the arcuate and ventromedial nuclei of the hypothalamus into the hypophyseal portal system. GHRH then acts on somatotropic cells in the anterior pituitary, where it stimulates the production and release of GH, which is then released in the general circulation and stimulates IGF1 mainly in the liver. IGF1 through negative feedback at the hypothalamus and pituitary reduces GH synthesis and release. Another hormone called somatostatin, which is secreted in the PVN of the hypothalamus, also acts on the pituitary and inhibits GH secretion. Between GHRH, somatostatin, and IGF1, the amount of GH secreted by the anterior pituitary is tightly regulated. Together GH and IGF1 regulate important physiologic processes in the body, such as postnatal growth and development, carbohydrate, and lipid metabolism.[96] Numerous studies in both humans and experimental animals have shown that acute and chronic alcohol exposure reduces circulating GH and IGF1 levels. Acute exposure of healthy men to ethanol (1.5 g/kg) was shown to reduce the nightly peak of GH secretion.[97] This effect did not seem to be mediated through a direct action of ethanol on the pituitary, rendering it less sensitive to GHRH, because intravenous injection of exogenous GHRH induced an increase in GH secretion in both groups of ethanol-treated (1 g/kg) and control men.[98] However, an acute exposure of healthy women to ethanol had no significant effects on GH secretion.[99] Sonntag and Boyd[100] found that, in rats exposed to 5% ethanol in a liquid diet for 4.5 months, ethanol induced a significant decrease in circulating IGF1 levels. Soszynski and Frohman[101] reported that a 6-day administration of 5% ethanol to chronically cannulated unanesthetized rats resulted in 75% to 90% decrease in spontaneous GH secretion. In addition, IGF1 serum levels and GHRH mRNA levels were significantly decreased with no change in somatostatin or GH mRNA levels after ethanol treatments.[102] These results suggest that chronic ethanol affects GH secretion primarily at the hypothalamic level, where it induces impairments in GHRH gene expression.

Chronic alcohol consumption was shown to induce muscle wasting,[103] and because IGF1 is a potent anabolic agent that regulates muscle protein balance, this next study showed that rats fed ethanol for 8 weeks had significantly lower IGF1 level in plasma, liver and skeletal muscle compared with pair-fed control.[104] The IGF1 mRNA level was also lower in liver and skeletal muscle. However, the concentration of IGF-binding protein 1 (IGFBP-1) was increased in plasma, liver, and muscle; and no changes in glucocorticoids or insulin or GH were reported in these ethanol-fed rats compared with controls.[104] These results suggest that the ethanol mediated-changes in IGF1 and IGFBP-1 concentrations are mediated through mechanisms that are independent of classic hormonal regulators of the IGF system (ie, GH, high glucocorticoid levels, and low insulin-induced hypoglycemia).

Alcohol and Circadian Rhythm

In all organisms, especially in mammals, a time-keeping system called the master circadian pacemaker located in the suprachiasmatic nucleus (SCN) of the anterior hypothalamus synchronizes biological rhythms in response to external cues. The circadian rhythm generated in the SCN, in response to external cues such as daylight, is converted into neuronal or hormonal signals that affect the entire body's physiologic and metabolic processes, thereby optimizing the interaction of the organism with changing environmental conditions. The circadian clockwork involves the interaction of specific clock genes, including Period (Per1, Per2, Per3), Clock, Bmal1, and Cryptochrome (Cry1, Cry2) genes, within 2 tightly interlocked transcriptional and translational feedback loops that sustain a near 24-hour period of cellular activity and regulate the expression of downstream clock-controlled genes. These processes occur not only in the master pacemaker (the SCN) but also in other regions of the brain as well as in the peripheral cells in the entire body.[105,106]

Numerous studies in both human and animal models showed that chronic exposure to alcohol induces alterations in the activity of clock genes, resulting in severe desynchronizations of physiologic clock systems such as sleep, body temperature, blood pressure, and hormonal secretions; and vice versa, clock genes influence alcohol use and abuse behavior.[107] Our own work has shown that chronic exposure of prenatal or postnatal rats to ethanol induces alterations in the circadian expression of POMC and the clock genes rPer1, rPer2 and rPer3 in the arcuate nucleus and rPer1 and rPer2 levels in SCN during the adult period.[108]

The circadian clock and clock gene activity not only controls the sleep/wake and feeding/fasting behavior but it also influences hormone release. The function of different endocrine axes is under tight circadian control, and dysregulations in the activity of clock genes might therefore affect the oscillatory characteristic of hormone secretion. Jimenez and colleagues,[109] in a study on peripubertal male rats, showed that chronic alcohol exposure for 4 weeks not only induced significant changes in hypothalamic-pituitary hormone levels but also affected their 24-hour secretory pattern. Two peaks of FSH during the inactive phase of the daily cycle appeared instead of 1, no LH plasma surge during the first part of the inactive phase, a second peak of testosterone and PRL during the second part of the inactive phase, and a second peak of plasma TSH during the first part of the active phase were observed. In addition, an interaction between circadian clock and responsiveness of the HPA axis to stress has been consistently linked to alcohol abuse and dependence. Stress is regarded as a major environmental risk factor for both heavy drinking[110] and disturbed circadian rhythmicity.[110,111] In a study on 268 young adults (126 men, 142 women) 19 years of age, a positive association between the major A allele of PER2 rs56013859 and alcohol consumption was found in homozygote individuals.[112] Moreover, under conditions of stress, carriers of the G allele drank less than those homozygous for the A allele. These findings suggest a role of a PER2 gene variant in both drinking patterns and stress responsiveness. In another study, Per3 gene was also linked to stress/anxiety traits, and its basal expression correlated with addiction-related phenotypes. Exposure to alcohol increased Per3 expression in the hippocampus, and this was shown to affect stress response.[113] In animal studies, it was shown that Per2 mutant mice had impairments in the glutamate transporter Eaat1, resulting in decreased glutamate uptake by astrocytes and its accumulation in the extracellular milieu; this finding was associated with increased alcohol intake in these Per2 mutant mice.[114] These researchers found that treating these Per2 mutant mice with acamprosate, a drug used in relapse prevention of alcoholism that is believed to attenuate the hyperglutamatergic state, reduced the increased glutamate levels and normalized alcohol intake in these mice. A significant association between a single nucleotide polymorphism variation in the human Per2 gene, PER2 SNP 10870 (A/G substitution), and regulation of alcohol consumption was shown in a clinical sample of severe alcoholics.[114] In addition to this interaction between the stress and circadian rhythm, many data suggest that the disruption in the mechanism of the circadian clocks negatively affects the function of the immune system and promotes susceptibility to cancer.[115,116] Taken together, these studies suggest the important role that clock genes play in the alcohol-mediated dysregulation of the circadian nature of endocrine function as well as in alcohol preference and abuse behaviors.

Alcohol and Pancreatic Function

The pancreas is one of the most important organs of the endocrine system and is involved in the tight control of blood glucose concentration through synthesis and secretion of a peptide hormone called insulin from β cells. Diabetes mellitus (DM) is a syndrome of dysregulated metabolism with high blood glucose levels (hyperglycemia) caused by either an abnormal insulin secretion or signaling in peripheral tissues.

DM is characterized by either a β-cell deficit such as in insulin-dependent type 1 diabetes or reduced peripheral insulin sensitivity, as in type 2 diabetes. Type 2 diabetes is recognized clinically as a complication that often occurs in alcoholics.[117,118] However, it has been shown that the relationship between alcohol consumption and the risk of type 2 diabetes is U shaped.

Low or moderate alcohol consumption shows protective effects against type 2 diabetes in some patients through enhanced peripheral insulin sensitivity.[119] A 30% reduced risk of type 2 diabetes was observed in patients with moderate alcohol consumption, whereas no risk reduction was observed in consumers of amounts of alcohol equal to or more than 48 g/d. Whether moderate alcohol consumption affects insulin secretion is still controversial. Some studies[120] show that moderate alcohol consumption improves insulin action without affecting its secretion, whereas others[121] show a reduced basal insulin secretion rate associated with a lower fasting plasma glucagon concentration. Avogaro and colleagues[120] have also shown that the enhanced insulin sensitivity observed may be in part caused by the inhibitory effect of alcohol on lipolysis. The beneficial metabolic effects of moderate alcohol consumption on insulin sensitivity and glucose tolerance may explain the significant reduction in the development of type 2 diabetes and the risk of cardiovascular disorders reported in several epidemiologic studies.[120,122]

Heavy alcohol consumption, on the other hand, is an independent risk factor for the development of type 2 DM.[123] In addition to its effects on peripheral tissues, such as adipose tissue and liver, where it induces insulin resistance, heavy alcohol consumption was also proposed to negatively affect pancreatic β-cell function. Patto and colleagues,[124] in a study of 16 healthy volunteer nonalcohol consumers and 10 chronic alcohol consumers, found that there was a decrease in insulin response in the chronic alcohol consumers compared with the control group. These investigators measured total integrated response (TIR) values for insulin and c-peptide after oral or intravenous glucose loads in these 2 groups. They found that the insulin and c-peptide TIR values were both significantly lower in the alcoholic group compared with the control group. In addition, in both groups, the insulin TIR values after the oral glucose load were significantly higher than those after the intravenous glucose load, suggesting an enhancing incretin effect on insulin secretion. These investigators concluded that the decreased insulin response observed in alcoholics was caused by a β-cell dysfunction, not to an enteroinsular axis dysfunction, because the decrease was also observed when a glucose load was given intravenously. In another study by Kim and colleagues,[125] it was shown that in mice exposed for 8 to 10 weeks to chronic alcohol, there was a significant increase in the impairment of fasting glucose and an increase in β-cell apoptosis, which were associated with a reduction in insulin secretion. These effects of chronic ethanol seemed to be mediated through a downregulation and inactivation by tyrosine nitration of the enzyme glucokinase, a critical player in glucose metabolism that leads to increased production of adenosine triphosphate and therefore to insulin secretion by β cells. These effects were also associated with a decrease in Glut2 and insulin expression, which exacerbates alcohol action. In an in vitro study on the RINm5F β-cell line,[126] it was suggested that ethanol generates ROS and induces β-cell apoptosis. All of these studies suggest that heavy alcohol consumption has deleterious effects on pancreatic β-cell function and on glucose homeostasis.

Alcohol and Immune System

The neuroendocrine and immune systems are highly interrelated. A bidirectional interaction between both systems has long been recognized; especially the sensitivity of the immune system to stress and its interaction with the HPA axis, which was primarily shown by the immunosuppressive actions of glucocorticoids, especially cortisol, which on binding to its specific receptor (GR) can interfere with signaling pathways of other transcription factors such as nuclear factor κB and AP-1 to repress transcription of many inflammatory molecules. In addition, CRH and ACTH were also shown to have immunopotentiating and proinflammatory properties, whereas, for example, interleukins and cytokines produced by activated macrophages, in an adaptive feedback mechanism, can act on the HPA axis and induce CRH and ACTH secretion. For example, interleukin 2 (IL-2) was shown to stimulate cholinergic neurons and activate neural NOS, which releases NO. After release, NO diffuses into CRH producing neurons and induces CRH secretion, which leads to ACTH release from anterior pituitary and cortisol from adrenal glands. This bidirectional interaction between HPA axis and immune system is essential for survival and for maintenance of the body's homeostasis. However, in alcohol abuse conditions, HPA axis and immune system function is compromised and contributes to a worsened state. Glucocorticoids, at excessive amounts, have serious negative effects; first, through their immunosuppressive action and second, through induced acute and chronic metabolic abnormalities.[127,128]

In recent years, a body of evidence from human as well as animal studies has established a link between long-term alcohol use and alterations of both HPA axis and immune system functions. Alcohol abuse disorders are often associated with chronic systemic inflammation and high circulating proinflammatory cytokine levels as well as high circulating cortisol levels. Two mechanisms through which alcohol induces inflammation have been proposed; first, the gut microflora-derived lipopolysaccharides (LPS) were suggested as key players in alcohol-mediated inflammation,[129] and second, alcohol metabolism through production of ROS and cell damage triggers the production of proinflammatory cytokines such as tumor necrosis factor α (TNF-α) and IL-6.[130] An alcohol-induced systemic inflammation that persists, in the case of alcohol abuse, has far-reaching damaging actions on every organ of the body. In the brain, alcohol has neurotoxic effects that result in neuronal death and neurodegeneration.[131,132] Alcoholics have been shown to have reduced brain mass, cortical neuronal loss, and impaired cognitive functions.[133,134] Studies from our laboratory as well as from others have clearly shown that ethanol exposure during the developmental period induces neurotoxicity and permanent impairments in the stress axis as well as the immune function.[131,135,136] Microglial cells, the macrophage cells in the brain, were shown to play an important role in these neurotoxic effects of alcohol on neuronal cells.[137–139]

Acute or chronic alcohol exposures have both been shown to induce immunosuppression through dysregulation in all branches of the immune system. Alcohol exposure reduces neutrophil (macrophage) infiltration and migration to sites of infection as well as production of new neutrophils in response to infection and their phagocytic activity.[140,141] Chronic alcohol exposure also decreases monocyte phagocytic activity, even though the number of these cells is increased.[142] Furthermore, chronic alcohol exposure decreases the number and activity of dendritic and natural killer cells.[143–145] The effect of alcohol on cytokine production depends on the length of exposure. For example, acute exposure to ethanol is associated with suppression of cytokine production (ie, TNF-α and IL-1β).[146] However, chronic exposure to alcohol induces an increase in proinflammatory cytokine production such as that of TNF-α.[147,148] In addition, alcohol exposure suppresses chemokine production, such as that of macrophage inflammatory protein 2 and interferon γ, which were shown to be suppressed after acute exposure to ethanol.[149,150] All these studies clearly suggest that ethanol disruption of cytokines and inflammation contributes in a multitude of ways to a diversity of alcoholic disorders. These alcohol-induced suppressive effects on the immune function were shown to be primarily caused by a blunted response of the HPA axis to external stressors such as infections. In this context, stress axis dysfunction is positively connected with not only immune incompetence but also promotion of various cancers.[11,151] More studies are needed to further understand and identify the mechanisms that underlie the bidirectional interactions between the immune and endocrine system in the case of alcohol-related disorders, which will help in the management and treatment of these disorders.

REFERENCES

1. Grant BF, Dawson DA, Stinson FS, et al. The 12-month prevalence and trends in DSM-IV alcohol abuse and dependence: United States, 1991-1992 and 2001-2002. Drug Alcohol Depend 2004;74:223–34.
2. Dick DM, Bierut LJ. The genetics of alcohol dependence. Curr Psychiatry Rep 2006;8:151–7.
3. Ducci F, Goldman D. Genetic approaches to addiction: genes and alcohol. Addiction 2008;103:1414–28.
4. Corbin WR, Farmer NM, Nolen-Hoekesma S. Relations among stress, coping strategies, coping motives, alcohol consumption and related problems: a mediated moderation model. Addict Behav 2013;38:1912–9.
5. Edwards G, Anderson P, Babor TF, et al. Alcohol policy and the public good: a good public debate. Addiction 1996;91:477–81.
6. Rehm JT, Bondy SJ, Sempos CT, et al. Alcohol consumption and coronary heart disease morbidity and mortality. Am J Epidemiol 1997;146:495–501.
7. Berger K, Ajani UA, Kase CS, et al. Light-to-moderate alcohol consumption and risk of stroke among U.S. male physicians. N Engl J Med 1999;341: 1557–64.
8. Calabrese G. Nonalcoholic compounds of wine: the phytoestrogen resveratrol and moderate red wine consumption during menopause. Drugs Exp Clin Res 1999;25:111–4.
9. Emanuele N, Emanuele MA. The endocrine system: alcohol alters critical hormonal balance. Alcohol Health Res World 1997;21:53–64.
10. Kusnecov A, Anisman H, editors. The Wiley-Blackwell handbook of psychoneuroimmunology. Oxford (United Kingdom): Wiley-Blackwell; 2013.
11. Wynne O, Sarker DK. Stress and neuroendocrine-immune interaction: a therapeutic role for â-endorphin. In: Kusnecov A, Anisman H, editors. The Wiley-Blackwell handbook of psychoneuroimmunology. Oxford (United Kingdom): Wiley-Blackwell; 2013.
12. Rivier C, Lee S. Acute alcohol administration stimulates the activity of hypothalamic neurons that express corticotropin-releasing factor and vasopressin. Brain Res 1996;726:1–10.
13. Rivier C, Bruhn T, Vale W. Effect of ethanol on the hypothalamic-pituitary-adrenal axis in the rat: role of corticotropin-releasing factor (CRF). J Pharmacol Exp Ther 1984;229:127–31.
14. Ogilvie KM, Lee S, Rivier C. Role of arginine vasopressin and corticotropin-releasing factor in mediating alcohol-induced adrenocorticotropin and vasopressin secretion in male rats bearing lesions of the paraventricular nuclei. Brain Res 1997;744:83–95.
15. Jenkins JS, Connolly J. Adrenocortical response to ethanol in man. Br Med J 1968;2:804–5.

16. Thayer JF, Hall M, Sollers JJ III, et al. Alcohol use, urinary cortisol, and heart rate variability in apparently healthy men: evidence for impaired inhibitory control of the HPA axis in heavy drinkers. Int J Psychophysiol 2006;59: 244–50.

17. Richardson HN, Lee SY, O'Dell LE, et al. Alcohol self-administration acutely stimulates the hypothalamic-pituitary-adrenal axis, but alcohol dependence leads to a dampened neuroendocrine state. Eur J Neurosci 2008;28:1641–53.

18. Rasmussen DD, Boldt BM, Bryant CA, et al. Chronic daily ethanol and withdrawal: 1. Long-term changes in the hypothalamo-pituitary-adrenal axis. Alcohol Clin Exp Res 2000;24:1836–49.

19. Sarnyai Z, Shaham Y, Heinrichs SC. The role of corticotropin-releasing factor in drug addiction. Pharmacol Rev 2001;53:209–43.

20. Olive MF, Mehmert KK, Koenig HN, et al. A role for corticotropin releasing factor (CRF) in ethanol consumption, sensitivity, and reward as revealed by CRF-deficient mice. Psychopharmacology (Berl) 2003;165:181–7.

21. Barr CS, Dvoskin RL, Gupte M, et al. Functional CRH variation increases stress-induced alcohol consumption in primates. Proc Natl Acad Sci U S A 2009;106: 14593–8.

22. Sillaber I, Rammes G, Zimmermann S, et al. Enhanced and delayed stress-induced alcohol drinking in mice lacking functional CRH1 receptors. Science 2002;296:931–3.

23. Holter SM, Danysz W, Spanagel R. Novel uncompetitive N-methyl-D-aspartate (NMDA)-receptor antagonist MRZ 2/579 suppresses ethanol intake in long-term ethanol-experienced rats and generalizes to ethanol cue in drug discrimination procedure. J Pharmacol Exp Ther 2000;292:545–52.

24. Koob GF. Brain stress systems in the amygdala and addiction. Brain Res 2009; 1293:61–75.

25. Koob GF, Le Moal M. Drug abuse: hedonic homeostatic dysregulation. Science 1997;278:52–8.

26. Roberts AJ, Heyser CJ, Cole M, et al. Excessive ethanol drinking following a history of dependence: animal model of allostasis. Neuropsychopharmacology 2000;22:581–94.

27. Krishnan S, Maickel RP. The effect of Hoe-427 (an ACTH4-9 analog) on free-choice ethanol consumption in male and female rats. Life Sci 1991;49: 2005–11.

28. Fahlke C, Eriksson CJ. Effect of adrenalectomy and exposure to corticosterone on alcohol intake in alcohol-preferring and alcohol-avoiding rat lines. Alcohol Alcohol 2000;35:139–44.

29. Fahlke C, Hansen S. Effect of local intracerebral corticosterone implants on alcohol intake in the rat. Alcohol Alcohol 1999;34:851–61.

30. Oswald LM, Wand GS. Opioids and alcoholism. Physiol Behav 2004;81:339–58.

31. Calogero AE. Neurotransmitter regulation of the hypothalamic corticotropin-releasing hormone neuron. Ann N Y Acad Sci 1995;771:31–40.

32. Gianoulakis C. Influence of the endogenous opioid system on high alcohol consumption and genetic predisposition to alcoholism. J Psychiatry Neurosci 2001; 26:304–18.

33. Wand GS, Mangold D, Ali M, et al. Adrenocortical responses and family history of alcoholism. Alcohol Clin Exp Res 1999;23:1185–90.

34. Schuckit MA. Subjective responses to alcohol in sons of alcoholics and control subjects. Arch Gen Psychiatry 1984;41:879–84.

35. Cintra A, Zoli M, Rosen L, et al. Mapping and computer assisted morphometry and microdensitometry of glucocorticoid receptor immunoreactive neurons and glial cells in the rat central nervous system. Neuroscience 1994;62:843–97.

36. Fahlke C, Hard E, Thomasson R, et al. Metyrapone-induced suppression of corticosterone synthesis reduces ethanol consumption in high-preferring rats. Pharmacol Biochem Behav 1994;48:977–81.

37. Sarkar DK, Chiappa SA, Fink G, et al. Gonadotropin-releasing hormone surge in pro-oestrous rats. Nature 1976;264:461–3.

38. Prendergast K, Heras-Herzig A, Dalkin A. GNRH-gonadotrophins physiology and pathology. 2008. Available at: Endotext.com.

39. Imai Y, Youn MY, Kondoh S, et al. Estrogens maintain bone mass by regulating expression of genes controlling function and life span in mature osteoclasts. Ann N Y Acad Sci 2009;1173(Suppl 1):E31–9.

40. Seifert-Klauss V, Schmidmayr M, Hobmaier E, et al. Progesterone and bone: a closer link than previously realized. Climacteric 2012;15(Suppl 1):26–31.

41. Oury F. A crosstalk between bone and gonads. Ann N Y Acad Sci 2012;1260: 1–7.

42. Patrelli TS, Gizzo S, Franchi L, et al. A prospective, case-control study on the lipid profile and the cardiovascular risk of menopausal women on oestrogen plus progestogen therapy in a northern Italy province. Arch Gynecol Obstet 2013. [Epub ahead of print].

43. Seftel A. Male hypogonadism. Part II: etiology, pathophysiology, and diagnosis. Int J Impot Res 2006;18:223–8.

44. Ackermann S, Spalek K, Rasch B, et al. Testosterone levels in healthy men are related to amygdala reactivity and memory performance. Psychoneuroendocrinology 2012;37:1417–24.

45. Sarkar DK, Fink G. Mechanism of the first spontaneous gonadotrophin surge and that induced by pregnant mare serum and effects of neonatal androgen in rats. J Endocrinol 1979;83:339–54.

46. Ojeda SR, Prevot V, Heger S, et al. The neurobiology of female puberty. Horm Res 2003;60(Suppl 3):15–20.

47. Ojeda SR, Lomniczi A, Sandau U, et al. New concepts on the control of the onset of puberty. Endocr Dev 2010;17:44–51.

48. Terasawa E, Fernandez DL. Neurobiological mechanisms of the onset of puberty in primates. Endocr Rev 2001;22:111–51.

49. Block GD, Yamamoto ME, Mallick A, et al. Effects on pubertal hormones by ethanol abuse in adolescents. Alcohol Clin Exp Res 1993;17:505.

50. Diamond F Jr, Ringenberg L, MacDonald D, et al. Effects of drug and alcohol abuse upon pituitary-testicular function in adolescent males. J Adolesc Health Care 1986;7:28–33.

51. Bo WJ, Krueger WA, Rudeen PK, et al. Ethanol-induced alterations in the morphology and function of the rat ovary. Anat Rec 1982;202:255–60.

52. Emanuele N, Ren J, Lapaglia N, et al. EtOH disrupts female mammalian puberty: age and opiate dependence. Endocrine 2002;18:247–54.

53. Hiney JK, Dees WL. Ethanol inhibits luteinizing hormone-releasing hormone release from the median eminence of prepubertal female rats in vitro: investigation of its actions on norepinephrine and prostaglandin-E2. Endocrinology 1991; 128:1404–8.

54. Dees WL, Skelley CW. Effects of ethanol during the onset of female puberty. Neuroendocrinology 1990;51:64–9.

55. Dees WL, Srivastava V, Hiney JK. Actions and interactions of alcohol and insulin-like growth factor-1 on female pubertal development. Alcohol Clin Exp Res 2009;33:1847–56.
56. Dees WL, Dissen GA, Hiney JK, et al. Alcohol ingestion inhibits the increased secretion of puberty-related hormones in the developing female rhesus monkey. Endocrinology 2000;141:1325–31.
57. Srivastava VK, Dissen GA, Ojeda SR, et al. Effects of alcohol on intraovarian nitric oxide synthase and steroidogenic acute regulatory protein in the prepubertal female rhesus monkey. J Stud Alcohol Drugs 2007;68:182–91.
58. Mauras N, Rogol AD, Haymond MW, et al. Sex steroids, growth hormone, insulin-like growth factor-1: neuroendocrine and metabolic regulation in puberty. Horm Res 1996;45:74–80.
59. Hiney JK, Srivastava V, Lara T, et al. Ethanol blocks the central action of IGF-1 to induce luteinizing hormone secretion in the prepubertal female rat. Life Sci 1998;62:301–8.
60. Jensen TK, Hjollund NH, Henriksen TB, et al. Does moderate alcohol consumption affect fertility? Follow up study among couples planning first pregnancy. BMJ 1998;317:505–10.
61. Mendelson JH, Lukas SE, Mello NK, et al. Acute alcohol effects on plasma estradiol levels in women. Psychopharmacology (Berl) 1988;94:464–7.
62. Mendelson JH, Mello NK. Chronic alcohol effects on anterior pituitary and ovarian hormones in healthy women. J Pharmacol Exp Ther 1988;245:407–12.
63. Muti P, Trevisan M, Micheli A, et al. Alcohol consumption and total estradiol in premenopausal women. Cancer Epidemiol Biomarkers Prev 1998;7:189–93.
64. Emanuele NV, Lapaglia N, Steiner J, et al. Effect of chronic ethanol exposure on female rat reproductive cyclicity and hormone secretion. Alcohol Clin Exp Res 2001;25:1025–9.
65. Li N, Fu S, Zhu F, et al. Alcohol intake induces diminished ovarian reserve in childbearing age women. J Obstet Gynaecol Res 2013;39:516–21.
66. Faut M, Rodríguez de Castro C, Bietto FM, et al. Metabolism of ethanol to acetaldehyde and increased susceptibility to oxidative stress could play a role in the ovarian tissue cell injury promoted by alcohol drinking. Toxicol Ind Health 2009;25:525–38.
67. Longnecker MP, Tseng M. Alcohol, hormones, and postmenopausal women. Alcohol Health Res World 1998;22:185–9.
68. Muthusami KR, Chinnaswamy P. Effect of chronic alcoholism on male fertility hormones and semen quality. Fertil Steril 2005;84:919–24.
69. Martinez-Riera A, Santolaria-Fernandez F, Gonzalez RE, et al. Alcoholic hypogonadism: hormonal response to clomiphene. Alcohol 1995;12:581–7.
70. Purohit V. Can alcohol promote aromatization of androgens to estrogens? A review. Alcohol 2000;22:123–7.
71. Castilla-Cortazar I, Quiroga J, Prieto J. Insulin-like growth factor-I, liver function, and hypogonadism in rats with experimentally induced cirrhosis. Hepatology 2000;31:1379.
72. Roser JF. Regulation of testicular function in the stallion: an intricate network of endocrine, paracrine and autocrine systems. Anim Reprod Sci 2008;107:179–96.
73. Ren JC, Zhu Q, Lapaglia N, et al. Ethanol-induced alterations in Rab proteins: possible implications for pituitary dysfunction. Alcohol 2005;35:103–12.
74. Ren JC, Banan A, Keshavarzian A, et al. Exposure to ethanol induces oxidative damage in the pituitary gland. Alcohol 2005;35:91–101.

75. Chiao YB, Van Thiel DH. Biochemical mechanisms that contribute to alcohol-induced hypogonadism in the male. Alcohol Clin Exp Res 1983;7:131–4.

76. Anderson RA Jr, Quigg JM, Oswald C, et al. Demonstration of a functional blood-testis barrier to acetaldehyde. Evidence for lack of acetaldehyde effect on ethanol-induced depression of testosterone in vivo. Biochem Pharmacol 1985;34:685–95.

77. Adams ML, Nock B, Truong R, et al. Nitric oxide control of steroidogenesis: endocrine effects of NG-nitro-L-arginine and comparisons to alcohol. Life Sci 1992;50:L35–40.

78. Sarkar DK. Hyperprolactinemia following chronic alcohol administration. Front Horm Res 2010;38:32–41.

79. Valimaki M, Pelkonen R, Harkonen M, et al. Pituitary-gonadal hormones and adrenal androgens in non-cirrhotic female alcoholics after cessation of alcohol intake. Eur J Clin Invest 1990;20:177–81.

80. Seki M, Yoshida K, Okamura Y. A study on hyperprolactinemia in female patients with alcoholics. Arukoru Kenkyuto Yakubutsu Ison 1991;26:49–59.

81. Teoh SK, Lex BW, Mendelson JH, et al. Hyperprolactinemia and macrocytosis in women with alcohol and polysubstance dependence. J Stud Alcohol 1992;53: 176–82.

82. Gavaler JS. Aging and alcohol: the hormonal status of postmenopausal women. In: Sarkar DK, Barnes C, editors. Reproductive neuroendocrinology of aging and drug abuse. Boca Raton (FL): CRC Press; 1994. p. 365–78.

83. Ida Y, Tsujimaru S, Nakamaura K, et al. Effects of acute and repeated alcohol ingestion on hypothalamic-pituitary-gonadal and hypothalamic-pituitary-adrenal functioning in normal males. Drug Alcohol Depend 1992;31:57–64.

84. Soyka M, Gorig E, Naber D. Serum prolactin increase induced by ethanol–a dose-dependent effect not related to stress. Psychoneuroendocrinology 1991; 16:441–6.

85. Mello NK, Mendelson JH, Bree MP, et al. Alcohol effects on naloxone-stimulated luteinizing hormone, follicle-stimulating hormone and prolactin plasma levels in female rhesus monkeys. J Pharmacol Exp Ther 1988;245:895–904.

86. Mello NK, Bree MP, Mendelson JH, et al. Alcohol self-administration disrupts reproductive function in female macaque monkeys. Science 1983; 221:677–9.

87. De A, Boyadjieva N, Oomizu S, et al. Ethanol induces hyperprolactinemia by increasing prolactin release and lactotrope growth in female rats. Alcohol Clin Exp Res 2002;26:1420–9.

88. De A, Boyadjieva N, Pastorcic M, et al. Potentiation of the mitogenic effect of estrogen on the pituitary-gland by alcohol-consumption. Int J Oncol 1995;7: 643–8.

89. Costa-e-Sousa RH, Hollenberg AN. Minireview: the neural regulation of the hypothalamic-pituitary-thyroid axis. Endocrinology 2012;153:4128–35.

90. Hegedus L, Rasmussen N, Ravn V, et al. Independent effects of liver disease and chronic alcoholism on thyroid function and size: the possibility of a toxic effect of alcohol on the thyroid gland. Metabolism 1988;37:229–33.

91. Pienaar WP, Roberts MC, Emsley RA, et al. The thyrotropin releasing hormone stimulation test in alcoholism. Alcohol Alcohol 1995;30:661–7.

92. Liappas I, Piperi C, Malitas PN, et al. Interrelationship of hepatic function, thyroid activity and mood status in alcohol-dependent individuals. In Vivo 2006;20: 293–300.

93. Mason GA, Stanley DA, Walker CH, et al. Chronic alcohol ingestion decreases pituitary-thyroid axis measures in Fischer-344 rats. Alcohol Clin Exp Res 1988; 12:731–4.

94. Zoeller RT, Fletcher DL, Simonyl A, et al. Chronic ethanol treatment reduces the responsiveness of the hypothalamic-pituitary-thyroid axis to central stimulation. Alcohol Clin Exp Res 1996;20:954–60.

95. Baumgartner A, Eravci M, Pinna G, et al. Thyroid hormone metabolism in the rat brain in an animal model of 'behavioral dependence' on ethanol. Neurosci Lett 1997;227:25–8.

96. Moller N, Jorgensen JO. Effects of growth hormone on glucose, lipid, and protein metabolism in human subjects. Endocr Rev 2009;30:152–77.

97. Valimaki M, Tuominen JA, Huhtaniemi I, et al. The pulsatile secretion of gonadotropins and growth hormone, and the biological activity of luteinizing hormone in men acutely intoxicated with ethanol. Alcohol Clin Exp Res 1990;14:928–31.

98. Valimaki M, Pelkonen R, Karonen SL, et al. Effect of ethanol on serum concentrations of somatomedin C and the growth hormone (GH) secretion stimulated by the releasing hormone (GHRH). Alcohol Alcohol Suppl 1987;1:557–9.

99. Valimaki M, Harkonen M, Ylikahri R. Acute effects of alcohol on female sex hormones. Alcohol Clin Exp Res 1983;7:289–93.

100. Sonntag WE, Boyd RL. Chronic ethanol feeding inhibits plasma levels of insulin-like growth factor-1. Life Sci 1988;43:1325–30.

101. Soszynski PA, Frohman LA. Inhibitory effects of ethanol on the growth hormone (GH)-releasing hormone-GH-insulin-like growth factor-I axis in the rat. Endocrinology 1992;131:2603–8.

102. Soszynski PA, Frohman LA. Interaction of ethanol with signal transduction mechanisms mediating growth hormone release by rat pituitary cells in vitro. Endocrinology 1992;131:173–80.

103. Fernandez-Sola J, Preedy VR, Lang CH, et al. Molecular and cellular events in alcohol-induced muscle disease. Alcohol Clin Exp Res 2007;31:1953–62.

104. Lang CH, Fan J, Lipton BP, et al. Modulation of the insulin-like growth factor system by chronic alcohol feeding. Alcohol Clin Exp Res 1998;22:823–9.

105. Ko CH, Takahashi JS. Molecular components of the mammalian circadian clock. Hum Mol Genet 2006;15(Spec No 2):R271–7.

106. Sarkar DK. Circadian genes, the stress axis, and alcoholism. Alcohol Res 2012; 34:362–6.

107. Perreau-Lenz S, Zghoul T, Spanagel R. Clock genes running amok. Clock genes and their role in drug addiction and depression. EMBO Rep 2007;8(Spec No): S20–3.

108. Chen CP, Kuhn P, Advis JP, et al. Chronic ethanol consumption impairs the circadian rhythm of pro-opiomelanocortin and period genes mRNA expression in the hypothalamus of the male rat. J Neurochem 2004;88:1547–54.

109. Jimenez V, Cardinali DP, Cano P, et al. Effect of ethanol on 24-hour hormonal changes in peripubertal male rats. Alcohol 2004;34:127–32.

110. Brady KT, Sonne SC. The role of stress in alcohol use, alcoholism treatment, and relapse. Alcohol Res Health 1999;23:263–71.

111. Young ME. Anticipating anticipation: pursuing identification of cardiomyocyte circadian clock function. J Appl Physiol 2009;107:1339–47.

112. Blomeyer D, Buchmann AF, Lascorz J, et al. Association of PER2 genotype and stressful life events with alcohol drinking in young adults. PLoS One 2013;8: e59136.

113. Wang X, Mozhui K, Li Z, et al. A promoter polymorphism in the Per3 gene is associated with alcohol and stress response. Transl Psychiatry 2012;2:e73.
114. Spanagel R, Pendyala G, Abarca C, et al. The clock gene Per2 influences the glutamatergic system and modulates alcohol consumption. Nat Med 2005;11:35–42.
115. Logan RW, Sarkar DK. Circadian nature of immune function. Mol Cell Endocrinol 2012;349:82–90.
116. Logan RW, Zhang C, Murugan S, et al. Chronic shift-lag alters the circadian clock of NK cells and promotes lung cancer growth in rats. J Immunol 2012; 188(6):2583–91.
117. Hodge AM, Dowse GK, Collins VR, et al. Abnormal glucose tolerance and alcohol consumption in three populations at high risk of non-insulin-dependent diabetes mellitus. Am J Epidemiol 1993;137:178–89.
118. Conigrave KM, Hu BF, Camargo CA Jr, et al. A prospective study of drinking patterns in relation to risk of type 2 diabetes among men. Diabetes 2001;50: 2390–5.
119. Koppes LL, Dekker JM, Hendriks HF, et al. Moderate alcohol consumption lowers the risk of type 2 diabetes: a meta-analysis of prospective observational studies. Diabetes Care 2005;28:719–25.
120. Avogaro A, Watanabe RM, Dall'Arche A, et al. Acute alcohol consumption improves insulin action without affecting insulin secretion in type 2 diabetic subjects. Diabetes Care 2004;27:1369–74.
121. Bonnet F, Disse E, Laville M, et al. Moderate alcohol consumption is associated with improved insulin sensitivity, reduced basal insulin secretion rate and lower fasting glucagon concentration in healthy women. Diabetologia 2012;55: 3228–37.
122. Bantle AE, Thomas W, Bantle JP. Metabolic effects of alcohol in the form of wine in persons with type 2 diabetes mellitus. Metabolism 2008;57:241–5.
123. Wei M, Gibbons LW, Mitchell TL, et al. Alcohol intake and incidence of type 2 diabetes in men. Diabetes Care 2000;23:18–22.
124. Patto RJ, Russo EK, Borges DR, et al. The enteroinsular axis and endocrine pancreatic function in chronic alcohol consumers: evidence for early beta-cell hypofunction. Mt Sinai J Med 1993;60:317–20.
125. Kim JY, Song EH, Lee HJ, et al. Chronic ethanol consumption-induced pancreatic {beta}-cell dysfunction and apoptosis through glucokinase nitration and its down-regulation. J Biol Chem 2010;285:37251–62.
126. Dembele K, Nguyen KH, Hernandez TA, et al. Effects of ethanol on pancreatic beta-cell death: interaction with glucose and fatty acids. Cell Biol Toxicol 2009; 25:141–52.
127. Barnes PJ. How corticosteroids control inflammation: Quintiles Prize Lecture 2005. Br J Pharmacol 2006;148:245–54.
128. Urbach-Ross D, Kusnecov AW. Impact of superantigenic molecules on central nervous system function. Front Biosci 2009;14:4416–26.
129. Wang HJ, Zakhari S, Jung MK. Alcohol, inflammation, and gut-liver-brain interactions in tissue damage and disease development. World J Gastroenterol 2010;16:1304–13.
130. Haorah J, Ramirez SH, Floreani N, et al. Mechanism of alcohol-induced oxidative stress and neuronal injury. Free Radic Biol Med 2008;45:1542–50.
131. De A, Boyadjieva NI, Pastorcic M, et al. Cyclic AMP and ethanol interact to control apoptosis and differentiation in hypothalamic beta-endorphin neurons. J Biol Chem 1994;269:26697–705.

132. Crews FT, Nixon K. Mechanisms of neurodegeneration and regeneration in alcoholism. Alcohol Alcohol 2009;44:115–27.
133. Pfefferbaum A, Sullivan EV, Mathalon DH, et al. Frontal lobe volume loss observed with magnetic resonance imaging in older chronic alcoholics. Alcohol Clin Exp Res 1997;21:521–9.
134. Mochizuki H, Masaki T, Matsushita S, et al. Cognitive impairment and diffuse white matter atrophy in alcoholics. Clin Neurophysiol 2005;116:223–8.
135. Hellemans KG, Sliwowska JH, Verma P, et al. Prenatal alcohol exposure: fetal programming and later life vulnerability to stress, depression and anxiety disorders. Neurosci Biobehav Rev 2010;34:791–807.
136. Sarkar DK, Kuhn P, Marano J, et al. Alcohol exposure during the developmental period induces beta-endorphin neuronal death and causes alteration in the opioid control of stress axis function. Endocrinology 2007;148:2828–34.
137. Boyadjieva NI, Sarkar DK. Role of microglia in ethanol's apoptotic action on hypothalamic neuronal cells in primary cultures. Alcohol Clin Exp Res 2010; 34:1835–42.
138. Crews FT, Mdzinarishvili A, Kim D, et al. Neurogenesis in adolescent brain is potently inhibited by ethanol. Neuroscience 2006;137:437–45.
139. Fernandez-Lizarbe S, Pascual M, Guerri C. Critical role of TLR4 response in the activation of microglia induced by ethanol. J Immunol 2009;183:4733–44.
140. Zhang P, Bagby GJ, Happel KI, et al. Alcohol abuse, immunosuppression, and pulmonary infection. Curr Drug Abuse Rev 2008;1:56–67.
141. Stoltz DA, Zhang P, Nelson S, et al. Ethanol suppression of the functional state of polymorphonuclear leukocytes obtained from uninfected and simian immuno-deficiency virus infected rhesus macaques. Alcohol Clin Exp Res 1999;23: 878–84.
142. Morland H, Johnsen J, Bjorneboe A, et al. Reduced IgG Fc-receptor-mediated phagocytosis in human monocytes isolated from alcoholics. Alcohol Clin Exp Res 1988;12:755–9.
143. Lau AH, Szabo G, Thomson AW. Antigen-presenting cells under the influence of alcohol. Trends Immunol 2009;30:13–22.
144. Arjona A, Boyadjieva N, Sarkar DK. Circadian rhythms of granzyme B, perforin, IFN-gamma, and NK cell cytolytic activity in the spleen: effects of chronic ethanol. J Immunol 2004;172(5):2811–7.
145. Boyadjieva NI, Chaturvedi K, Poplawski MM, et al. Opioid antagonist naltrexone disrupts feedback interaction between mu and delta opioid receptors in splenocytes to prevent alcohol inhibition of NK cell function. J Immunol 2004;173: 42–9.
146. Pruett SB, Schwab C, Zheng Q, et al. Suppression of innate immunity by acute ethanol administration: a global perspective and a new mechanism beginning with inhibition of signaling through TLR3. J Immunol 2004;173: 2715–24.
147. Mandrekar P, Bala S, Catalano D, et al. The opposite effects of acute and chronic alcohol on lipopolysaccharide-induced inflammation are linked to IRAK-M in human monocytes. J Immunol 2009;183:1320–7.
148. Nagy LE. Stabilization of tumor necrosis factor-alpha mRNA in macrophages in response to chronic ethanol exposure. Alcohol 2004;33:229–33.
149. Boe DM, Nelson S, Zhang P, et al. Alcohol-induced suppression of lung chemokine production and the host defense response to Streptococcus pneumoniae. Alcohol Clin Exp Res 2003;27:1838–45.

150. Zisman DA, Strieter RM, Kunkel SL, et al. Ethanol feeding impairs innate immunity and alters the expression of Th1- and Th2-phenotype cytokines in murine *Klebsiella* pneumonia. Alcohol Clin Exp Res 1998;22:621–7.

151. Sarkar DK, Murugan S, Zhang C, et al. Regulation of cancer progression by β-endorphin neuron. Cancer Res 2012;72:836–40.

Sleep Disorders and the Development of Insulin Resistance and Obesity

Omar Mesarwi, MD, Jan Polak, MD, PhD, Jonathan Jun, MD,
Vsevolod Y. Polotsky, MD, PhD*

KEYWORDS

- Obstructive sleep apnea • Metabolism • Diabetes • Sleep duration
- Glucose homeostasis

KEY POINTS

- Sleep is a physiologic state of decreased metabolism and likely serves a reparative role. Normal sleep is characterized by reduced glucose turnover by the brain and other metabolically active tissues. Circadian and sleep-related changes in glucose tolerance occur in normal subjects.
- Sleep duration has decreased over the past several decades. Cross-sectional and longitudinal data suggest a link between short sleep duration and type 2 diabetes. Forced decreased sleep duration in healthy individuals has also been linked to impaired glucose homeostasis.
- Obstructive sleep apnea is a disorder of sleep characterized by diminished or abrogated airflow, which results in intermittent hypoxia and sleep fragmentation. A large body of evidence suggests an association between this disorder and impaired glucose tolerance.
- The quality and quantity of sleep may have a profound effect on obesity and type 2 diabetes, and therefore should be routinely assessed in endocrine clinic.

METABOLIC CHANGES IN SLEEP

Sleep is a physiologic recurring state of reduced consciousness, absence of voluntary activity, and suspension of sensory activity. Approximately one-third of the human lifespan is spent asleep, yet its fundamental purpose remains a mystery.[1] However, it has been recognized for decades that sleep is necessary for optimal cognitive, motor, and metabolic function.[2,3] The drive to sleep is controlled by homeostatic regulation,

Funded by: NIH; Grant number(s): HL080105; HL109475.
The authors disclose no financial relationships relevant to the authorship of this article.
Division of Pulmonary and Critical Care Medicine, Johns Hopkins University School of Medicine, 5501 Hopkins Bayview Circle, Baltimore, MD 21224, USA
* Corresponding author.
E-mail address: vpolots1@jhmi.edu

Endocrinol Metab Clin N Am 42 (2013) 617–634
http://dx.doi.org/10.1016/j.ecl.2013.05.001
0889-8529/13/$ – see front matter © 2013 Elsevier Inc. All rights reserved.

endo.theclinics.com

whereby sleep propensity increases with time awake, and circadian regulation, where sleep propensity waxes and wanes according to the time of day.[4]

According to a standardized scoring system by the American Academy of Sleep Medicine,[5] adult sleep is divided into two electroencephalographic stages: non–rapid eye movement (NREM) and rapid-eye movement (REM) sleep. NREM sleep is further subdivided into progressively deeper sleep stages referred to as N1, N2, and N3 (or slow-wave) sleep. During sleep, sympathetic tone, blood pressure, heart rate, and metabolic rate decrease, with a more marked suppression of these parameters in NREM compared with REM stages.[6] In fact, REM is often described as "active" sleep, as neural activity during REM bears a resemblance to wakefulness. Respiratory, hemodynamic, and metabolic changes are also more erratic during REM sleep. A typical sleep period in adults consists mostly of NREM sleep with REM periods occurring at 60-minute to 90-minute intervals. Slow-wave sleep usually occurs in the first few hours of sleep, whereas periods of REM lengthen toward the latter hours of sleep.

One of the functions ascribed to sleep is that of energy conservation and cellular repair. Sleep induces a fall in core body temperature, and oxygen consumption decreases by approximately 10%. These changes were first described in the mid-twentieth century[7] and were reaffirmed by subsequent studies,[8] some of which showed trends of progressively lower metabolic rate from REM to N3 sleep.[9,10] Glycogen stores,[11] ATP levels,[12] and peptide synthesis[13] increase in the brain during mammalian sleep. Several hormonal changes that foster growth and repair also occur during NREM sleep. For example, growth hormone (GH) is secreted in the first few hours of a usual sleep period, coinciding with slow-wave sleep.[14–16] This surge in GH induces peripheral lipolysis and insulin resistance, which may serve to spare the catabolism of protein and glucose stores.[17] Conversely, most hypothalamic-pituitary-adrenocortical hormones are suppressed during NREM sleep.[18]

In parallel with decreased metabolic demand, glucose turnover decreases during sleep. The changes in energy requirements during sleep are driven by a decrease in the high glucose demands of the brain.[19–21] During NREM sleep, the uptake of glucose in the brain falls progressively, while hepatic glucose output decreases, commensurate with reductions in cerebral blood flow.[22,23] Other metabolically active tissues, such as skeletal muscle, exhibit reduced blood flow and glucose uptake.[24,25] The underlying mechanisms involved in lowered glucose turnover during sleep are not known. Patterns of insulin, cortisol, and glucagon secretion make these hormones unlikely mediators.[26] Substrate availability does not limit brain metabolism, as glucose levels are usually unchanged during sleep.[22,26]

Increases in glucose during sleep have been reported, but in the setting of specialized research or clinical conditions. Frank and colleagues[27] infused glucose continuously in volunteers as they slept, either at night or during the day. This protocol revealed a rise in evening glucose and a superimposed glucose elevation during sleep, regardless of the time of day that sleep occurred. Thus, circadian and sleep-related changes in glucose tolerance occur in healthy subjects. This physiologic glucose intolerance may play a role in the "dawn phenomenon," which describes hyperglycemia in the early morning in diabetic subjects.[28] This phenomenon was also later reported to a lesser degree in individuals who did not have diabetes.[29] The pathogenesis of the dawn phenomenon is not known, but it is associated with increased catecholamines[29,30] and GH,[31–33] both of which induce insulin resistance.

Lipid metabolism during sleep has received comparatively less scrutiny. Glycerol and free fatty acids (FFA) decreased progressively during sleep in one study,[26] and the investigators speculated that reduced adipose tissue lipolysis may signal a reduction in hepatic gluconeogenesis. However, another study showed that lipid turnover decreases during early sleep, then subsequently rises in a GH-dependent manner.[34] Discrepancies between these studies may relate to the extent and distribution of slow-wave sleep, when GH is primarily secreted. In fact, a "rebound" in slow-wave sleep that occurs after sleep deprivation is accompanied by significant elevations of GH, plasma glycerol, and FFA.[35]

Circadian rhythms, independent of sleep, also affect hormone profiles and metabolism. For example, cortisol levels peak early in the morning, regardless of sleep-wake state.[36,37] Ghrelin, a peptide synthesized in multiple tissues and which stimulates appetite, is secreted in a pulsatile fashion in anticipation of daily meals.[25] However, ghrelin is also secreted in early sleep, suggesting a correlation with GH.[38] Closer analysis of the interacting influences of sleep and circadian rhythm require protocols that disrupt the timing of cues that ordinarily serve to delineate a 24-hour day. Scheer and colleagues[39] subjected volunteers to a week of 28-hour "days" to parse the effects of sleep and circadian rhythm on glucose metabolism. This study showed that, independent of the time of day, glucose and insulin increased following meals, and both decreased during sleep. Mild diurnal fluctuations in glucose also occurred, without changes in insulin. More striking, they found that circadian misalignment caused significant insulin resistance and elevations of blood pressure.[40] In the sections that follow, we examine how altered quantity, timing, or quality of sleep can affect glucose metabolism and obesity.

Key points:
- Sleep, particularly NREM sleep, is a physiologic state of decreased global metabolism that likely serves a reparative role.
- Normal NREM sleep is characterized by decreased glucose turnover, but there are conflicting data regarding lipid metabolism during sleep.
- Brain metabolism in REM sleep is similar to wakefulness.

THE METABOLIC EFFECTS OF SLEEP DURATION

Today's "around-the-clock" society, characterized by demands for high work performance, prolonged daily commutes, and leisure activity, has significantly compromised sleep duration. Self-reported sleep times have decreased from more than 8 hours in the 1960s to approximately 6.5 hours in 2012. Up to 30% of middle-aged Americans sleep fewer than 6 hours a night.[41–46] Similar results were reported in other countries[47,48] and were confirmed in population-based cohorts in which sleep duration was objectively measured.[49,50] Sleep duration is also compromised by sleep disorders, such as insomnia and obstructive sleep apnea (OSA). Whether it is voluntarily or involuntarily compromised, sleep loss has significant health consequences. These consequences range from impaired cognitive function[51,52] to increased all-cause morbidity and mortality.[53–56] Derangements in sleep also affect glucose homeostasis and appetite control. Impaired sleep thus might contribute to the rising prevalence of type 2 diabetes (T2DM) and obesity in modern society. In the following section we examine evidence linking short sleep duration to decreased glucose tolerance, insulin sensitivity, and insulin secretion. Of note, excessive sleep has also been associated with metabolic dysfunction[57,58]; however, this association has not been adequately explored, and may be confounded by medical comorbidities (eg, sleep apnea, depression) that can lengthen sleep time.

Cross-sectional studies suggest that short sleep duration is associated with an increased prevalence of T2DM or impaired glucose homeostasis. Data from large cohorts (Sleep Heart Health Study, Finnish Type 2 Diabetes Study, Quebec Family study, Behavioral Risk Factor Surveillance System, National Health Interview Study, and Isfahan Healthy Heart Program) have demonstrated that middle-aged to elderly subjects with self-reported short sleep duration are approximately twice as likely to be diagnosed with T2DM, and are at higher risk for impaired glucose tolerance. These results were independent of common T2DM risk factors in all studies[58–62] but one.[63] Similar associations between short sleep and T2DM have been observed in patients in a hypertension clinic,[64] young subjects with a family history of T2DM,[65] obese adolescents,[66] and pregnant women.[67,68] Interestingly, the association may be statistically stronger in women than men.[59,60] However, a smaller study conducted in middle-aged adults observed no association between sleep duration and diabetes.[69] Self-perceived insufficient, poor, or short sleep is also associated with prediabetic metabolic impairments, such as elevated glucose and insulin levels, HbA1c, or whole-body insulin resistance.[61,67,69–77] Moreover, inadequate sleep has been shown to worsen glucose control in patients with preexisting T2DM.[78,79] Despite various definitions of short sleep time among cross-sectional studies, outcomes of these studies are rather uniform, suggesting a significant association between short sleep duration and worsened glucose homeostasis. However, cross-sectional studies cannot establish causality. In fact, it has been reported that T2DM negatively impacts sleep architecture, making an inverse or bi-directional relationship between sleep and glucose regulation plausible.[80–82]

Stronger evidence for a causal link between short sleep duration and diabetes is provided by prospective studies following diabetes-free individuals with various sleep durations over time. Twelve published studies have been conducted in the United States, Japan, Germany, Sweden, and South Korea, investigating 661 to 70,026 adult subjects for incident diabetes over a 4-year to 32-year follow-up period.[83–94] All of these studies, except the two most recent,[93,94] were included in a meta-analysis of 90,623 subjects,[57] which showed an increased relative risk (RR) of developing diabetes in subjects with short (RR = 1.28) as well as long sleep duration (RR = 1.48), compared with subjects with normal sleep duration (typically 7–8 hours), after adjusting for known confounding variables. Similarly, more recent studies confirmed short sleep as a risk factor for newly developed diabetes[79,93]; however, this association became insignificant in one study after adjusting for multiple confounding variables.[93] Limitations of these prospective studies include differing definitions of short sleep duration, reliance on self-reported data, and the potential for residual confounding bias. Nonetheless, prospective and cross-sectional studies provide strong circumstantial evidence for the independent role of short sleep in the development of T2DM.

Experiments in human volunteers demonstrate how short-term changes in sleep duration can directly impact glucose homeostasis. After total sleep deprivation lasting from 24 hours to 5 days, studies report decreased insulin sensitivity[95–97] and impaired fasting or postprandial glucose levels.[98–102] Additionally, sleep deprivation reduced postprandial insulin secretion,[98] suggesting impaired pancreatic β-cell function. However, not all parameters of glucose metabolism were affected equally across studies and some investigators did not find impairments in glucose homeostasis after total sleep deprivation,[103] probably due to methodological differences and interindividual variability. Still, no study to date has reported *improved* glucose metabolism after sleep loss. Some studies have restricted sleep to 4 to 5 hours per night, more closely modeling the sleep habits of today's society. Although a few studies have not observed impairments in glucose metabolism,[104,105] most studies show that glucose tolerance and/or insulin sensitivity are substantially impaired when sleep is restricted for a few days to several weeks in a laboratory or in the home environment.[106–113] The metabolic phenotype induced by partial sleep deprivation is characterized by features typically observed in T2DM, such as diminished muscle glucose uptake, enhanced hepatic glucose output, and inadequate glucose-induced insulin secretion.[106,108,109,114]

Mechanisms inducing impairments in insulin sensitivity and glucose metabolism during acute sleep deprivation are complex and poorly understood. The suggested endocrine and molecular mediators are typically supported by limited and often indirect evidence. For example, sleep deprivation increases circulating levels of cortisol (elevated evening cortisol and 24-hour profile)[102,106–108,115–117] and induces sympathetic activation,[107] accompanied by elevated catecholamine levels.[111] However, metabolic impairments were also reported in studies in which cortisol or catecholamine levels remained unchanged.[108–110,114] Moreover, sleep restriction was reported to reduce thyroid-stimulating hormone and testosterone levels,[107,118] disrupt the pattern of GH secretion,[119] and elevate levels of proinflammatory cytokines.[120] These complex endocrine changes might contribute to impaired insulin signaling in peripheral tissues. In adipocytes, changes in production of circulating adipokines occurred after short sleep duration.[97,121,122] Although mechanisms are not fully understood, metabolic impairments induced by experimental sleep deprivation are reversible after sleep recovery in young and older individuals.[109]

Sleep loss also affects appetite and food intake, thereby promoting obesity. Following partial sleep deprivation, subjects increase caloric intake by approximately 20%,[104,123–126] with a preference for foods rich in carbohydrates and fat.[124,126–130] Additionally, a meta-analysis of several studies confirmed that short sleep increases appetite.[131] Among many factors that regulate food intake,[132] leptin (which suppresses appetite) and ghrelin (which stimulates appetite) have been investigated extensively under conditions of sleep restriction. Considering the numerous interacting factors that affect food intake, it is not surprising that results are mixed. Decreased leptin and increased ghrelin levels were observed in some studies following sleep deprivation[107,127,133–136] and in some cross-sectional studies,[137,138] but opposite results or no changes have also been reported elsewhere.[102,104,112,117,125,135,139,140] Although methodological differences might be responsible for inconsistent results, it is also possible that other mechanisms, such as decreased levels of satiety promoting peptide YY,[141] might contribute to increased food intake. If these appetite-stimulating effects of acute sleep loss are extrapolated to chronic sleep loss, one might expect obesity to develop in those with reduced sleep time. Indeed, cross-sectional and prospective studies have linked short sleep with weight gain and abdominal fat accumulation.[142,143] Interestingly, short sleep was associated with lower fat loss during caloric restriction in overweight subjects.[135] Some mechanistic studies of sleep loss and energy regulation have been attempted in animals. In rodents, sleep deprivation appears to lead to weight loss and energy catabolism, culminating in death. However, dramatic metabolic differences between species and stressful sleep deprivation protocols have limited the clinical applicability of these findings.[144]

There is evidence that the timing of sleep, in addition to the duration, may be a critical factor for metabolic health. Approximately 20% of workers in the United States perform their jobs under flexible or shift schedules,[145,146] which misaligns sleep timing with circadian rhythms. Shift work induces profound and sustained misalignment between circadian and homeostatic or behavioral rhythms.[39,147,148] As previously noted, an acute circadian misalignment is associated with impaired glucose tolerance and pancreatic β-cell dysfunction, leading to elevated postprandial glucose excursions,[39] independent of sleep duration. Furthermore, decreased leptin levels and an inverted cortisol profile across sleep and wake might further deteriorate glucose regulation and food intake. Thus, adequate and properly timed sleep may be important for normal glucose and weight regulation.

Key points:
- Pressures of modern society have resulted in decreased sleep duration over the past several decades.
- Cross-sectional studies suggest a link between short sleep duration and the prevalence of T2DM. These results are echoed by longitudinal studies that have even described a worsening of preexisting glucose intolerance.
- Short-term studies in healthy volunteers also demonstrate a variety of measures of impaired glucose homeostasis with short sleep time.
- Decreased sleep duration is associated with the development of obesity, although the mechanisms that underlie this are not clear.

EFFECTS OF OSA ON INSULIN RESISTANCE AND OBESITY

One sleep disorder with a potential impact on metabolic health is OSA. OSA is a common sleep disorder with an estimated prevalence of 4% to 5% in the general population. It is about twice as common in men as in women.[149] OSA is characterized by repeated collapse of the upper airway during sleep, causing intermittent oxygen desaturations and arousals from sleep. During sleep, a patient or bed partner may recall snoring, gasping, or witnessed pauses in breathing. While awake, the patient may complain of excessive daytime sleepiness, fatigue, or morning headaches. A patient may also describe poor workplace performance or impaired vigilance during driving or other monotonous activity. When OSA is suspected, a polysomnogram (PSG) should be performed, a test that monitors a patient's sleep architecture, breathing patterns, and gas exchange during sleep. A diagnosis of OSA is made by an examination of airflow and breathing effort during sleep. Obstructive *apneas* are noted when oronasal airflow ceases for more than 10 seconds despite continued breathing effort. Obstructive *hypopneas* are noted when airflow decreases significantly (but does not completely cease), leading to a fall in oxygen level or an arousal from sleep. The combined rate of apneas and hypopneas per hour, or the apnea-hypopnea index (AHI), is used to classify OSA severity. An AHI of 5 to 15, 15 to 30, or more than 30 events per hour describes mild, moderate, or severe OSA, respectively. The first-line treatment for OSA is a nasal mask which delivers continuous positive airway pressure (CPAP), thereby splinting the airway open. This often results in much more restful sleep, markedly reduced daytime symptoms, and improved gas exchange. Besides its more obvious impact on quality of life,[150,151] OSA is associated with significant long-term health consequences. Sleep apnea is a risk factor for cardiovascular disease,[152,153] and more recently an association has also been shown between OSA and a variety of metabolic disorders, including hypertension, dyslipidemia, nonalcoholic fatty liver disease, glucose intolerance, and T2DM. In this section, we briefly examine the evidence supporting links between OSA and insulin resistance and obesity.

Theoretically, OSA is a plausible cause of insulin resistance and T2DM, as it can induce sleep loss and hypoxia, each of which can impact glucose metabolism. The nature of sleep loss in OSA is best described as "sleep fragmentation," whereby deeper stages of sleep are replaced by less restful, lighter stages of sleep. When healthy volunteers are frequently awakened from sleep with acoustic and mechanical stimulation, they exhibit decreased morning insulin sensitivity, and increased morning cortisol levels and sympathetic activity.[154] Tasali and colleagues[155] showed qualitatively similar results when slow-wave sleep was specifically interrupted, and that the effect was "dose dependent"; that is, the magnitude of the disruption correlated with the magnitude of the blunting of insulin sensitivity. Acute hypoxia also causes glucose intolerance,[156–159] and one study showed that intermittent hypoxia in healthy volunteers decreased insulin sensitivity and increased sympathetic tone.[160] Mouse models of OSA that involve exposures to intermittent hypoxia have further implicated reactive oxygen species,[161] increased sympathetic tone,[161,162] inflammation,[163] and pancreatic beta cell apoptosis[164,165] as possible causes of glucose intolerance and impaired insulin secretion. Additionally, intermittent hypoxia induced arousals in mice,[166] which demonstrates the interconnectedness between the two defining characteristics of OSA.

Biologic plausibility itself is insufficient proof that sleep apnea *causes* worsened insulin resistance, however, so we must examine the clinical evidence as well. Cross-sectional studies have provided some of the support for an association between the two. In diabetic individuals, the average prevalence of OSA has been reported at 71%[167] and as high as 86% among obese diabetic patients in one recent study, with most having moderate to severe OSA.[168] This suggests that considerably more diabetic patients have OSA than are diagnosed. Twenty years ago, Levinson and colleagues[169] showed that men with OSA had twofold the expected prevalence of impaired glucose tolerance compared with published data from a control population. Subsequent studies attempted to account for the confounding influence of obesity, which is an obvious shared risk factor for OSA and T2DM. Ip and colleagues[170] showed that OSA was associated with a higher degree of insulin resistance as measured by HOMA-IR, even after correction for body mass index (BMI). Similar results were shown in another study that examined oral glucose tolerance among apneic individuals after adjusting for BMI and body fat, and hypoxia appeared to drive the association between OSA and impaired glucose tolerance.[171] McArdle and colleagues[172] showed that men with OSA had a significantly higher HOMA-IR when compared with controls matched for age, BMI, and smoking status. Numerous other cross-sectional studies support a robust association between OSA and insulin resistance.[167,173]

Longitudinal studies have the potential to provide stronger evidence for a causal association between OSA and T2DM. Reichmuth and colleagues[174] examined the baseline prevalence and incidence of T2DM in a cohort of 1387 patients from Wisconsin, some with OSA. OSA was associated with a higher prevalence of T2DM, but the incidence of T2DM over 4 years was not increased by OSA when adjusted for waist girth. A Swedish study found that OSA (defined only by nocturnal intermittent hypoxia) was associated with increased incidence of T2DM over 16 years in women, but not men, although this increase was not statistically significant.[175] However, the Busselton Health Study found that subjects with moderate to severe OSA were more likely to develop T2DM over 4 years after adjusting for age, gender, waist circumference, and BMI, but only 9 of the subjects developed T2DM during the study, resulting in wide confidence intervals.[176] A larger study of Veterans Affairs patients identified OSA as an independent risk factor for incident diabetes over 2.7 years, and CPAP appeared to attenuate this risk in those with more severe OSA.[177] A recent longitudinal study of 141 men over 11 years showed a fourfold increased risk of T2DM in those with nocturnal hypoxia.[178] Collectively, these studies point to an impact of OSA on glucose metabolism, but they are limited by sample size, and difficulties in accounting for effects of CPAP treatment during the trail periods.

Does CPAP treatment improve glucose metabolism in OSA? This finding would provide the strongest degree of evidence for a causal link between OSA and T2DM. To date, 9 randomized controlled trials have examined the effect of CPAP (compared with sham CPAP) on glucose metabolism.[167] The studies ranged in duration from 1 week to 3 months and examined various markers of insulin sensitivity, including fasting glucose, HOMA, HbA1c, and hyperinsulinemic euglycemic clamp testing. Four studies showed a beneficial effect of therapeutic CPAP, whereas the other five did not. The largest study randomized 86 patients with OSA to 3 months of CPAP or sham, and then crossed patients over to the other treatment group after a 1-month washout period. Several components of the metabolic syndrome were improved after CPAP, including a significant but modest absolute reduction in HbA1c (0.2%). However, CPAP did not alter fasting glucose, insulin, or HOMA.[179] It appears that most studies showing a benefit of CPAP were characterized by subjects with more severe OSA,[180] or who were more adherent to CPAP.[181] Hence, although some studies show improvements in markers of insulin sensitivity with CPAP use, no firm conclusions can be drawn from the available evidence. Moreover, even if CPAP attenuates diabetes risks, poor adherence to this therapy remains a significant clinical problem.

Much clearer is the relationship between obesity and the development of OSA. Approximately 70% of patients with OSA are obese,[182] whereas 60% of obese patients have OSA; this figure is nearly 100% of the morbidly obese (BMI $\geq$40).[183] Young and colleagues[184] examined a cohort of 600 patients who underwent PSG and determined that a single standard deviation higher of any measure of body habitus was associated with a threefold increased risk of having an AHI of 5 or higher. Moreover, weight loss has been shown both to decrease the AHI in patients with OSA,[185] and to decrease the collapsibility of the upper airway.[186] However, one study found that some patients who lose weight and subsequently achieve a cure of their sleep apnea may later develop an increased AHI on repeat PSG after long-term follow-up, despite maintaining their weight loss.[187] This suggests that although obesity clearly contributes to the development of OSA, it is indeed a complex, multifactorial illness.

Because of mounting evidence linking OSA to the development of other facets of the metabolic syndrome, there has also been speculation that OSA itself can cause obesity; however, the data supporting this reciprocal relationship are scant. A small study by Loube and colleagues[188] showed that patients who were compliant with CPAP use (>4 hours per night) were more likely than noncompliant patients to have significant weight loss (10 pounds or greater) on follow-up after 6 months; in fact, none of the 11 patients who were nonadherent to CPAP achieved this degree of weight loss. However, other studies have not replicated this finding, and at least one study has demonstrated no weight loss, and some weight gain in a subset of patients compliant with CPAP.[189] Intriguingly, there is evidence that CPAP may reduce visceral body fat even if overall weight is not significantly altered.[190] Therefore, no clear conclusion can be drawn about the possibility of OSA causing obesity based on the currently available evidence.

Key points:

- A growing body of evidence, including data from cross-sectional and longitudinal studies, links OSA with the development of insulin resistance.
- The effect of CPAP on insulin resistance and type 2 diabetes has not been consistent in several randomized clinical trials; large randomized clinical trials should be conducted to better assess this effect.
- Though a multifactorial illness, obesity clearly is a major risk factor for the development of OSA. The effect of OSA on obesity is not well defined.

In conclusion, sleep is a necessary human activity, and although the exact functions are unclear, it is associated with a state of decreased metabolism and energy conservation. Impairments in the timing and particularly the duration of sleep seem to be associated with worsened glucose tolerance and perhaps the development of T2DM. Sleep disorders, such as OSA, may predispose to the development and the progression of T2DM. Because of disturbing worldwide trends in sleep habits, obesity, and T2DM, it will be critical for clinicians and researchers to recognize and address the potential impact of sleep disorders on metabolic health.

REFERENCES

1. Rechtschaffen A. Current perspectives on the function of sleep. Perspect Biol Med 1998;41(3):359–90.
2. Siegel JM. The REM sleep-memory consolidation hypothesis. Science 2001; 294(5544):1058–63.
3. Siegel JM. Clues to the functions of mammalian sleep. Nature 2005;437(7063): 1264–71.
4. Daan S, Beersma DG, Borbely AA. Timing of human sleep: recover process gated by a circadian pacemaker. Am J Physiol 1984;246:R161–83.
5. Berry R, Brooks R, Gamaldo C, et al. AASM Manual for the scoring of sleep and associated events: rules, terminology and technical specifications version 2.0. Darien (IL): American Academy of Sleep Medicine; 2012.
6. Coote JH. Respiratory and circulatory control during sleep. J Exp Biol 1982;100: 223–44.
7. Kreider MB, Buskirk ER, Bass DE. Oxygen consumption and body temperatures during the night. J Appl Physiol 1958;12(3):361–6.
8. Ravussin E, Lillioja S, Anderson TE, et al. Determinants of 24-hour energy expenditure in man. Methods and results using a respiratory chamber. J Clin Invest 1986;78(6):1568–78.
9. Brebbia DR, Altshuler KZ. Oxygen consumption rate and electroencephalographic stage of sleep. Science 1965;150(3703):1621–3.
10. White DP, Weil JV, Zwillich CW. Metabolic rate and breathing during sleep. J Appl Physiol 1985;59(2):384–91.
11. Kong J, Shepel PN, Holden CP, et al. Brain glycogen decreases with increased periods of wakefulness: implications for homeostatic drive to sleep. J Neurosci 2002;22(13):5581–7.
12. Dworak M, McCarley RW, Kim T, et al. Sleep and brain energy levels: ATP changes during sleep. J Neurosci 2010;30(26):9007–16.
13. Nakanishi H, Sun Y, Nakamura RK, et al. Positive correlations between cerebral protein synthesis rates and deep sleep in Macaca mulatta. Eur J Neurosci 1997; 9(2):271–9.
14. Takahashi Y, Kipnis DM, Daughaday WH. Growth hormone secretion during sleep. J Clin Invest 1968;47(9):2079–90.
15. Van CE, Kerkhofs M, Caufriez A, et al. A quantitative estimation of growth hormone secretion in normal man: reproducibility and relation to sleep and time of day. J Clin Endocrinol Metab 1992;74(6):1441–50.
16. Van CE, Latta F, Nedeltcheva A, et al. Reciprocal interactions between the GH axis and sleep. Growth Horm IGF Res 2004;14(Suppl A):S10–7.
17. Moller N, Jorgensen JO. Effects of growth hormone on glucose, lipid, and protein metabolism in human subjects. Endocr Rev 2009;30(2):152–77.
18. Friess E, Wiedemann K, Steiger A, et al. The hypothalamic-pituitary-adrenocortical system and sleep in man. Adv Neuroimmunol 1995;5(2):111–25.
19. Sherwin RS. Role of the liver in glucose homeostasis. Diabetes Care 1980;3(2): 261–5.

20. Biggers DW, Myers SR, Neal D, et al. Role of brain in counterregulation of insulin-induced hypoglycemia in dogs. Diabetes 1989;38(1):7–16.

21. Peters A. The selfish brain: competition for energy resources. Am J Human Biol 2011;23(1):29–34.

22. Boyle PJ, Scott JC, Krentz AJ, et al. Diminished brain glucose metabolism is a significant determinant for falling rates of systemic glucose utilization during sleep in normal humans. J Clin Invest 1994;93(2):529–35.

23. Sawaya R, Ingvar DH. Cerebral blood flow and metabolism in sleep. Acta Neurol Scand 1989;80(6):481–91.

24. Zoccoli G, Cianci T, Lenzi P, et al. Shivering during sleep: relationship between muscle blood flow and fiber type composition. Experientia 1992;48(3):228–30.

25. Morris CJ, Aeschbach D, Scheer FA. Circadian system, sleep and endocrinology. Mol Cell Endocrinol 2012;349(1):91–104.

26. Clore JN, Nestler JE, Blackard WG. Sleep-associated fall in glucose disposal and hepatic glucose output in normal humans. Putative signaling mechanism linking peripheral and hepatic events. Diabetes 1989;38(3):285–90.

27. Frank SA, Roland DC, Sturis J, et al. Effects of aging on glucose regulation during wakefulness and sleep. Am J Physiol 1995;269(6 Pt 1):E1006–16.

28. Bolli GB, Gerich JE. The "dawn phenomenon"—a common occurrence in both non-insulin-dependent and insulin-dependent diabetes mellitus. N Engl J Med 1984;310(12):746–50.

29. Bolli GB, De FP, De CS, et al. Demonstration of a dawn phenomenon in normal human volunteers. Diabetes 1984;33(12):1150–3.

30. Schmidt MI, Lin QX, Gwynne JT, et al. Fasting early morning rise in peripheral insulin: evidence of the dawn phenomenon in nondiabetes. Diabetes Care 1984;7(1):32–5.

31. Rizza RA, Mandarino LJ, Gerich JE. Effects of growth hormone on insulin action in man. Mechanisms of insulin resistance, impaired suppression of glucose production, and impaired stimulation of glucose utilization. Diabetes 1982; 31(8 Pt 1):663–9.

32. Carroll KF, Nestel PJ. Diurnal variation in glucose tolerance and in insulin secretion in man. Diabetes 1973;22(5):333–48.

33. Boyle PJ, Avogaro A, Smith L, et al. Absence of the dawn phenomenon and abnormal lipolysis in type 1 (insulin-dependent) diabetic patients with chronic growth hormone deficiency. Diabetologia 1992;35(4):372–9.

34. Boyle PJ, Avogaro A, Smith L, et al. Role of GH in regulating nocturnal rates of lipolysis and plasma mevalonate levels in normal and diabetic humans. Am J Physiol 1992;263(1 Pt 1):E168–72.

35. Cooper BG, White JE, Ashworth LA, et al. Hormonal and metabolic profiles in subjects with obstructive sleep apnea syndrome and the acute effects of nasal continuous positive airway pressure (CPAP) treatment. Sleep 1995;18(3):172–9.

36. Weitzman ED. Circadian rhythms and episodic hormone secretion in man. Annu Rev Med 1976;27:225–43.

37. Halberg F, Frank G, Harner R, et al. The adrenal cycle in men on different schedules of motor and mental activity. Experientia 1961;17:282–4.

38. Dzaja A, Dalal MA, Himmerich H, et al. Sleep enhances nocturnal plasma ghrelin levels in healthy subjects. Am J Physiol Endocrinol Metab 2004;286(6): E963–7.

39. Scheer FA, Hilton MF, Mantzoros CS, et al. Adverse metabolic and cardiovascular consequences of circadian misalignment. Proc Natl Acad Sci U S A 2009; 106(11):4453–8.

40. Bass J, Takahashi JS. Circadian integration of metabolism and energetics. Science 2010;330(6009):1349–54.
41. Kripke DF, Simons RN, Garfinkel L, et al. Short and long sleep and sleeping pills. Is increased mortality associated? Arch Gen Psychiatry 1979;36(1):103–16.
42. Schoenborn CA, Adams PE. Health behaviors of adults: United States, 2005-2007. Vital Health Stat 10 2010;(245):1–132.
43. Krueger PM, Friedman EM. Sleep duration in the United States: a cross-sectional population-based study. Am J Epidemiol 2009;169(9):1052–63.
44. Centers for Disease Control and Prevention. Short Sleep Duration Among Workers—United States, 2010. MMWR Morb Mortal Wkly Rep 2012;61(16): 281–5.
45. National Sleep Foundation. NSF Bedroom Poll 2012. National Sleep Foundation 2012;1–56.
46. Centers for Disease Control and Prevention. Effect of short sleep duration on daily activities—United States, 2005-2008. MMWR Morb Mortal Wkly Rep 2011;60(8):239–42.
47. Shankar A, Koh WP, Yuan JM, et al. Sleep duration and coronary heart disease mortality among Chinese adults in Singapore: a population-based cohort study. Am J Epidemiol 2008;168(12):1367–73.
48. Tamakoshi A, Ohno Y. Self-reported sleep duration as a predictor of all-cause mortality: results from the JACC study, Japan. Sleep 2004;27(1):51–4.
49. Lauderdale DS, Knutson KL, Yan LL, et al. Objectively measured sleep characteristics among early-middle-aged adults: the CARDIA study. Am J Epidemiol 2006;164(1):5–16.
50. Redline S, Kirchner HL, Quan SF, et al. The effects of age, sex, ethnicity, and sleep-disordered breathing on sleep architecture. Arch Intern Med 2004; 164(4):406–18.
51. Stickgold R, Walker MP. Sleep-dependent memory consolidation and reconsolidation. Sleep Med 2007;8(4):331–43.
52. Walker MP. The role of sleep in cognition and emotion. Ann N Y Acad Sci 2009; 1156:168–97.
53. Cappuccio FP, D'Elia L, Strazzullo P, et al. Sleep duration and all-cause mortality: a systematic review and meta-analysis of prospective studies. Sleep 2010;33(5):585–92.
54. Chien KL, Chen PC, Hsu HC, et al. Habitual sleep duration and insomnia and the risk of cardiovascular events and all-cause death: report from a community-based cohort. Sleep 2010;33(2):177–84.
55. Punjabi NM, Caffo BS, Goodwin JL, et al. Sleep-disordered breathing and mortality: a prospective cohort study. PLoS Med 2009;6(8):e1000132.
56. Ikehara S, Iso H, Date C, et al. Association of sleep duration with mortality from cardiovascular disease and other causes for Japanese men and women: the JACC study. Sleep 2009;32(3):295–301.
57. Cappuccio FP, D'Elia L, Strazzullo P, et al. Quantity and quality of sleep and incidence of type 2 diabetes: a systematic review and meta-analysis. Diabetes Care 2010;33(2):414–20.
58. Buxton OM, Marcelli E. Short and long sleep are positively associated with obesity, diabetes, hypertension, and cardiovascular disease among adults in the United States. Soc Sci Med 2010;71(5):1027–36.
59. Gottlieb DJ, Punjabi NM, Newman AB, et al. Association of sleep time with diabetes mellitus and impaired glucose tolerance. Arch Intern Med 2005; 165(8):863–7.

60. Tuomilehto H, Peltonen M, Partinen M, et al. Sleep duration is associated with an increased risk for the prevalence of type 2 diabetes in middle-aged women—the FIN-D2D survey. Sleep Med 2008;9(3):221–7.

61. Chaput JP, Despres JP, Bouchard C, et al. Association of sleep duration with type 2 diabetes and impaired glucose tolerance. Diabetologia 2007;50(11):2298–304.

62. Najafian J, Mohamadifard N, Siadat ZD, et al. Association between sleep duration and diabetes mellitus: Isfahan Healthy Heart Program. Niger J Clin Pract 2013;16(1):59–62.

63. Altman NG, Izci-Balserak B, Schopfer E, et al. Sleep duration versus sleep insufficiency as predictors of cardiometabolic health outcomes. Sleep Med 2012; 13(10):1261–70.

64. Fiorentini A, Valente R, Perciaccante A, et al. Sleep's quality disorders in patients with hypertension and type 2 diabetes mellitus. Int J Cardiol 2007;114(2):E50–2.

65. Darukhanavala A, Booth JN III, Bromley L, et al. Changes in insulin secretion and action in adults with familial risk for type 2 diabetes who curtail their sleep. Diabetes Care 2011;34(10):2259–64.

66. Koren D, Levitt Katz LE, Brar PC, et al. Sleep architecture and glucose and insulin homeostasis in obese adolescents. Diabetes Care 2011;34(11):2442–7.

67. Qiu C, Enquobahrie D, Frederick IO, et al. Glucose intolerance and gestational diabetes risk in relation to sleep duration and snoring during pregnancy: a pilot study. BMC Womens Health 2010;10:17.

68. Facco FL, Grobman WA, Kramer J, et al. Self-reported short sleep duration and frequent snoring in pregnancy: impact on glucose metabolism. Am J Obstet Gynecol 2010;203(2):142–5.

69. Knutson KL, Van CE, Zee P, et al. Cross-sectional associations between measures of sleep and markers of glucose metabolism among subjects with and without diabetes: the Coronary Artery Risk Development in Young Adults (CARDIA) Sleep Study. Diabetes Care 2011;34(5):1171–6.

70. Jennings JR, Muldoon MF, Hall M, et al. Self-reported sleep quality is associated with the metabolic syndrome. Sleep 2007;30(2):219–23.

71. Flint J, Kothare SV, Zihlif M, et al. Association between inadequate sleep and insulin resistance in obese children. J Pediatr 2007;150(4):364–9.

72. Matthews KA, Dahl RE, Owens JF, et al. Sleep duration and insulin resistance in healthy black and white adolescents. Sleep 2012;35(10):1353–8.

73. Hung HC, Yang YC, Ou HY, et al. The association between self-reported sleep quality and metabolic syndrome. PLoS One 2013;8(1):e54304.

74. Hung HC, Yang YC, Ou HY, et al. The relationship between impaired fasting glucose and self-reported sleep quality in a Chinese population. Clin Endocrinol (Oxf) 2013;78(4):518–24.

75. Nakajima H, Kaneita Y, Yokoyama E, et al. Association between sleep duration and hemoglobin A1c level. Sleep Med 2008;9(7):745–52.

76. Hall MH, Muldoon MF, Jennings JR, et al. Self-reported sleep duration is associated with the metabolic syndrome in midlife adults. Sleep 2008;31(5):635–43.

77. Reutrakul S, Zaidi N, Wroblewski K, et al. Sleep disturbances and their relationship to glucose tolerance in pregnancy. Diabetes Care 2011;34(11):2454–7.

78. Knutson KL, Ryden AM, Mander BA, et al. Role of sleep duration and quality in the risk and severity of type 2 diabetes mellitus. Arch Intern Med 2006;166(16): 1768–74.

79. Ohkuma T, Fujii H, Iwase M, et al. Impact of sleep duration on obesity and the glycemic level in patients with type 2 diabetes mellitus: the Fukuoka Diabetes Registry. Diabetes Care 2013;36(3):611–7.

80. Song Y, Ye X, Ye L, et al. Disturbed subjective sleep in Chinese females with type 2 diabetes on insulin therapy. PLoS One 2013;8(1):e54951.
81. Pallayova M, Donic V, Gresova S, et al. Do differences in sleep architecture exist between persons with type 2 diabetes and nondiabetic controls? J Diabetes Sci Technol 2010;4(2):344–52.
82. Nakanishi-Minami T, Kishida K, Funahashi T, et al. Sleep-wake cycle irregularities in type 2 diabetics. Diabetol Metab Syndr 2012;4(1):18.
83. Ayas NT, White DP, Al-Delaimy WK, et al. A prospective study of self-reported sleep duration and incident diabetes in women. Diabetes Care 2003;26(2):380–4.
84. Nilsson PM, Roost M, Engstrom G, et al. Incidence of diabetes in middle-aged men is related to sleep disturbances. Diabetes Care 2004;27(10):2464–9.
85. Bjorkelund C, Bondyr-Carlsson D, Lapidus L, et al. Sleep disturbances in midlife unrelated to 32-year diabetes incidence: the prospective population study of women in Gothenburg. Diabetes Care 2005;28(11):2739–44.
86. Mallon L, Broman JE, Hetta J. High incidence of diabetes in men with sleep complaints or short sleep duration: a 12-year follow-up study of a middle-aged population. Diabetes Care 2005;28(11):2762–7.
87. Yaggi HK, Araujo AB, McKinlay JB. Sleep duration as a risk factor for the development of type 2 diabetes. Diabetes Care 2006;29(3):657–61.
88. Gangwisch JE, Heymsfield SB, Boden-Albala B, et al. Sleep duration as a risk factor for diabetes incidence in a large U.S. sample. Sleep 2007;30(12): 1667–73.
89. Beihl DA, Liese AD, Haffner SM. Sleep duration as a risk factor for incident type 2 diabetes in a multiethnic cohort. Ann Epidemiol 2009;19(5):351–7.
90. Hayashino Y, Fukuhara S, Suzukamo Y, et al. Relation between sleep quality and quantity, quality of life, and risk of developing diabetes in healthy workers In Japan: the High-risk and Population Strategy for Occupational Health Promotion (HIPOP-OHP) Study. BMC Public Health 2007;7:129.
91. Kawakami N, Takatsuka N, Shimizu H. Sleep disturbance and onset of type 2 diabetes. Diabetes Care 2004;27(1):282–3.
92. Meisinger C, Heier M, Loewel H. Sleep disturbance as a predictor of type 2 diabetes mellitus in men and women from the general population. Diabetologia 2005;48(2):235–41.
93. von RA, Weikert C, Fietze I, et al. Association of sleep duration with chronic diseases in the European Prospective Investigation into Cancer and Nutrition (EPIC)-Potsdam study. PLoS One 2012;7(1):e30972.
94. Kita T, Yoshioka E, Satoh H, et al. Short sleep duration and poor sleep quality increase the risk of diabetes in Japanese workers with no family history of diabetes. Diabetes Care 2012;35(2):313–8.
95. Gonzalez-Ortiz M, Martinez-Abundis E, Balcazar-Munoz BR, et al. Effect of sleep deprivation on insulin sensitivity and cortisol concentration in healthy subjects. Diabetes Nutr Metab 2000;13(2):80–3.
96. VanHelder T, Symons JD, Radomski MW. Effects of sleep deprivation and exercise on glucose tolerance. Aviat Space Environ Med 1993;64(6):487–92.
97. Broussard JL, Ehrmann DA, Van CE, et al. Impaired insulin signaling in human adipocytes after experimental sleep restriction: a randomized, crossover study. Ann Intern Med 2012;157(8):549–57.
98. Benedict C, Hallschmid M, Lassen A, et al. Acute sleep deprivation reduces energy expenditure in healthy men. Am J Clin Nutr 2011;93(6):1229–36.
99. Kuhn E, Brodan V, Brodanova M, et al. Metabolic reflection of sleep deprivation. Act Nerv Super (Praha) 1969;11(3):165–74.

100. Vondra K, Brodan V, Bass A, et al. Effects of sleep deprivation on the activity of selected metabolic enzymes in skeletal muscle. Eur J Appl Physiol Occup Physiol 1981;47(1):41–6.

101. Wehrens SM, Hampton SM, Finn RE, et al. Effect of total sleep deprivation on postprandial metabolic and insulin responses in shift workers and non-shift workers. J Endocrinol 2010;206(2):205–15.

102. Reynolds AC, Dorrian J, Liu PY, et al. Impact of five nights of sleep restriction on glucose metabolism, leptin and testosterone in young adult men. PLoS One 2012;7(7):e41218.

103. Schmid SM, Hallschmid M, Jauch-Chara K, et al. Sleep loss alters basal metabolic hormone secretion and modulates the dynamic counterregulatory response to hypoglycemia. J Clin Endocrinol Metab 2007;92(8):3044–51.

104. Bosy-Westphal A, Hinrichs S, Jauch-Chara K, et al. Influence of partial sleep deprivation on energy balance and insulin sensitivity in healthy women. Obes Facts 2008;1(5):266–73.

105. Zielinski MR, Kline CE, Kripke DF, et al. No effect of 8-week time in bed restriction on glucose tolerance in older long sleepers. J Sleep Res 2008;17(4):412–9.

106. Spiegel K, Leproult R, Van CE. Impact of sleep debt on metabolic and endocrine function. Lancet 1999;354(9188):1435–9.

107. Spiegel K, Leproult R, L'hermite-Baleriaux M, et al. Leptin levels are dependent on sleep duration: relationships with sympathovagal balance, carbohydrate regulation, cortisol, and thyrotropin. J Clin Endocrinol Metab 2004;89(11):5762–71.

108. Buxton OM, Pavlova M, Reid EW, et al. Sleep restriction for 1 week reduces insulin sensitivity in healthy men. Diabetes 2010;59(9):2126–33.

109. Buxton OM, Cain SW, O'Connor SP, et al. Adverse metabolic consequences in humans of prolonged sleep restriction combined with circadian disruption. Sci Transl Med 2012;4(129):129ra43.

110. Schmid SM, Hallschmid M, Jauch-Chara K, et al. Disturbed glucoregulatory response to food intake after moderate sleep restriction. Sleep 2011;34(3):371–7.

111. Nedeltcheva AV, Kessler L, Imperial J, et al. Exposure to recurrent sleep restriction in the setting of high caloric intake and physical inactivity results in increased insulin resistance and reduced glucose tolerance. J Clin Endocrinol Metab 2009;94(9):3242–50.

112. van Leeuwen WM, Hublin C, Sallinen M, et al. Prolonged sleep restriction affects glucose metabolism in healthy young men. Int J Endocrinol 2010;2010:108641.

113. Robertson MD, Russell-Jones D, Umpleby AM, et al. Effects of three weeks of mild sleep restriction implemented in the home environment on multiple metabolic and endocrine markers in healthy young men. Metabolism 2013;62(2):204–11.

114. Donga E, van DM, van Dijk JG, et al. A single night of partial sleep deprivation induces insulin resistance in multiple metabolic pathways in healthy subjects. J Clin Endocrinol Metab 2010;95(6):2963–8.

115. Leproult R, Copinschi G, Buxton O, et al. Sleep loss results in an elevation of cortisol levels the next evening. Sleep 1997;20(10):865–70.

116. Kumari M, Badrick E, Ferrie J, et al. Self-reported sleep duration and sleep disturbance are independently associated with cortisol secretion in the Whitehall II study. J Clin Endocrinol Metab 2009;94(12):4801–9.

117. Omisade A, Buxton OM, Rusak B. Impact of acute sleep restriction on cortisol and leptin levels in young women. Physiol Behav 2010;99(5):651–6.

118. Leproult R, Van CE. Effect of 1 week of sleep restriction on testosterone levels in young healthy men. JAMA 2011;305(21):2173–4.
119. Spiegel K, Leproult R, Colecchia EF, et al. Adaptation of the 24-h growth hormone profile to a state of sleep debt. Am J Physiol Regul Integr Comp Physiol 2000;279(3):R874–83.
120. Patel SR, Zhu X, Storfer-Isser A, et al. Sleep duration and biomarkers of inflammation. Sleep 2009;32(2):200–4.
121. Hayes AL, Xu F, Babineau D, et al. Sleep duration and circulating adipokine levels. Sleep 2011;34(2):147–52.
122. Al-Disi D, Al-Daghri N, Khanam L, et al. Subjective sleep duration and quality influence diet composition and circulating adipocytokines and ghrelin levels in teen-age girls. Endocrinol Jpn 2010;57(10):915–23.
123. Brondel L, Romer MA, Nougues PM, et al. Acute partial sleep deprivation increases food intake in healthy men. Am J Clin Nutr 2010;91(6):1550–9.
124. St-Onge MP, Roberts AL, Chen J, et al. Short sleep duration increases energy intakes but does not change energy expenditure in normal-weight individuals. Am J Clin Nutr 2011;94(2):410–6.
125. Nedeltcheva AV, Kilkus JM, Imperial J, et al. Sleep curtailment is accompanied by increased intake of calories from snacks. Am J Clin Nutr 2009;89(1):126–33.
126. Calvin AD, Carter RE, Adachi T, et al. Effects of experimental sleep restriction on caloric intake and activity energy expenditure. Chest 2013. [Epub ahead of print].
127. Spiegel K, Tasali E, Penev P, et al. Brief communication: sleep curtailment in healthy young men is associated with decreased leptin levels, elevated ghrelin levels, and increased hunger and appetite. Ann Intern Med 2004;141(11): 846–50.
128. Santana AA, Pimentel GD, Romualdo M, et al. Sleep duration in elderly obese patients correlated negatively with intake fatty. Lipids Health Dis 2012;11:99.
129. Weiss A, Xu F, Storfer-Isser A, et al. The association of sleep duration with adolescents' fat and carbohydrate consumption. Sleep 2010;33(9):1201–9.
130. Grandner MA, Kripke DF, Naidoo N, et al. Relationships among dietary nutrients and subjective sleep, objective sleep, and napping in women. Sleep Med 2010; 11(2):180–4.
131. Chapman CD, Benedict C, Brooks SJ, et al. Lifestyle determinants of the drive to eat: a meta-analysis. Am J Clin Nutr 2012;96(3):492–7.
132. Suzuki K, Jayasena CN, Bloom SR. Obesity and appetite control. Exp Diabetes Res 2012;2012:824305.
133. Guilleminault C, Powell NB, Martinez S, et al. Preliminary observations on the effects of sleep time in a sleep restriction paradigm. Sleep Med 2003;4(3): 177–84.
134. St-Onge MP, O'Keeffe M, Roberts AL, et al. Short sleep duration, glucose dysregulation and hormonal regulation of appetite in men and women. Sleep 2012; 35(11):1503–10.
135. Nedeltcheva AV, Kilkus JM, Imperial J, et al. Insufficient sleep undermines dietary efforts to reduce adiposity. Ann Intern Med 2010;153(7):435–41.
136. Schmid SM, Hallschmid M, Jauch-Chara K, et al. A single night of sleep deprivation increases ghrelin levels and feelings of hunger in normal-weight healthy men. J Sleep Res 2008;17(3):331–4.
137. Taheri S, Lin L, Austin D, et al. Short sleep duration is associated with reduced leptin, elevated ghrelin, and increased body mass index. PLoS Med 2004;1(3):e62.

138. Chaput JP, Despres JP, Bouchard C, et al. Short sleep duration is associated with reduced leptin levels and increased adiposity: results from the Quebec family study. Obesity (Silver Spring) 2007;15(1):253–61.
139. Schmid SM, Hallschmid M, Jauch-Chara K, et al. Short-term sleep loss decreases physical activity under free-living conditions but does not increase food intake under time-deprived laboratory conditions in healthy men. Am J Clin Nutr 2009;90(6):1476–82.
140. Simpson NS, Banks S, Dinges DF. Sleep restriction is associated with increased morning plasma leptin concentrations, especially in women. Biol Res Nurs 2010; 12(1):47–53.
141. Magee CA, Huang XF, Iverson DC, et al. Acute sleep restriction alters neuroendocrine hormones and appetite in healthy male adults. Sleep Biol Rhythm 2009; 7(2):125–7.
142. Morselli LL, Guyon A, Spiegel K. Sleep and metabolic function. Pflugers Arch 2012;463(1):139–60.
143. Knutson KL. Sleep duration and cardiometabolic risk: a review of the epidemiologic evidence. Best Pract Res Clin Endocrinol Metab 2010;24(5):731–43.
144. Jun JC, Polotsky VY. Sleep and sleep loss: an energy paradox? Sleep 2012; 35(11):1447–8.
145. Luyster FS, Strollo PJ Jr, Zee PC, et al. Sleep: a health imperative. Sleep 2012; 35(6):727–34.
146. U.S. Department of Labor. Workers on flexible and shift schedules in 2004. Washington, DC: Bureau of Labor Statistics; 2005.
147. Folkard S. Do permanent night workers show circadian adjustment? A review based on the endogenous melatonin rhythm. Chronobiol Int 2008;25(2):215–24.
148. Sack RL, Blood ML, Lewy AJ. Melatonin rhythms in night shift workers. Sleep 1992;15(5):434–41.
149. Jennum P, Riha RL. Epidemiology of sleep apnoea/hypopnoea syndrome and sleep-disordered breathing. Eur Respir J 2009;33(4):907–14.
150. Meslier N, Lebrun T, Grillier-Lanoir V, et al. A French survey of 3,225 patients treated with CPAP for obstructive sleep apnoea: benefits, tolerance, compliance and quality of life. Eur Respir J 1998;12(1):185–92.
151. Kawahara S, Akashiba T, Akahoshi T, et al. Nasal CPAP improves the quality of life and lessens the depressive symptoms in patients with obstructive sleep apnea syndrome. Intern Med 2005;44(5):422–7.
152. Lopez-Jimenez F, Sert Kuniyoshi FH, Gami A, et al. Obstructive sleep apnea: implications for cardiac and vascular disease. Chest 2008;133(3):793–804.
153. Caples SM, Garcia-Touchard A, Somers VK. Sleep-disordered breathing and cardiovascular risk. Sleep 2007;30(3):291–303.
154. Stamatakis KA, Punjabi NM. Effects of sleep fragmentation on glucose metabolism in normal subjects. Chest 2010;137(1):95–101.
155. Tasali E, Leproult R, Ehrmann DA, et al. Slow-wave sleep and the risk of type 2 diabetes in humans. Proc Natl Acad Sci U S A 2008;105(3):1044–9.
156. Larsen JJ, Hansen JM, Olsen NV, et al. The effect of altitude hypoxia on glucose homeostasis in men. J Physiol 1997;504(Pt 1):241–9.
157. Barnholt KE, Hoffman AR, Rock PB, et al. Endocrine responses to acute and chronic high-altitude exposure (4,300 meters): modulating effects of caloric restriction. Am J Physiol Endocrinol Metab 2006;290(6):E1078–88.
158. Braun B, Rock PB, Zamudio S, et al. Women at altitude: short-term exposure to hypoxia and/or alpha(1)-adrenergic blockade reduces insulin sensitivity. J Appl Physiol 2001;91(2):623–31.

159. Oltmanns KM, Gehring H, Rudolf S, et al. Hypoxia causes glucose intolerance in humans. Am J Respir Crit Care Med 2004;169(11):1231–7.

160. Louis M, Punjabi NM. Effects of acute intermittent hypoxia on glucose metabolism in awake healthy volunteers. J Appl Physiol 2009;106(5):1538–44.

161. Peng YJ, Yuan G, Ramakrishnan D, et al. Heterozygous HIF-1alpha deficiency impairs carotid body-mediated systemic responses and reactive oxygen species generation in mice exposed to intermittent hypoxia. J Physiol 2006; 577(Pt 2):705–16.

162. Fletcher EC. Sympathetic over activity in the etiology of hypertension of obstructive sleep apnea. Sleep 2003;26(1):15–9.

163. Ryan S, Taylor CT, McNicholas WT. Selective activation of inflammatory pathways by intermittent hypoxia in obstructive sleep apnea syndrome. Circulation 2005;112(17):2660–7.

164. Yokoe T, Alonso LC, Romano LC, et al. Intermittent hypoxia reverses the diurnal glucose rhythm and causes pancreatic beta-cell replication in mice. J Physiol 2008;586(3):899–911.

165. Xu J, Long YS, Gozal D, et al. Beta-cell death and proliferation after intermittent hypoxia: role of oxidative stress. Free Radic Biol Med 2009;46(6):783–90.

166. Polotsky VY, Rubin AE, Balbir A, et al. Intermittent hypoxia causes REM sleep deficits and decreases EEG delta power in NREM sleep in the C57BL/6J mouse. Sleep Med 2006;7(1):7–16.

167. Pamidi S, Tasali E. Obstructive sleep apnea and type 2 diabetes: is there a link? Front Neurol 2012;3:126.

168. Foster GD, Sanders MH, Millman R, et al. Obstructive sleep apnea among obese patients with type 2 diabetes. Diabetes Care 2009;32(6):1017–9.

169. Levinson PD, McGarvey ST, Carlisle CC, et al. Adiposity and cardiovascular risk factors in men with obstructive sleep apnea. Chest 1993;103(5):1336–42.

170. Ip MS, Lam B, Ng MM, et al. Obstructive sleep apnea is independently associated with insulin resistance. Am J Respir Crit Care Med 2002;165(5):670–6.

171. Punjabi NM, Sorkin JD, Katzel LI, et al. Sleep-disordered breathing and insulin resistance in middle-aged and overweight men. Am J Respir Crit Care Med 2002;165(5):677–82.

172. McArdle N, Hillman D, Beilin L, et al. Metabolic risk factors for vascular disease in obstructive sleep apnea: a matched controlled study. Am J Respir Crit Care Med 2007;175(2):190–5.

173. Punjabi NM. Do sleep disorders and associated treatments impact glucose metabolism? Drugs 2009;69(Suppl 2):13–27.

174. Reichmuth KJ, Austin D, Skatrud JB, et al. Association of sleep apnea and type II diabetes: a population-based study. Am J Respir Crit Care Med 2005;172(12): 1590–5.

175. Celen YT, Hedner J, Carlson J, et al. Impact of gender on incident diabetes mellitus in obstructive sleep apnea: a 16-year follow-up. J Clin Sleep Med 2010; 6(3):244–50.

176. Marshall NS, Wong KK, Phillips CL, et al. Is sleep apnea an independent risk factor for prevalent and incident diabetes in the Busselton Health Study? J Clin Sleep Med 2009;5(1):15–20.

177. Botros N, Concato J, Mohsenin V, et al. Obstructive sleep apnea as a risk factor for type 2 diabetes. Am J Med 2009;122(12):1122–7.

178. Lindberg E, Theorell-Haglow J, Svensson M, et al. Sleep apnea and glucose metabolism: a long-term follow-up in a community-based sample. Chest 2012; 142(4):935–42.

179. Sharma SK, Agrawal S, Damodaran D, et al. CPAP for the metabolic syndrome in patients with obstructive sleep apnea. N Engl J Med 2011;365(24):2277–86.

180. Weinstock TG, Wang X, Rueschman M, et al. A controlled trial of CPAP therapy on metabolic control in individuals with impaired glucose tolerance and sleep apnea. Sleep 2012;35(5):617–625B.

181. Lam JC, Lam B, Yao TJ, et al. A randomised controlled trial of nasal continuous positive airway pressure on insulin sensitivity in obstructive sleep apnoea. Eur Respir J 2010;35(1):138–45.

182. Malhotra A, White DP. Obstructive sleep apnoea. Lancet 2002;360(9328): 237–45.

183. Valencia-Flores M, Orea A, Castano VA, et al. Prevalence of sleep apnea and electrocardiographic disturbances in morbidly obese patients. Obes Res 2000;8(3):262–9.

184. Young T, Palta M, Dempsey J, et al. The occurrence of sleep-disordered breathing among middle-aged adults. N Engl J Med 1993;328(17):1230–5.

185. Smith PL, Gold AR, Meyers DA, et al. Weight loss in mildly to moderately obese patients with obstructive sleep apnea. Ann Intern Med 1985;103(6 (Pt 1)):850–5.

186. Schwartz AR, Gold AR, Schubert N, et al. Effect of weight loss on upper airway collapsibility in obstructive sleep apnea. Am Rev Respir Dis 1991;144(3 Pt 1): 494–8.

187. Sampol G, Munoz X, Sagales MT, et al. Long-term efficacy of dietary weight loss in sleep apnoea/hypopnoea syndrome. Eur Respir J 1998;12(5):1156–9.

188. Loube DI, Loube AA, Erman MK. Continuous positive airway pressure treatment results in weight less in obese and overweight patients with obstructive sleep apnea. J Am Diet Assoc 1997;97(8):896–7.

189. Redenius R, Murphy C, O'Neill E, et al. Does CPAP lead to change in BMI? J Clin Sleep Med 2008;4(3):205–9.

190. Chin K, Shimizu K, Nakamura T, et al. Changes in intra-abdominal visceral fat and serum leptin levels in patients with obstructive sleep apnea syndrome following nasal continuous positive airway pressure therapy. Circulation 1999; 100(7):706–12.

Index

Note: Page numbers of article titles are in **boldface** type.

A

ACTH. See *Corticotrophin (ACTH).*
ACTH-deficiency, in hypopituitarism, treatment perspectives of, 574–576
    with traumatic brain injury, 571–573
ACTH-secreting tumor, in Cushing disease, 478–479
Adolescence, anorexia nervosa prevalence related to, 516–517, 521
Adrenal hormones. See also *Corticotrophin (ACTH); Cortisol.*
  alcohol effects on, 594–598
Adrenergic receptors, in glucometabolic side effects of APDs, 552–554
Adults, anorexia nervosa in, 516–517, 521
Affect, in Cushing syndrome, 478–479
    response to treatment, 481
Alcohol, effects on endocrine system, **593–615**
    circadian rhythm and, 603–604
    communication function with nervous system, 594–595
    hormonal changes as, 593–595
    immune system and, 595, 605–607
    in GH-IGF1 axis, 594, 602–603
    in HPA axis, 594–598
    in HPG axis, 594–595, 598–602
    in HPT axis, 594–595, 602
    introduction to, 593–594
    pancreatic function and, 594, 604–605
  sexual dysfunction and, 586
Alcoholism, adverse health consequences of, 594–595
  anorexia nervosa and, 516
  human genome-wide association studies of, 593–594
  subclinical hyperthyroidism associated with, 466
Alendronate, for low bone mineral density, in anorexia nervosa, 523
Alzheimer disease (AD), spontaneous vs. exogenous Cushing disease and, 478, 485
  subclinical hyperthyroidism associated with, 465–466
  traumatic brain injury and, 566
  type 2 diabetes and, 489–495
    as risk factor, 490–491
    conclusions on, 495
    insulin levels association with, 491–492
    prevalence of, 489, 533
    treatment effects on, 491–495
      with glucagon-like peptide-1, 494
      with insulin administration, 491–493
      with metformin, 494–495
      with peroxisome proliferator-activated receptor-γ agonists, 493–494

Endocrinol Metab Clin N Am 42 (2013) 635–656
http://dx.doi.org/10.1016/S0889-8529(13)00074-1
0889-8529/13/$ – see front matter © 2013 Elsevier Inc. All rights reserved.

endo.theclinics.com

Printed and bound by CPI Group (UK) Ltd, Croydon, CR0 4YY

03/10/2024

01040465-0003